Illustrated Dermatology

Including Skin of Color

Illustrated Dermatology

Including Skin of Color

Fourth Edition

Yasaman Mansouri MD MRCP (UK) Dermatology
Attending
Department of Dermatology
NYC Health + Hospitals/Woodhull
Icahn School of Medicine at Mount Sinai
New York, New York, USA

Howard Maibach MD
Professor
Department of Dermatology
University of California School of Medicine
San Francisco, California, USA

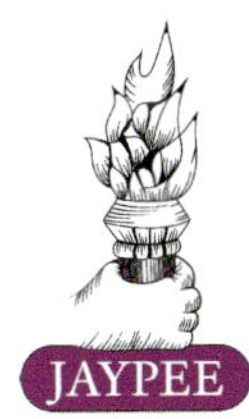

JAYPEE BROTHERS MEDICAL PUBLISHERS
The Health Sciences Publisher
New Delhi | London

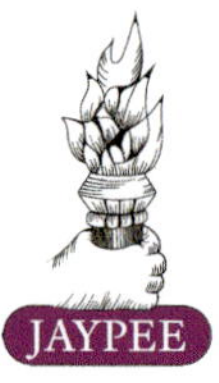

Jaypee Brothers Medical Publishers (P) Ltd

Headquarters
Jaypee Brothers Medical Publishers (P) Ltd
EMCA House, 23/23-B
Ansari Road, Daryaganj
New Delhi 110 002, India
Landline: +91-11-23272143, +91-11-23272703
+91-11-23282021, +91-11-23245672
Email: jaypee@jaypeebrothers.com

Corporate Office
Jaypee Brothers Medical Publishers (P) Ltd
4838/24, Ansari Road, Daryaganj
New Delhi 110 002, India
Phone: +91-11-43574357
Fax: +91-11-43574314
Email: jaypee@jaypeebrothers.com

Overseas Office
JP Medical Ltd
83 Victoria Street, London
SW1H 0HW (UK)
Phone: +44 20 3170 8910
Fax: +44 (0)20 3008 6180
Email: info@jpmedpub.com

Website: www.jaypeebrothers.com
Website: www.jaypeedigital.com

Inquiries for bulk sales may be solicited at: jaypee@jaypeebrothers.com

Illustrated Dermatology Including Skin of Color

Fourth Edition: **2023,** Reprint 2025

ISBN: 978-93-5465-757-3

Printed in India

Dedicated to

Susan,
my beloved mother,
who has a heart of gold.
Thank you for your love and support.

—Yasaman Mansouri

Preface

Since the previous edition of *Illustrated Dermatology* was published, dermatology has advanced substantially. Numerous new agents have been introduced for the management of psoriasis, including oral therapies such as a phosphodiesterase-4 enzyme inhibitor and injectable biologic agents. The therapeutic preferences for conditions such as tinea, candidiasis, and hair loss have changed, and new topical treatments have been developed for acne, rosacea, atopic dermatitis, and pigmentary disorders. We have revised each chapter carefully and tried to make this edition even more practical than the previous one and included any new treatments that are useful for the intended audience.

This book is intended for nondermatologists, such as physicians in primary care, medical students, nurses, and physician assistants, who wish to increase their knowledge of this vast field and is highly applicable to daily practice.

After realizing that many books, including our previous edition, contain mostly images of light skin, we have added numerous skin of color photographs highlighting how some dermatoses can appear very differently in different skin types.

Dr Howard Maibach and the new senior editor want to thank the staff at the M/s Jaypee Brothers Medical Publishers, New Delhi, India for their exceptional support throughout the preparation of this edition, particularly Ms Nikita Chauhan, Ms Harsha Madan, and Ms Chetna Malhotra.

We hope the book becomes one of your favorite references for any patient you encounter with a skin disease. The authors welcome comments, corrections, and suggestions for improvement.

Yasaman Mansouri
Howard Maibach
E-mail: Howard.Maibach@ucsf.edu

Acknowledgments

We would like to thank the following physicians for allowing us to use photographs from their collections: Drs Loren E Golitz, Steven A Davis, Axel Hoke, Peter Webb, and Timothy L Berger.

We are very thankful to Shri Jitendar P Vij (Group Chairman), Mr Ankit Vij (Managing Director), Ms Chetna Malhotra (Senior Director—Professional Publishing, Marketing and Business Development), Ms Nikita Chauhan (Senior Development Editor), and the team of M/s Jaypee Brothers Medical Publishers (P) Ltd, New Delhi, India, for putting efforts to bring this edition.

Contents

Introduction

Skin conditions have characteristic patterns, locations, and morphologies. The location or pattern leads experienced clinicians to markedly narrow their list of possible diagnoses. We present common skin conditions by anatomic location, starting from the scalp and working down, and outline their treatment. We have chosen to discuss in depth about 70 skin conditions and growths most commonly seen in clinical practice. For reasons of space you will not find rare skin disorders, such as pemphigus, even if they are interesting and possibly dangerous.

The Patient Guides, which have been limited to those we have found useful in our own experience, are suitable for photocopying and will help patients understand their disease and its management.

We hope that you will find this manual valuable in daily clinical practice.

CHAPTER 1
Scalp

Seborrheic Dermatitis

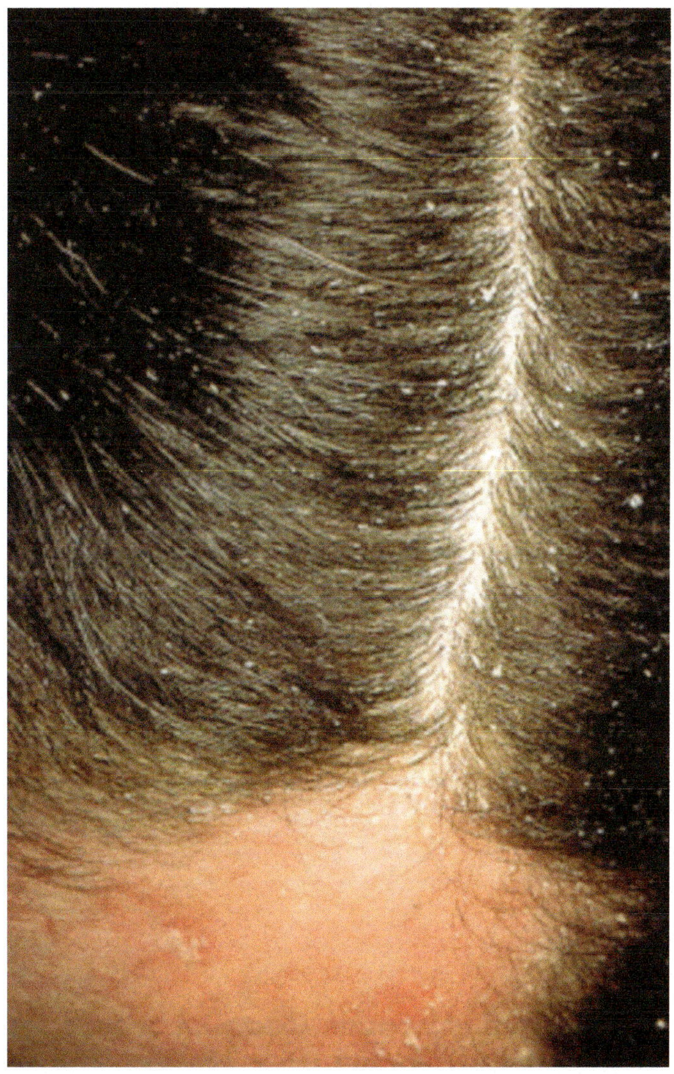

"Dandruff" or excessive scaling of the scalp. Redness in seborrheic dermatitis is faint, patchy, ill-defined, and difficult to see even with close inspection.

CLINICAL

- Occasional flakes of *dander* on the scalp are normal and should not precipitate attempts at therapy.
- Seborrheic dermatitis consists of excessive scaling, itching, and faint inflammation. *(Note: Seborrhea* merely means increased oil flow and is not synonymous with seborrheic dermatitis.)

- Seborrheic dermatitis occurs in areas of high-oil gland activity—scalp, face, upper chest, and, infrequently, axillae and pubis.
- This condition is chronic but intermittent, frequently flaring with physical and emotional stress.
- Seborrheic dermatitis is more common and severe in fair-skinned individuals.
- This condition is not seen in children. It may be seen in infants up to 3 and 4 months of age because of maternal hormones. It then appears as "cradle cap" and as a red, scaly rash of the skinfold areas of neck, axillae, and groins.
- Possibly contributing to the pathogenesis of seborrheic dermatitis is the yeast *Malassezia ovalis,* but this organism is present as part of the skin's normal flora. Antiyeast medications may help severe and refractory cases.

TREATMENT

This treatment is aimed at reducing scaling and inflammation, either of which may predominate in a given individual.

Shampoos (*See* page 242)

- Antidandruff activity has been demonstrated for shampoos containing:
  - Selenium sulfide
  - Sulfur and salicylic acid
  - Zinc pyrithione
  - Tar
  - Ketoconazole
- Selenium sulfide (2.5%) shampoos require prescriptions in some countries but may be more effective than less expensive over-the-counter products containing zinc pyrithione or sulfur and salicylic acid.
- Ketoconazole shampoo is available as 1% over the counter or 2% on prescription. Using this two or three times a week is about as effective as selenium sulfide shampoo and it also may take 6 weeks to reach maximum benefit. Anecdotally, it has worked in cases not responding to other shampoos.
- Shampoos vary considerably with respect to cosmetic texture, ease of lathering, and drying effect. Some are offered with protein or quaternary ammonium compounds added as a conditioner. Patients should be given a variety of samples or they should try many brands so that they can select one they like.

Dandruff shampoos usually work well. Failure may be due to:
- Infrequent use (may be required once daily to once weekly; often needed every 2–3 days)
- Inadequate duration (may take a week to work and may take 6 weeks to reach peak benefit)
- Inadequate scalp contact (the most common cause of "failure"); **leave on scalp several minutes**
- Natural fluctuations in disease (shampoos may not suppress all flares)

These points must be emphasized to the patient. (*See* Patient Guides, page 245, for specific instructions)

- If that regimen is not successful, then the patient may try lathering the scalp, covering it with a plastic shower cap, and leaving the shampoo on for 30 minutes before rinsing. This will usually remove even stubborn scale but may cause slight irritation.
- If dandruff shampoo leaves the hair dry, listless, or with an objectionable odor, the patient may perform a final shampoo with a scented cosmetic product, a rinse, or a conditioner.

Topical Corticosteroids

- Corticosteroids suppress the inflammatory component of the disease and result in reduced scaling. Mild preparations (hydrocortisone 1%) are usually adequate. Often, only a few applications of the medicine will cause a complete disappearance of the disease for several days or even weeks. If adequate shampooing and keratolytics do not suppress inflammation of the scalp, a corticosteroid may be used.
- Corticosteroids should be prescribed in a thin solution vehicle to minimize residue on the hair. Solutions are applied to the scalp in the following manner: The hair is parted in a continuous line along the scalp and 1 drop of solution is applied every few centimeters along this line and rubbed in. The hair is then parted 2 cm parallel to this line and solution again applied. Parting the hair and applying the solution every few centimeters allow application to all areas, with minimum residue. This technique is described in the Patient Guides, page 245.

- Hydrocortisone solutions are often effective, but more potent corticoids provide a brisker response and probably are not injurious to the scalp when used intermittently. Some corticoid-containing aerosols are available with a thin nozzle to facilitate application to the scalp. These are easier to apply but expensive.

Scale-removing Preparations

- These products are rubbed into the scalp, left for a prolonged period (usually several hours), and then shampooed out. It is convenient to apply them overnight under a shower cap (*See* page 244). They may be slightly irritating.
- Scale-removing preparations remove more scale than do shampoos and are usually effective even in the more severe cases of seborrheic dermatitis and often in psoriasis.
  - Mineral oil, "baby oil," olive oil, and other oils facilitate scale removal.
  - Salicylic acid may be compounded by the pharmacist, 10% in an oil.
  - *Tar*: Tar gels such as Betatar gel, DHS, or MG217 are readily available over the counter (*See* page 244).

Psoriasis

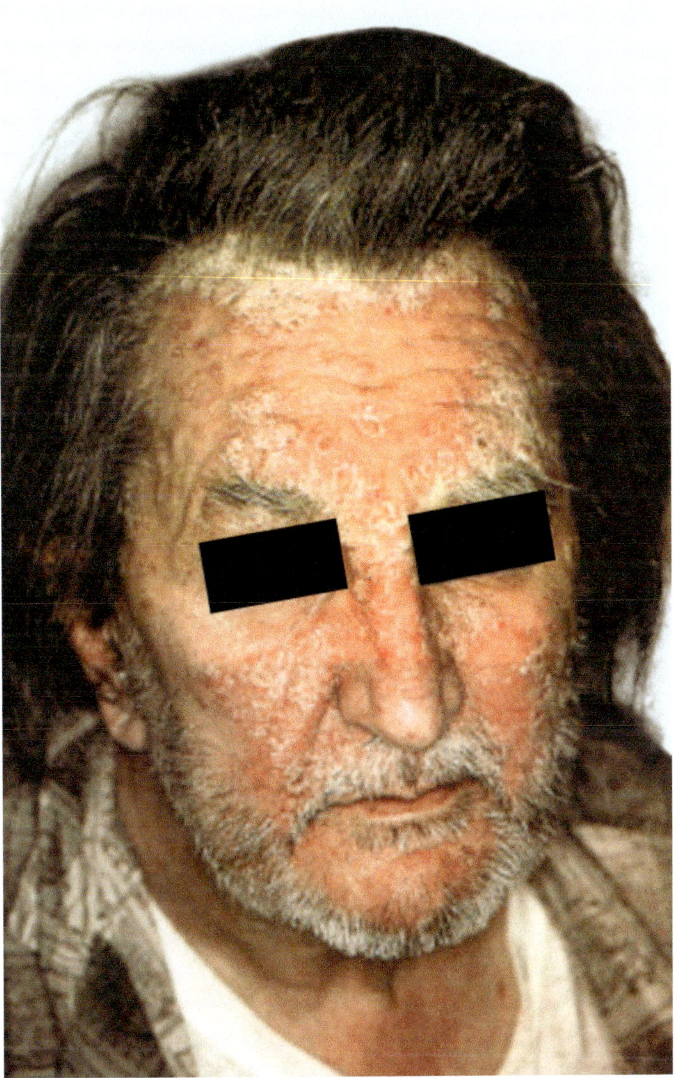

Neglected psoriasis showing marked involvement of the scalp and the much less common involvement of the face.

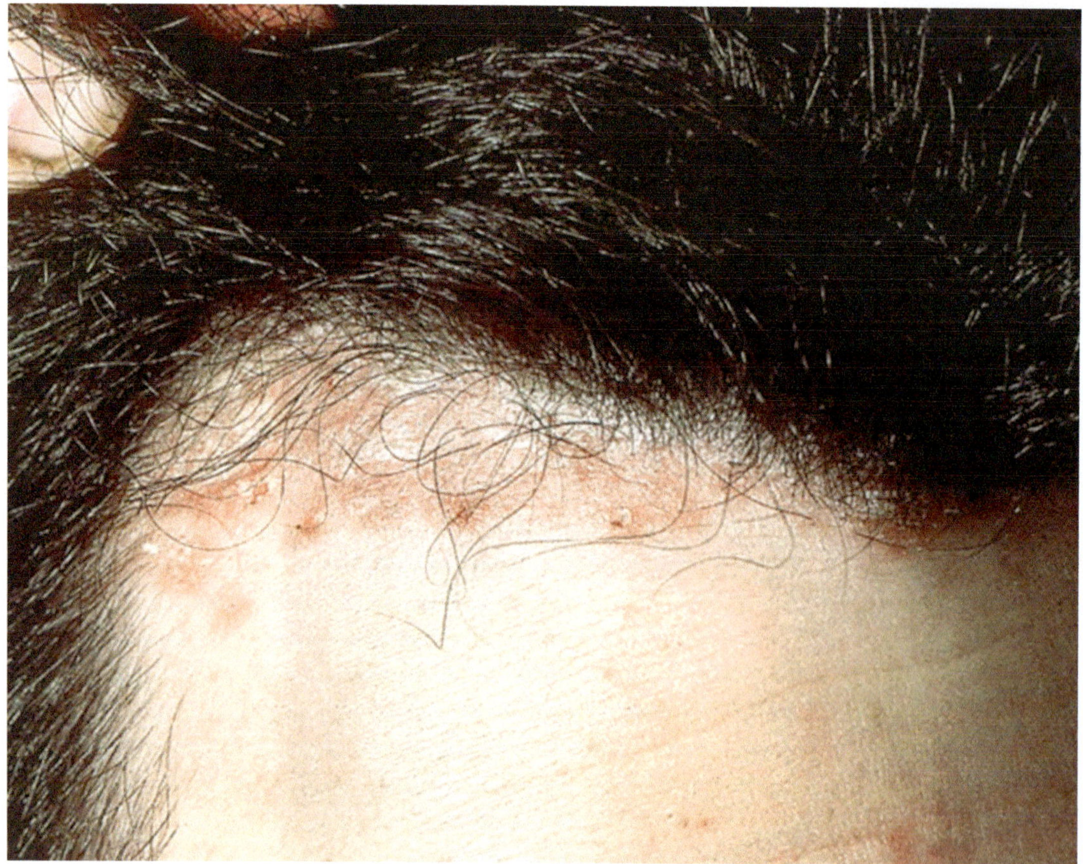

In contrast to seborrheic dermatitis, psoriasis occurs in well-defined plaques and usually has a thicker and caked scale.

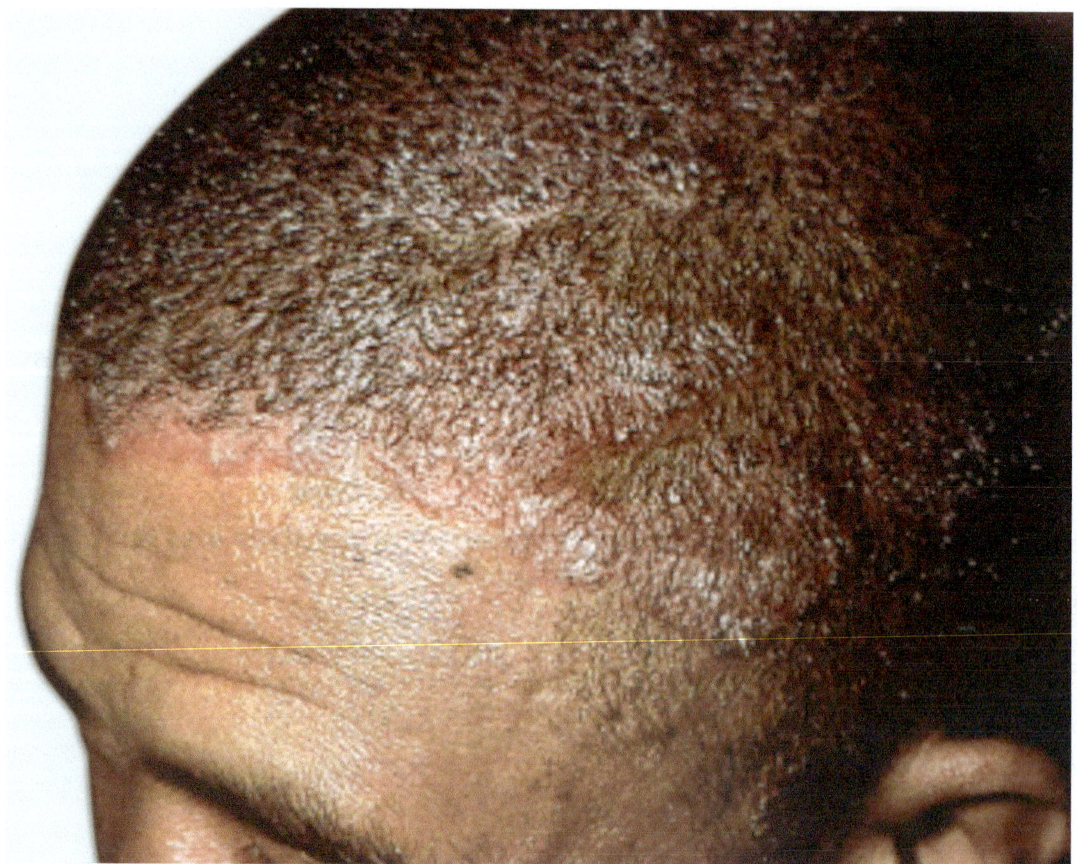

Well-defined pink, scaly plaques are typical of psoriasis.

CLINICAL

- Differs from seborrheic dermatitis (*See* page 1) in that:
  - The red areas are clearly demarcated, often elevated, and of a deep red color.
  - The scale is thicker and more profuse.
  - Involvement of the face, brows, and lashes is less common.
- Look for plaques of psoriasis elsewhere (*See* page 117), "pinking" of the skin of the intergluteal fold (*See* page 121), and nail changes (*See* page 122).

TREATMENT

Similar to seborrheic dermatitis (*See* page 2) except that:

- It is more often necessary to use topical tars, scale-removing oils, or potent corticosteroid solutions, especially under occlusion overnight.
- Calcipotriene (*See* page 123), a topical vitamin D analog, in a liquid form and foam for scalp application.
  - No more effective than midpotency corticosteroid betamethasone valerate
  - Irritating if it drips or bleeds slowly down onto the face, especially in facial skinfolds
- If the condition is widespread on the body, severe, or disabling, then referral to a dermatologist is indicated for phototherapy, treatment with oral antimetabolites (*See* page 124) or a biologic agent that may be required.

Tinea Capitis

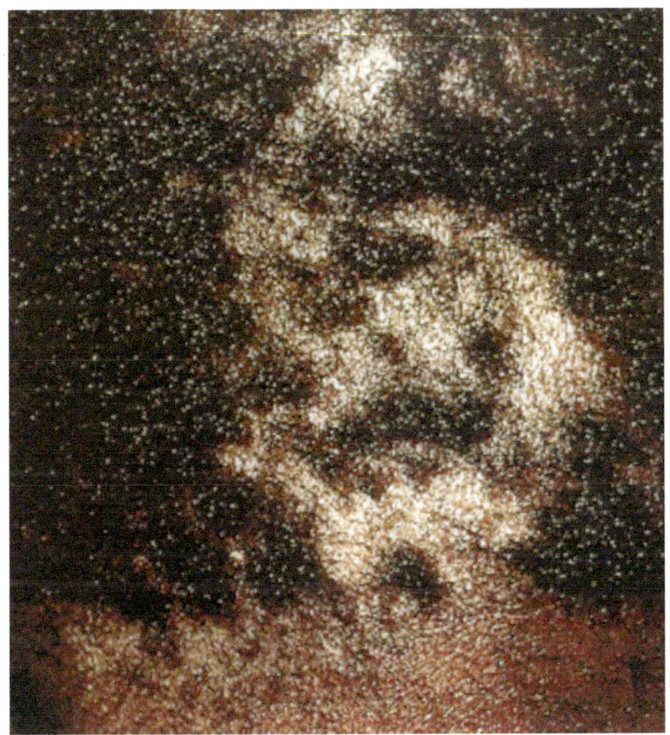

Early, noninflammatory tinea capitis. Spotty, "motheaten" pattern.

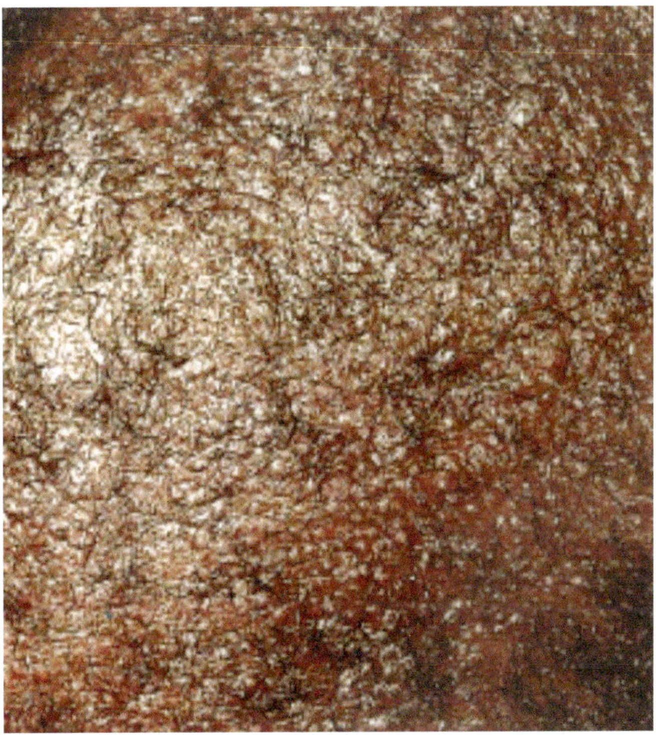

Noninflammatory tinea capitis causing well-demarcated area of hair loss with residual stumps of broken hairs.

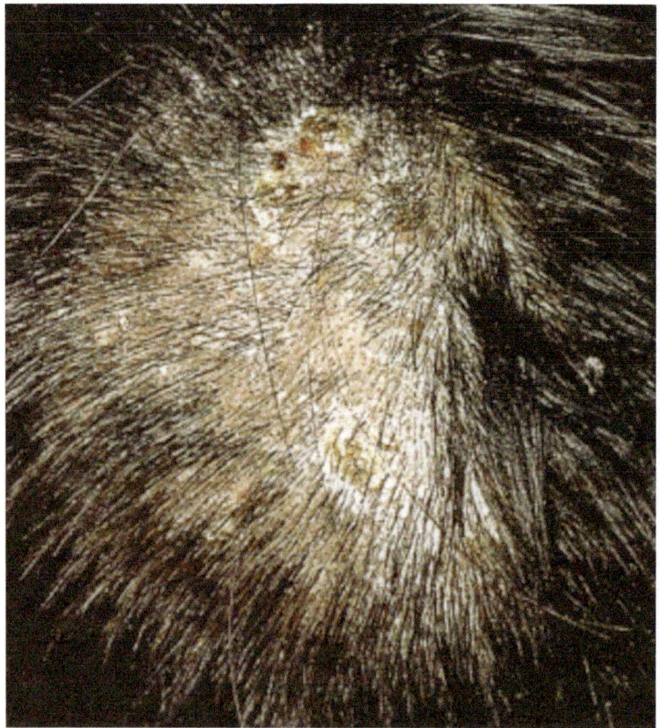

Patch of tinea capitis with broken hair stubs and spots of early inflammation or kerion formation.

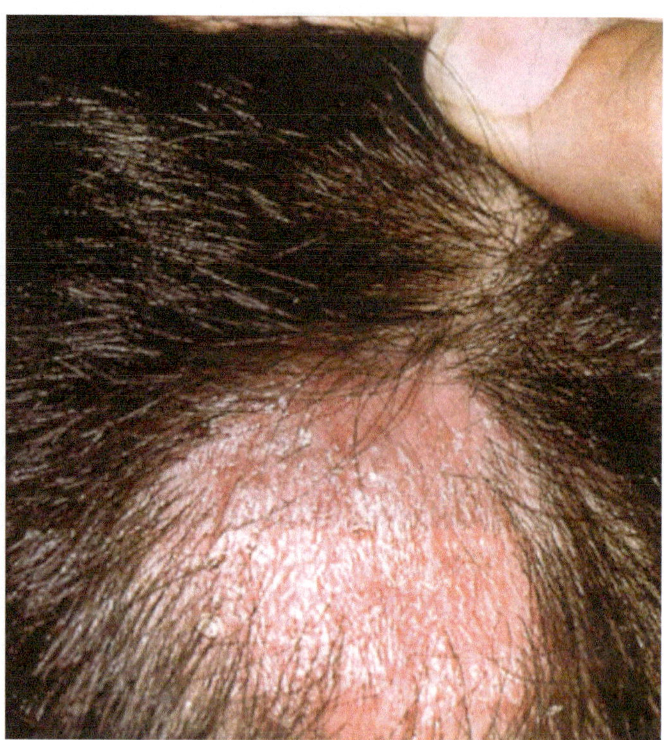

Marked inflammation of kerion in tinea capitis.

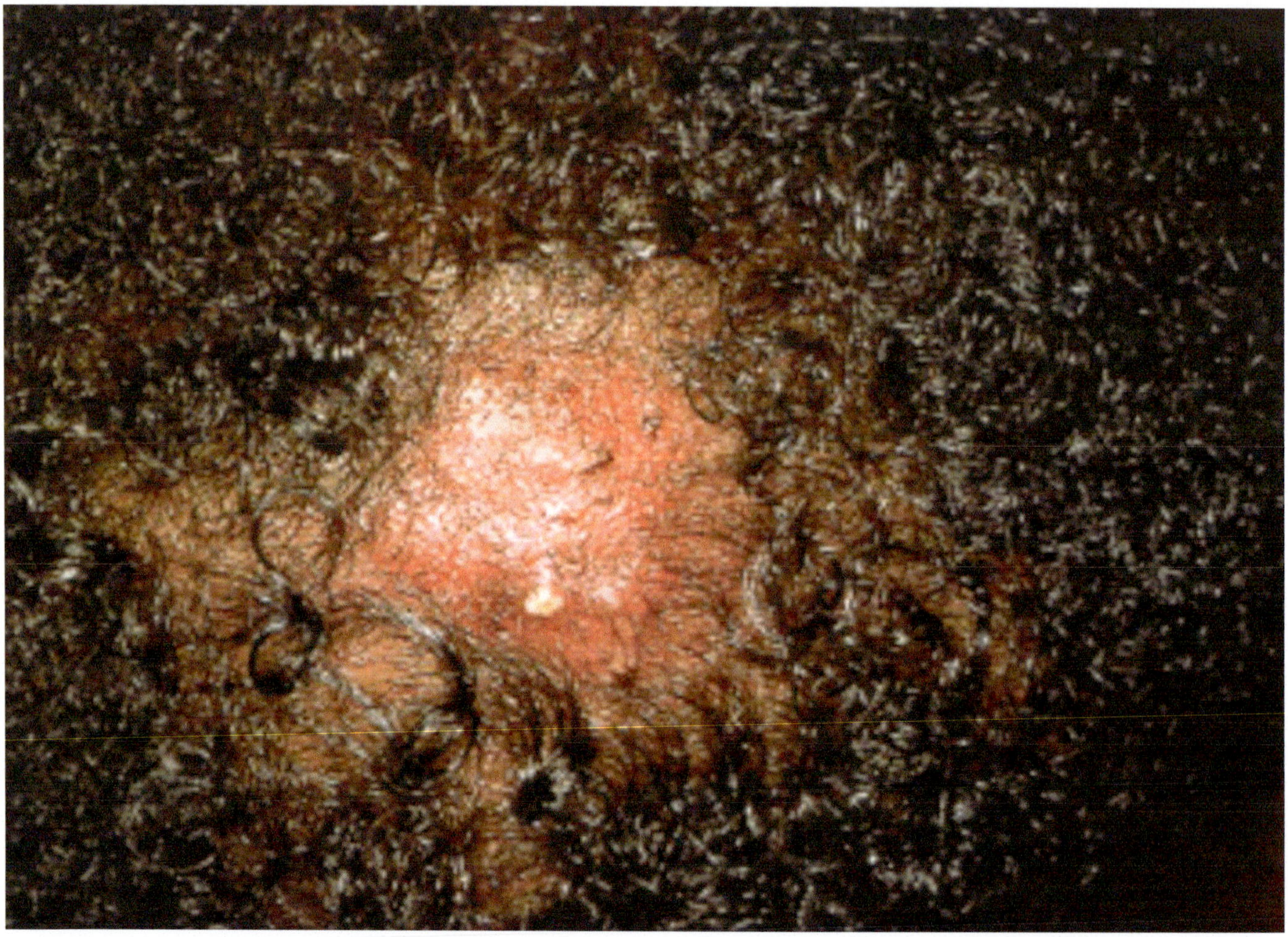

Extreme delayed hypersensitivity to fungal antigens in kerion with inflammatory (sterile) pustules.

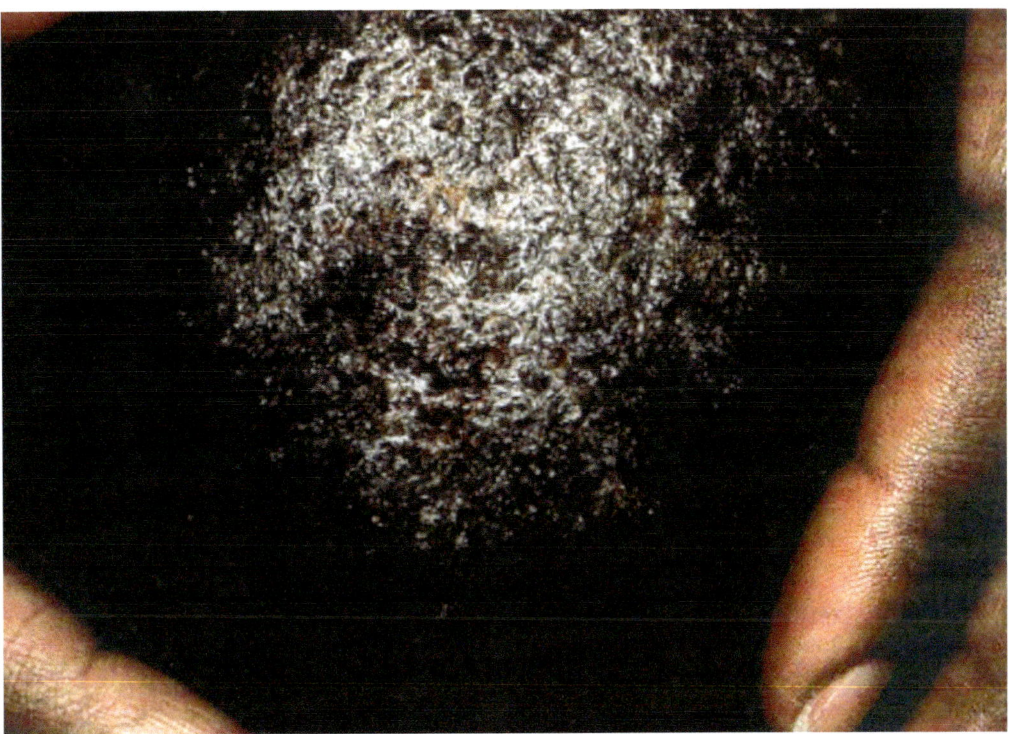

Heavily crusted kerion of long duration.

CLINICAL

- "Ringworm" of the scalp and hair appears as scattered, scaly patches containing broken hairs.
- Tinea capitis is asymptomatic to mildly itchy.
- This disorder does *not* result in permanent alopecia.

After several weeks, the lesion may suddenly become inflamed, swollen, and even surmounted by pustules. This is *kerion,* a delayed hypersensitivity reaction to fungal antigens, similar to a violent purified protein derivative (PPD) reaction. It may result in permanent alopecia.

- Kerion is often misdiagnosed as an acute bacterial process. However, in this case, bacterial culture results are negative, and antibacterial therapy is ineffective.
- The clinical tipoff is the serenity of the patient. Kerion is nearly asymptomatic, whereas the equivalent bacterial folliculitis is exquisitely tender with painful adenopathy.
- Plucking a hair and performing a potassium hydroxide (KOH) examination or fungal culture will confirm the diagnosis. (*See* Diagnosis of Fungal Infections, page 226).

TREATMENT

- Topical therapy does not work because hyphae may grow down into the follicles.
- Patients should receive appropriate oral therapy for 4–8 weeks or for at least 1 week after the apparent clearing of the lesion.
    - Therapy should continue for 4–8 weeks or for at least 1 week after the apparent clearing of the lesion.
        - An oral antifungal agent that has been shown to work is itraconazole 100 mg daily for 4–6 weeks. This treatment is not officially approved in the United States for dermatophyte infections or for children, although there are several reports of safe use in children. (*See* Treatment of Fungal Infections, page 235).
        - Alternatives are griseofulvin, terbinafine, and fluconazole. Treatment choice should be guided by the resistance pattern in the respective country.

Oral antifungals are given as treatment for kerion, but inflammation will not subside in the first few weeks because the fungal antigen will still be present during this time.

- Kerion inflammation should be treated promptly and vigorously to minimize the likelihood of permanent alopecia. Depot intralesional (*See* page 240) or oral corticosteroids (for 2 weeks) are required to promptly suppress the reaction. Topical corticosteroids are usually ineffective in this deep inflammation.
- Learn to diagnose kerion quickly to avoid frustrating, ineffective treatment with systemic antibiotics and incision and drainage, which postpones the administration of appropriate (corticosteroid) therapy.

Head Lice

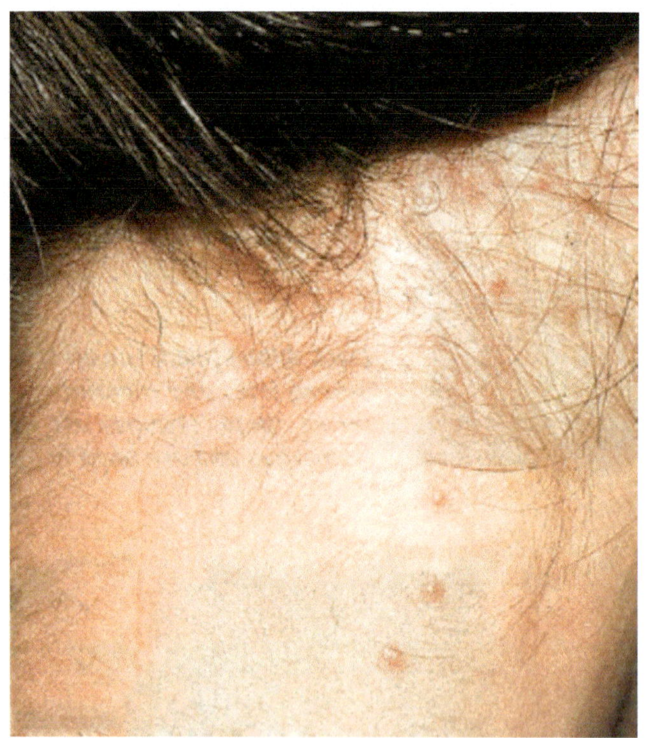

Typical bite papules at nape of neck in pediculosis capitis.

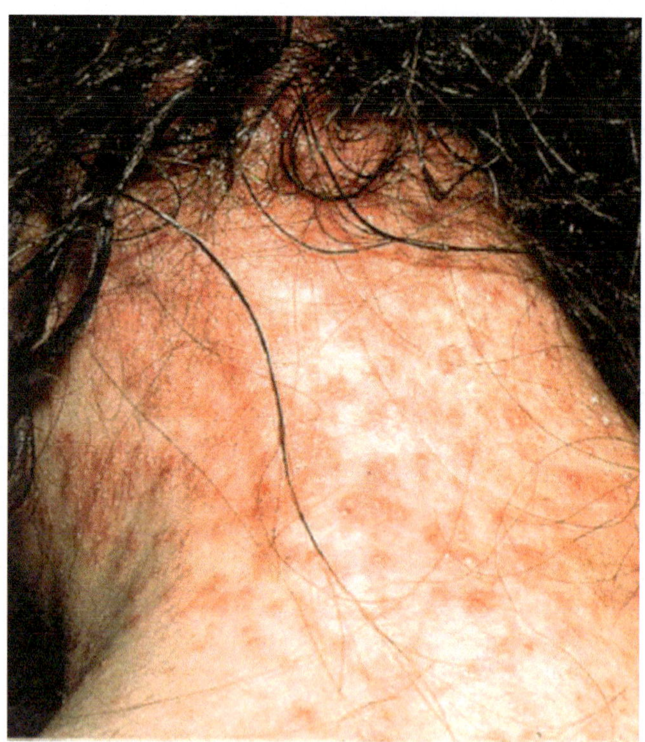

Marked bites with exudation, edema, and possible secondary infection in neglected pediculosis capitis.

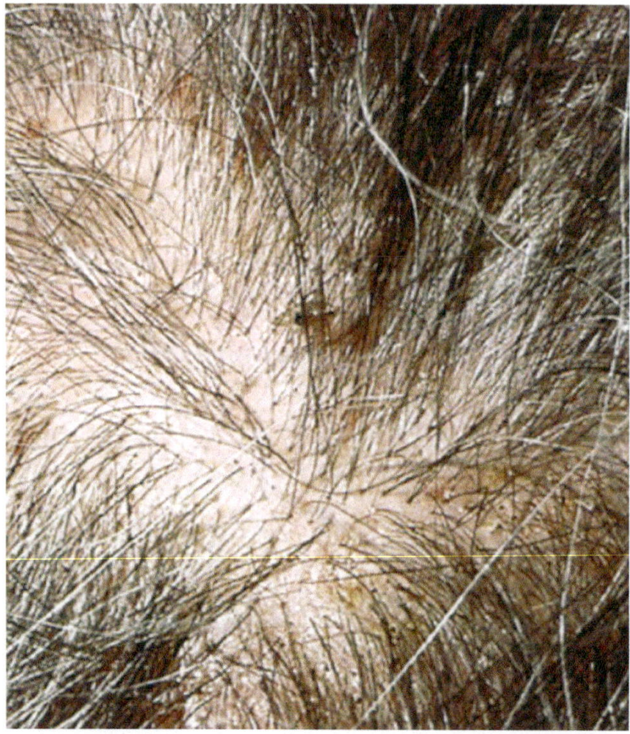

Dark (blood-filled) lice on scalp, among bites and excoriations. As a rule, these creatures are not numerous and are hard to find.

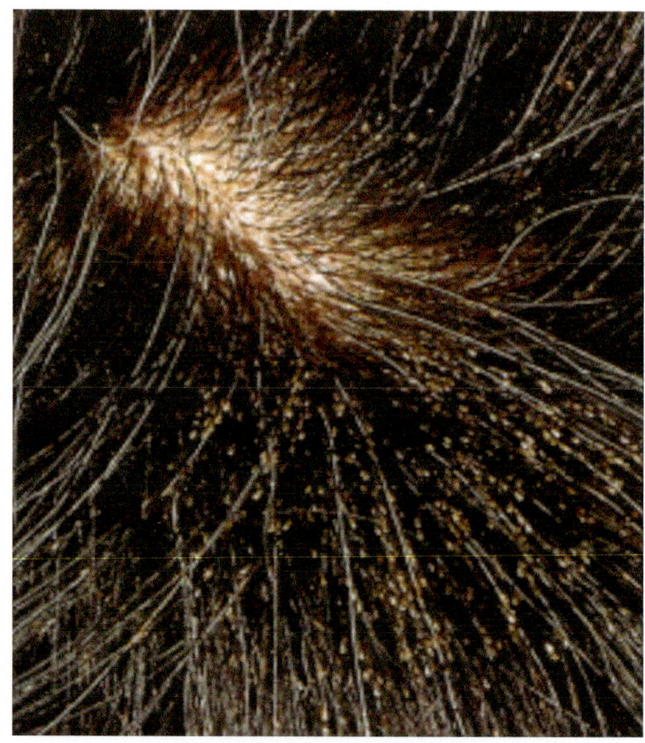

Profuse collection of nits attached to hairs in long-standing pediculosis capitis.

CLINICAL

- Minor to intense itching may occur, especially at the occiput, but not uncommonly this condition is asymptomatic.
- Occasionally, an exudative rash is seen.
- Several live adult insects, 2-mm long, and several to hundreds of white 1-mm nits (ova) may be seen adhering to hairs.
- This is quite contagious among children; less so in adults.

TREATMENT

Pediculocides (*See* page 237)

- Permethrin cream rinse is rubbed into the scalp and shampooed out in 10 minutes. This product is available over-the-counter.
- Over-the-counter products include pyrethrins with piperonyl butoxide and ivermectin 0.5% lotion, which are applied to dry hair and rinsed out after 10 minutes. Prescription products include malathion 0.5% lotion or gel, spinosad 0.9% cream rinse, ivermectin 0.5% lotion, and benzyl alcohol 5%. Oral ivermectin (off label for resistant cases) may be given at 200–400 μg/kg on days 1 and 8.

Nit Removal

The previously listed treatments kill the nits as well as the adult lice, but the devitalized nits continue to adhere tenaciously to the hair. Removal may be difficult. Two procedures are recommended:

1. Over-the-counter "nit removal system" (Step 2), using a soak containing 8% formic acid, followed by combing with the fine-toothed comb provided in the kit
2. The time-honored but somewhat less effective program, consisting of the following:
   - Soak hair in generous amounts of white vinegar diluted 1:1 with water; keep under shower cap or towel for 30 minutes.
   - Immediately comb out dripping hair with a fine-toothed flea comb (purchased in pet stores); then shampoo with mild shampoo.
   - This procedure may need to be repeated daily for a few days.

After adequate pediculocide treatment, the child is no longer contagious and may return to school even if (now dead) nits are still present. However, school policy may bar children from school until all nits are removed.

Preventing Reinfestation and Contagion

- Adult organisms may contaminate hats, collars, high-chair backs, bed clothes, combs, and brushes
- Wash, dry-clean, or hot-iron hats, coats, shirts, blankets, sheets, and pillow cases
- Thoroughly wash combs and brushes in hot, soapy water
- Vacuum or otherwise clean beds, pillows, and upholstered furniture used by the patient
- *See* Patient Guides, page 249.

Hair Loss (Alopecia)

Ascertain whether the patient's symptom is increased shedding of hair (most noticeable when combing or washing) or thinning and balding.

THINNING AND BALDING

Patchy Hair Loss (Bald Spots)

- Well-circumscribed patches of complete baldness with a normal scalp is usually alopecia areata.
  - Short, constricted, blunt-tipped "exclamation point" hairs may be seen at the periphery of the bald area.
  - White hairs may remain when pigmented hairs fall out.
  - Hair loss may involve brows, lashes, beard, and body hair.
  - Hair usually regrows spontaneously in several months but bald spots may remain or progress to intermittent or permanent alopecia.
- *Other:*
  - If the area is inflamed, the condition may be folliculitis or tinea capitis (*See* page 5).
  - A mass may indicate a cyst or metastatic lesion.

- Vague, scattered, and small areas of thinning may be "moth-eaten" alopecia of secondary syphilis.
- An area of short, blunt stubble on an otherwise normal scalp is trichotillomania, the nervous habit of pulling hair.

TREATMENT OF ALOPECIA AREATA

Corticosteroids

- Potent topical preparations under occlusion are occasionally effective.
- Intralesional injection of triamcinolone acetonide 5 mg/mL or other repository preparation (*See* page 240 for technique) is often at least temporarily effective. Repeat at monthly to bimonthly intervals.
- Systemic corticosteroids are occasionally given for long term, often on alternate days, to patients with total or disfiguring alopecia. Refer these patients to a specialist for such management.

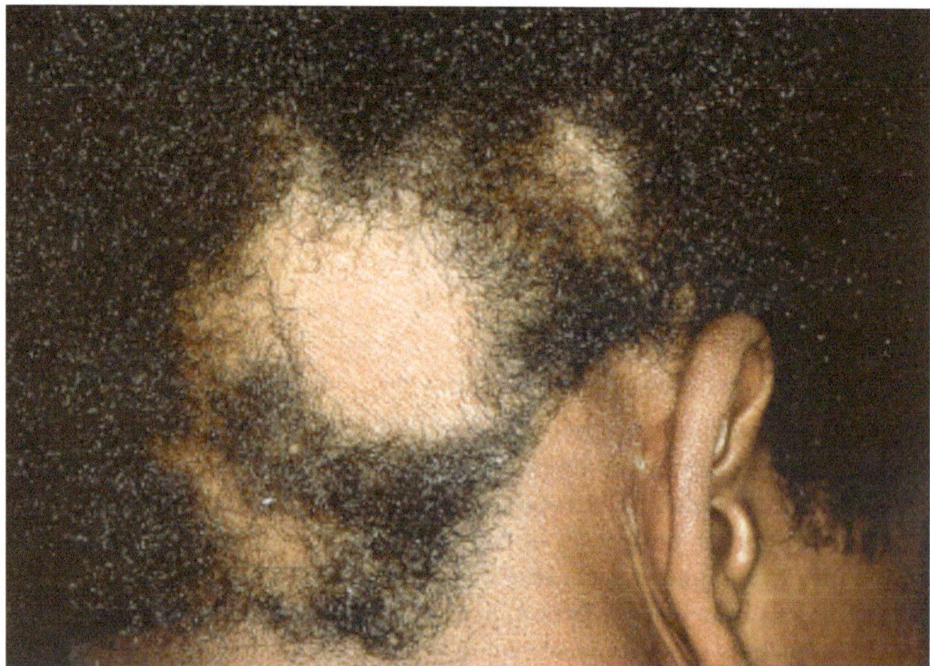

Typical well-defined areas of complete hair loss in alopecia areata.

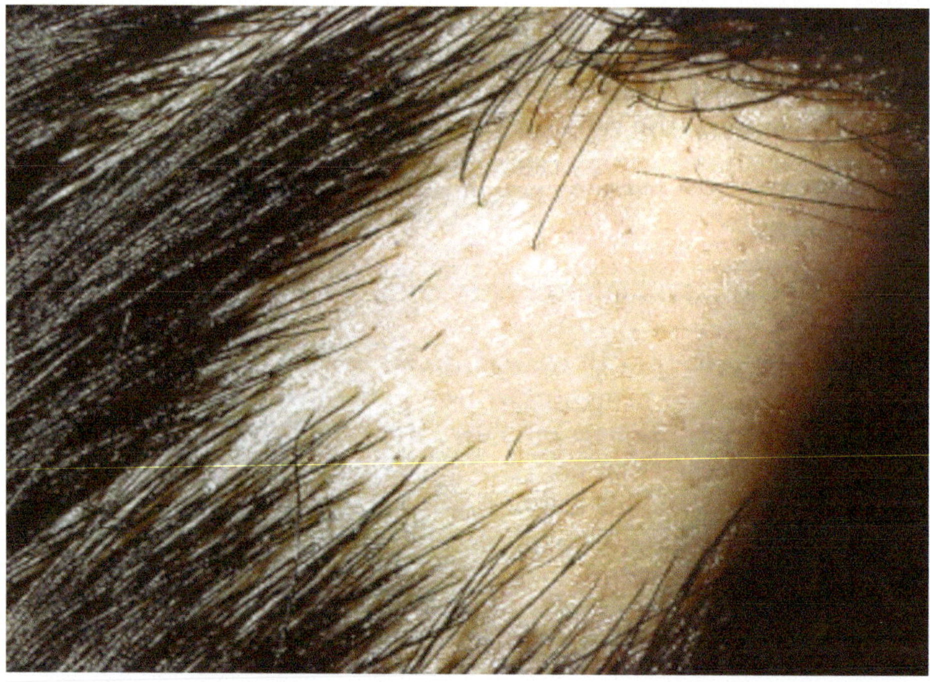

Short, blunt-ended, loose "exclamation-point" hairs may be seen at the edge of the bald area.

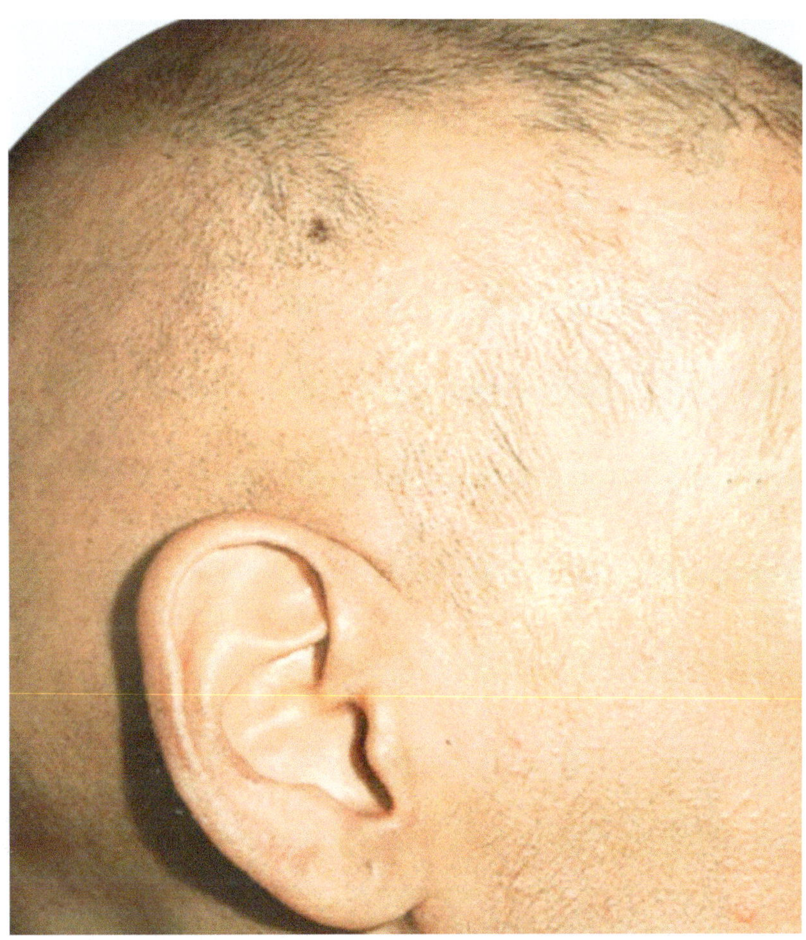

Alopecia can be extensive, having a poor prognosis.

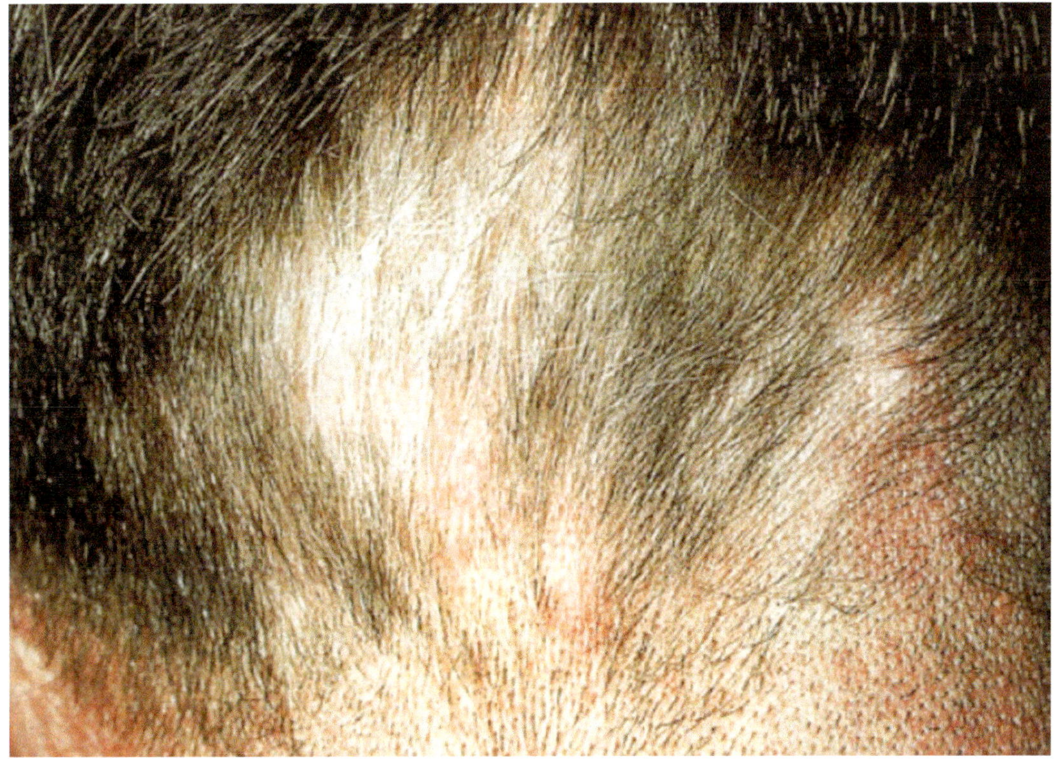

*Early regrowth in alopecia areata is often with nonpigmented hairs.
Later growth has normal pigmentation.*

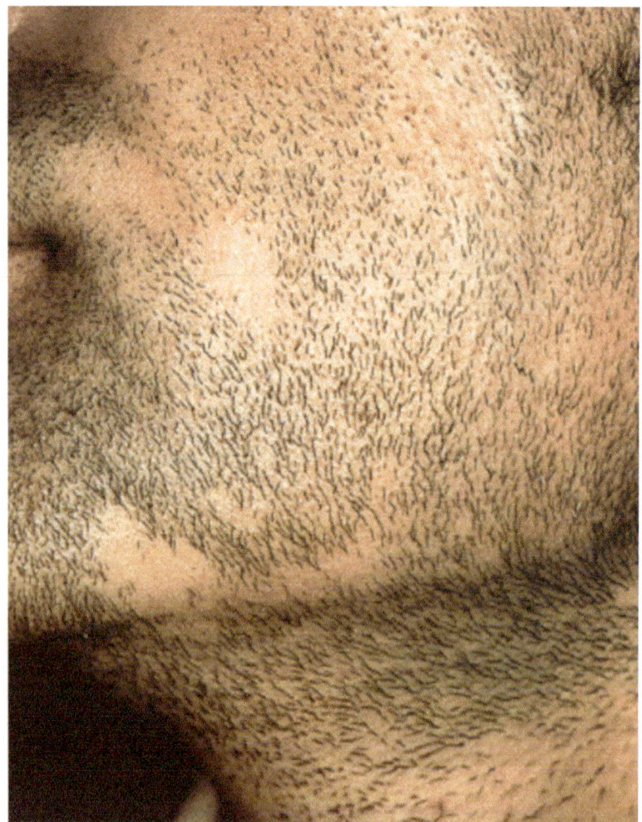

Any hair-bearing site can be affected by alopecia areata.

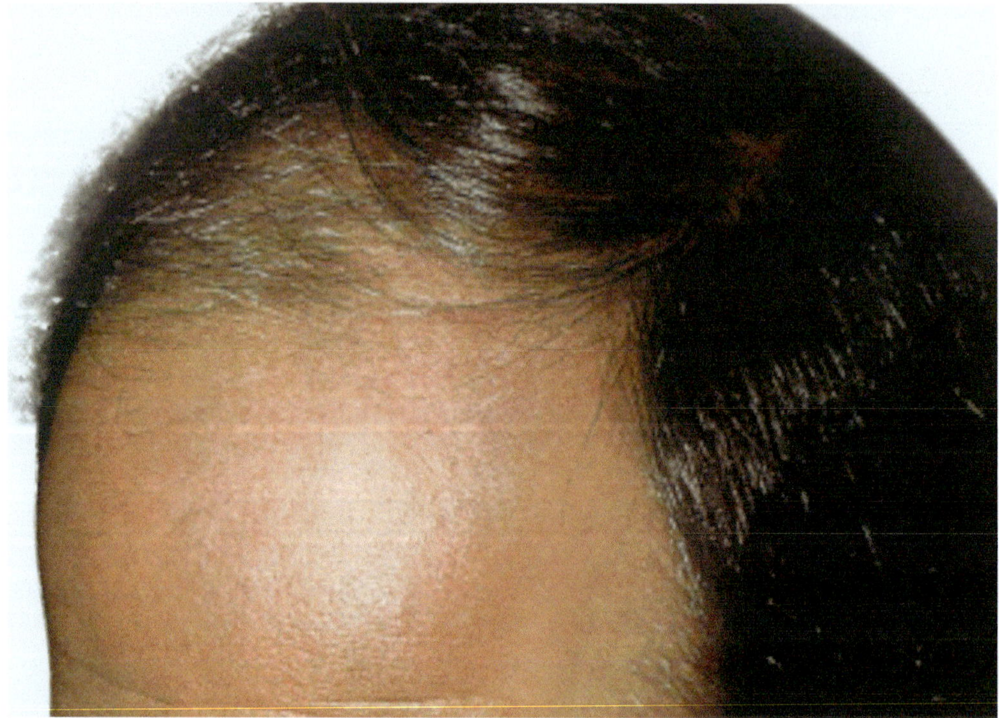

Androgenetic alopecia (male balding) has a temporofrontal pattern with fine, wispy hairs at the margin.

Other Treatments

- Minoxidil solution or foam (2% or 5%) applied topically is occasionally effective.
- Scalp-irritative treatments such as that caused by the application of anthralin, sensitization to and light application of a contact allergen, and psoralen–ultraviolet light therapy show promise. All have practical and theoretical drawbacks.

Diffuse Thinning of Hair

Thinning or bald patches at temples and crown are due to "androgenetic" alopecia, or inherited pattern balding.

- In men, this occurs at temples and crown.
- In women, diffuse thinning of entire top of scalp is usually seen.
- Immature, fine, short, and tapering hairs are present at edges of thinning area.

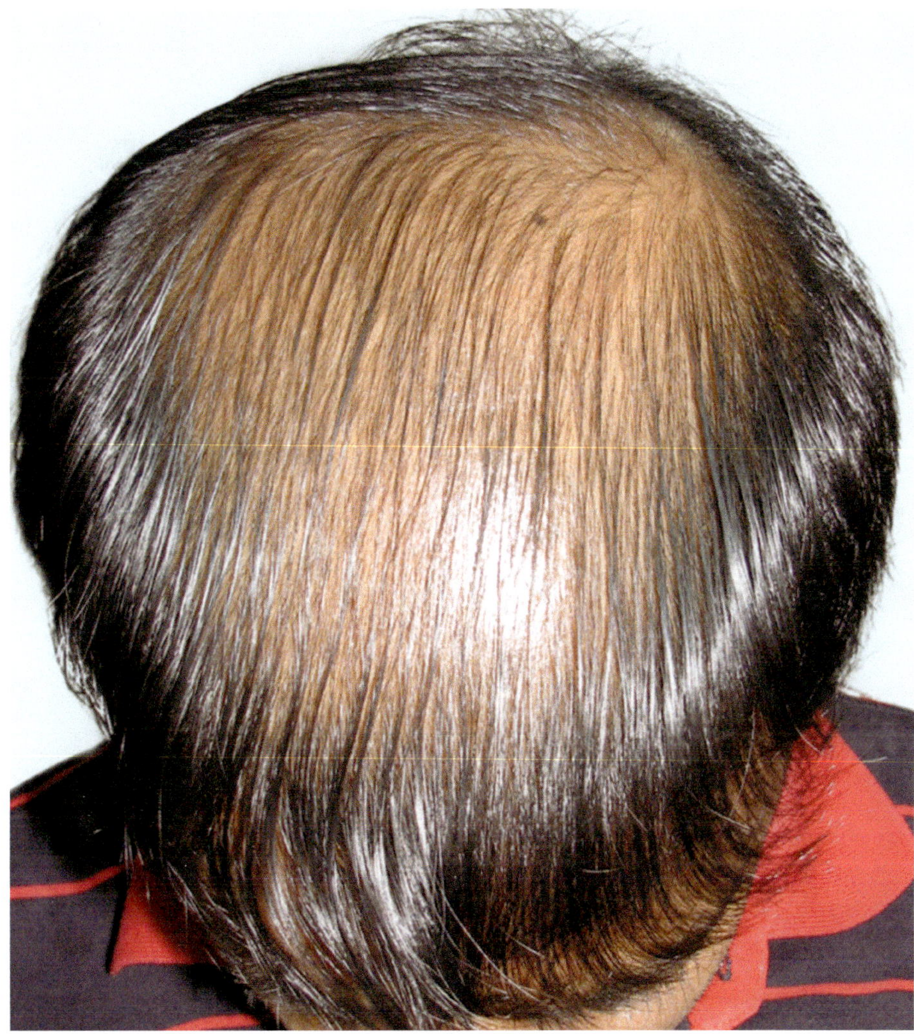

Diffuse hair loss.

Treatment of hereditary baldness:

- Minoxidil 2% or 5% solution applied twice daily results in cosmetically noticeable regrowth of hair in approximately 30% of men and a slightly higher percentage of women.
  - Younger men with thinning hair but not complete baldness respond best. This treatment is also effective in older women with thinning hair.
  - Treatment with minoxidil appears to be safe, except for occasional instances of contact dermatitis.
  - Hair growth reverses when treatment is stopped, so commitment is lifelong if successful.
- Vitamins, massage, and ultraviolet light are without benefit.
- Creative hairstyling may minimize the appearance of thinning.
- Wigs available today are lightweight, cool, and stay glued on in all conditions.
- Scalp plug transplants or flaps improve appearance in selected patients.
- Oral finasteride 1 mg daily may be given to men with male-pattern hair loss. Possible alterations in sexual function and depression are under evaluation.
- Laser caps or combs might be of benefit.

INCREASED SHEDDING OF HAIR

"Telogen effluvium" occurs 2–3 months after childbirth, fever, severe illness, injury, or surgery. Occasionally, it occurs during or after drug therapy (thyroxine, vitamin A, and anticancer drugs).

- Intact hairs, with tiny white bulbs on their proximal ends, are shed profusely.
- Scalp is normal.

Treatment of Telogen Effluvium

- No treatment is necessary; regrowth is bound to occur.
- Follicles are not damaged, just temporarily synchronized in a resting phase.
- Shedding occurs because new hairs are pushing out old ones.
- Growth will proceed at a normal rate of about 12 mm per month.

2 CHAPTER

Face and Neck

Seborrheic Dermatitis

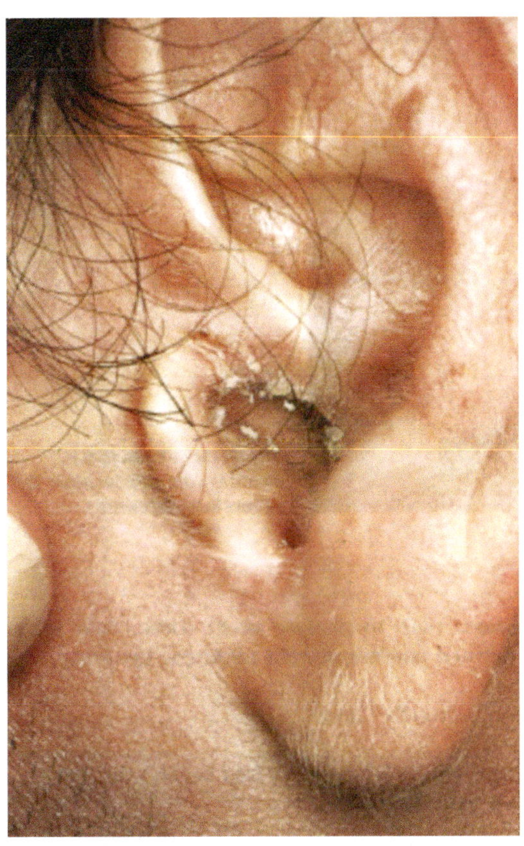

The ear is a common site of seborrheic dermatitis, seen here in the ear canal.

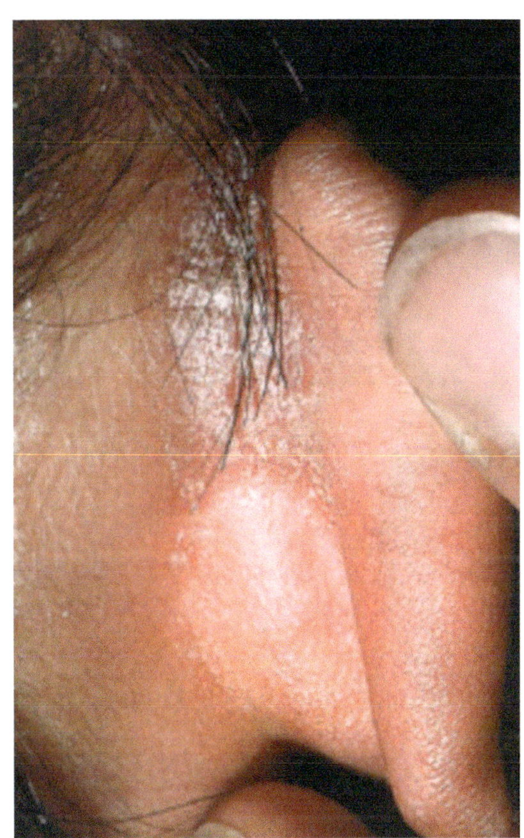

The posterior ear fold is another common location for seborrheic dermatitis.

CLINICAL

- This condition causes mild to profuse small, loose, flaky scales, often on poorly defined patches of mild pinkness, involving:
  - Brows and lashes
  - Nasolabial fold and "butterfly" area
  - Mustache and beard
  - Recesses of pinna, ear canal, and the fold behind the ear
- Mild itching, if any, may be present.
- Scalp itching and scaling are usually present.

- This condition is most common and severe in fair-skinned individuals, less common in the dark skinned.
- The yeast *Malassezia ovalis* may contribute to the pathogenesis of seborrheic dermatitis, but it is also a part of the skin's normal flora, so its role in this condition is unclear.

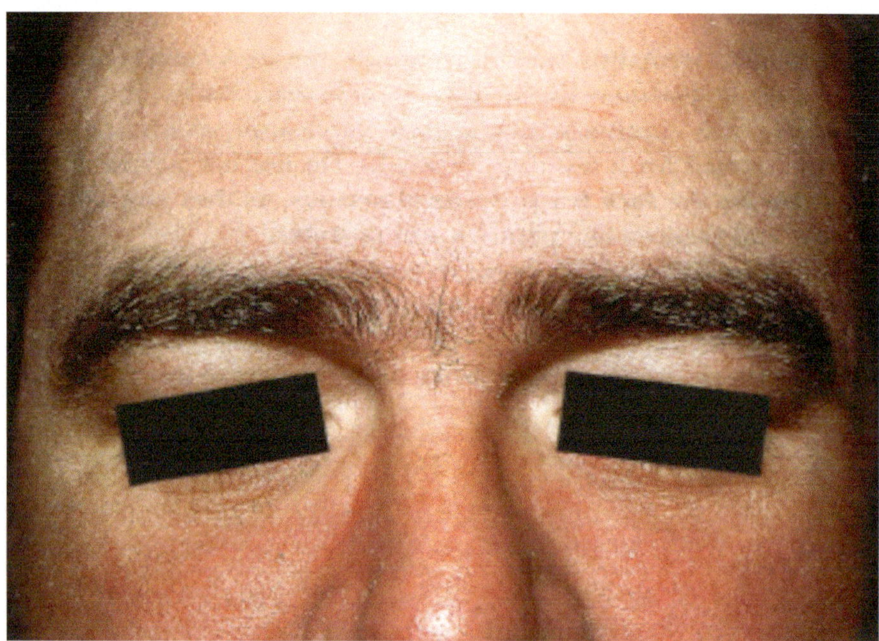

Mild redness and scaling between and in the eyebrows and on the cheeks, constituting the typical centrofacial distribution of seborrheic dermatitis.

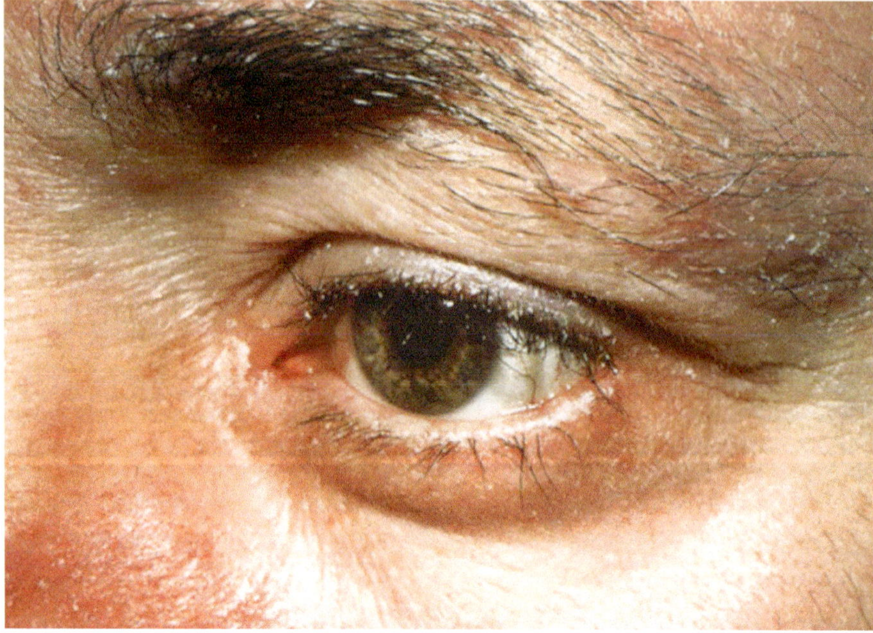

Seborrheic dermatitis of the brows and lashes.

TREATMENT

- Seborrheic dermatitis usually responds quickly to mild corticosteroid cream (hydrocortisone 1%) applied twice daily.
- If severe, this condition may require application of a more potent corticosteroid for a few days or weeks. **Do not use potent corticosteroids on the face for prolonged periods, as they may cause atrophy and rosacea-like papules and pustules.**
- *Alternative therapy:* Low-strength coal tar cream or gel (*See* page 244) or iodoquinol 1%, either alone or in combination with a mild corticosteroid.
- **Ketoconazole cream applied twice daily for days to weeks may benefit refractory cases.**

Pityriasis Alba

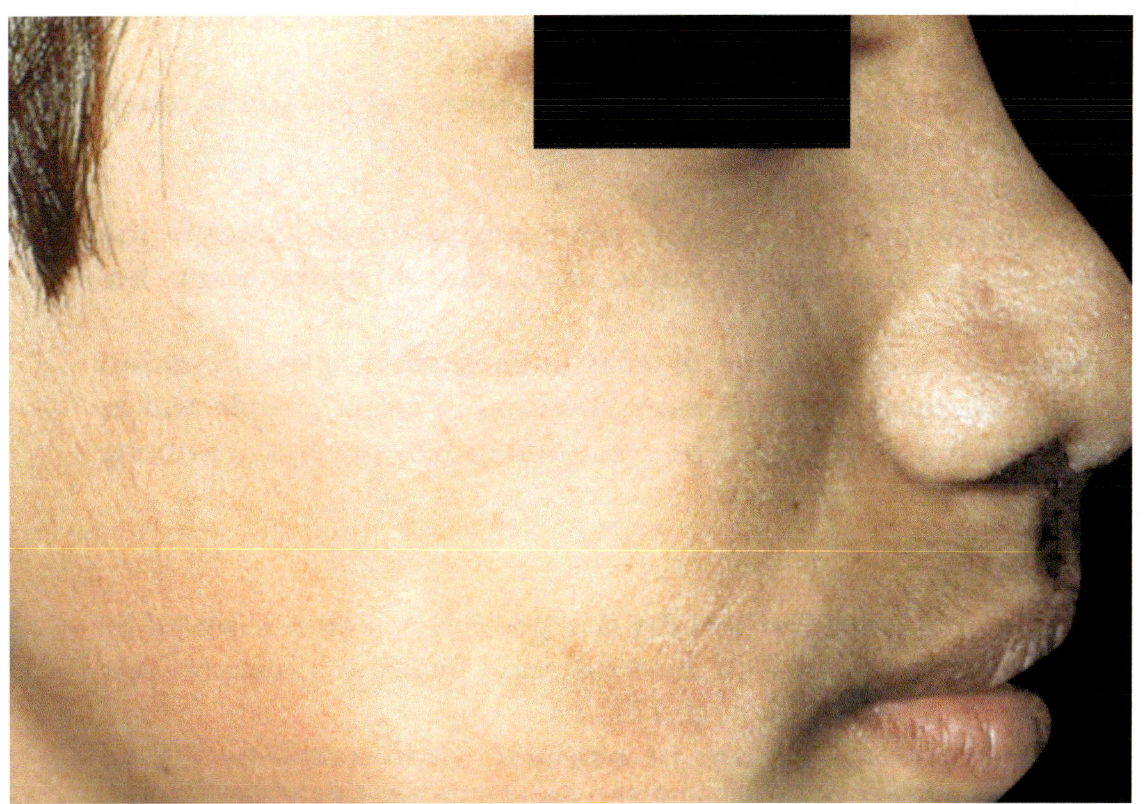

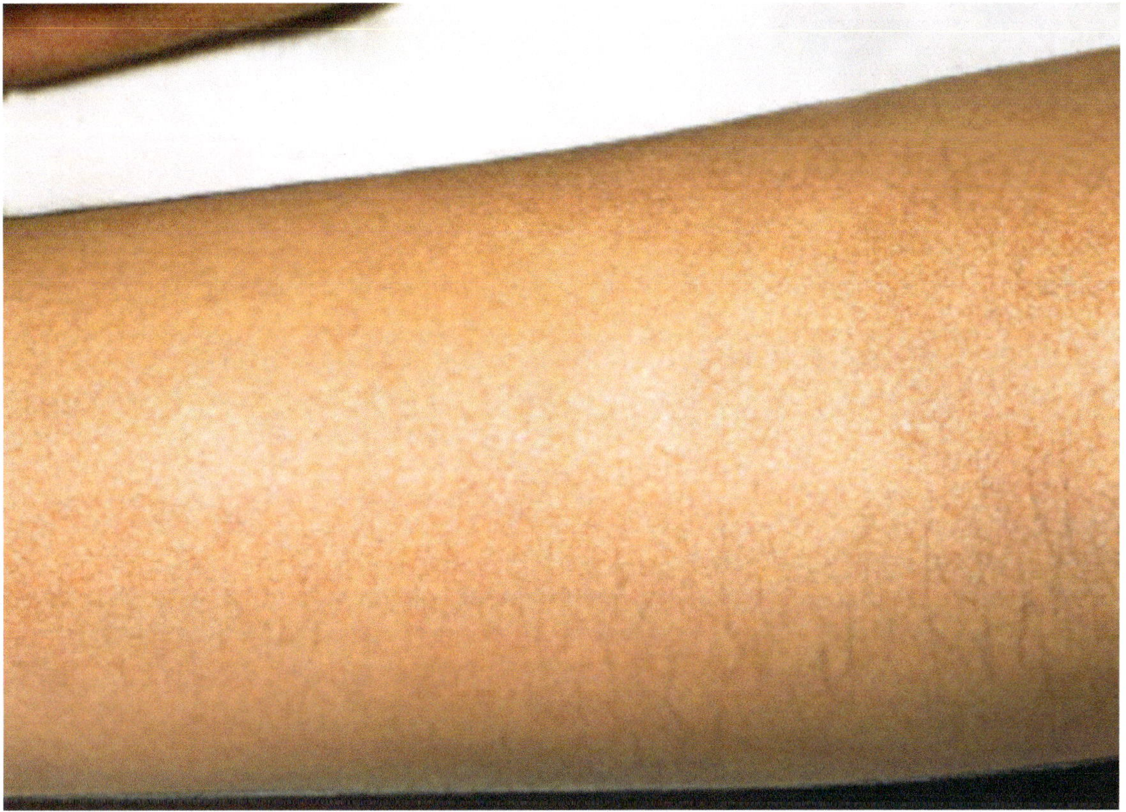

Poorly defined areas of faint hypopigmentation, often with mild scale, on the face and/or arms in pityriasis alba.

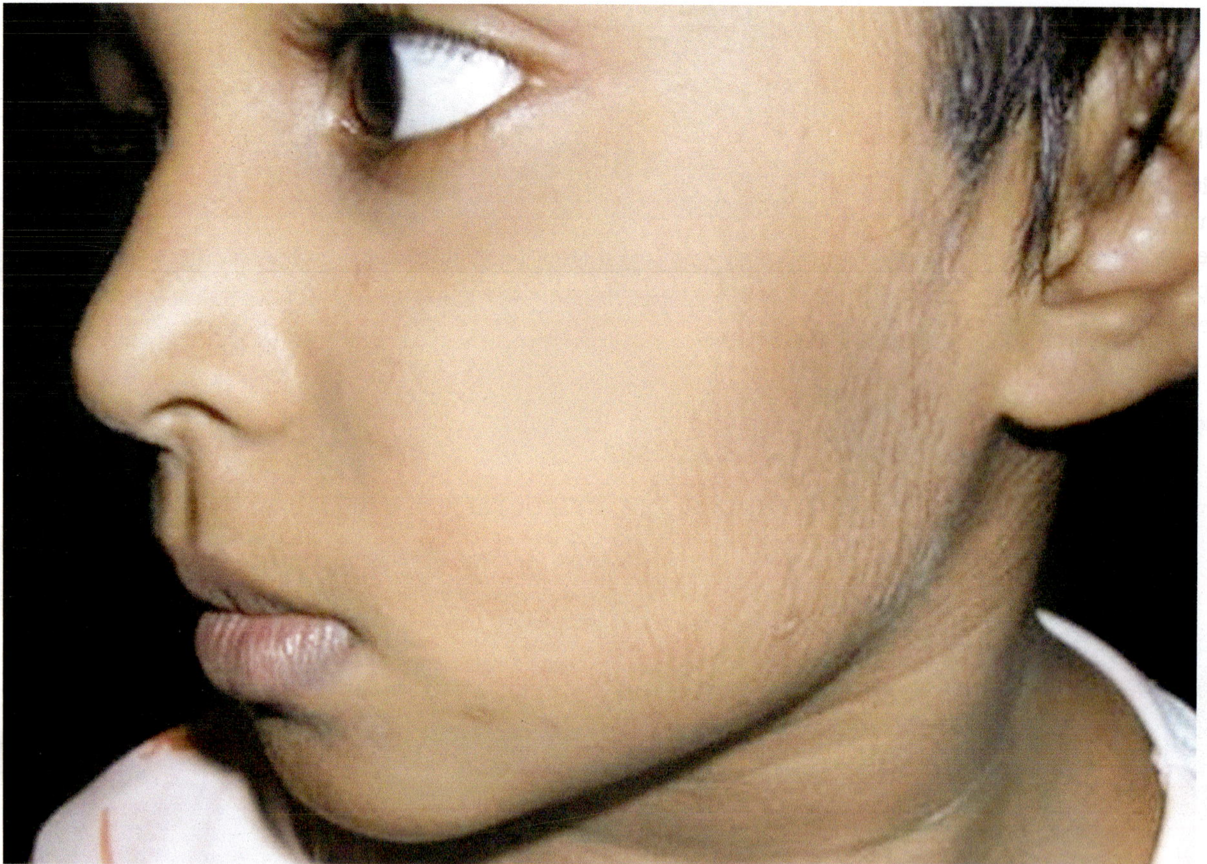

Pityriasis alba over the face.

CLINICAL

- In pityriasis alba, there are usually faint, poorly defined areas of hypopigmentation on the skin, often with fine, shiny scales or slightly glazed surface. The skin may be generally dry or chapped.
- The condition usually occurs on the cheeks and occasionally on the forehead, neck, and upper arms.
- Pityriasis alba occurs in children and young adults and is much more noticeable in the dark skinned.
- This condition is asymptomatic.
- It occurs in dry climates, more often during the dry times of the year (winter in temperate zones, when central heating lowers humidity).
- Hypopigmentation is due to mild inflammation, a manifestation of dry, chapped skin. It is more common in atopic people and in individuals with dry skin. The condition usually resolves at puberty when oil production starts.

TREATMENT

- The hypopigmentation and dry skin possibly can be minimized by washing infrequently with mild soap and by using lubricants (*See* Management of Dry Skin, page 111).
- Mild corticosteroid cream or ointment (hydrocortisone 1-2.5%) should be used twice daily, especially after washing. Repigmentation is not noticeable for at least 4-6 weeks, so **encourage persistence**.
- Total repigmentation from treatment may not occur in all patients but will resolve in adulthood.

Contact Dermatitis

CLINICAL

- **Irritant dermatitis:** Skin irritated by excessive washing with any type of soap or detergent, astringents, medications (e.g., benzoyl peroxides for acne), industrial exposure, or cosmetics.
- **Allergic dermatitis:** Occasional allergy to cosmetics (especially on the eyelids), perfumes, tanning lotions, medications (topical antibiotics, anesthetics), industrial agents (hair dye allergy usually involves the face and ears as well as the scalp)

The thinness of eyelid and facial skin may cause it to react exclusively upon general exposure to an allergen [e.g., *Rhus* (poison ivy, poison oak) dermatitis].

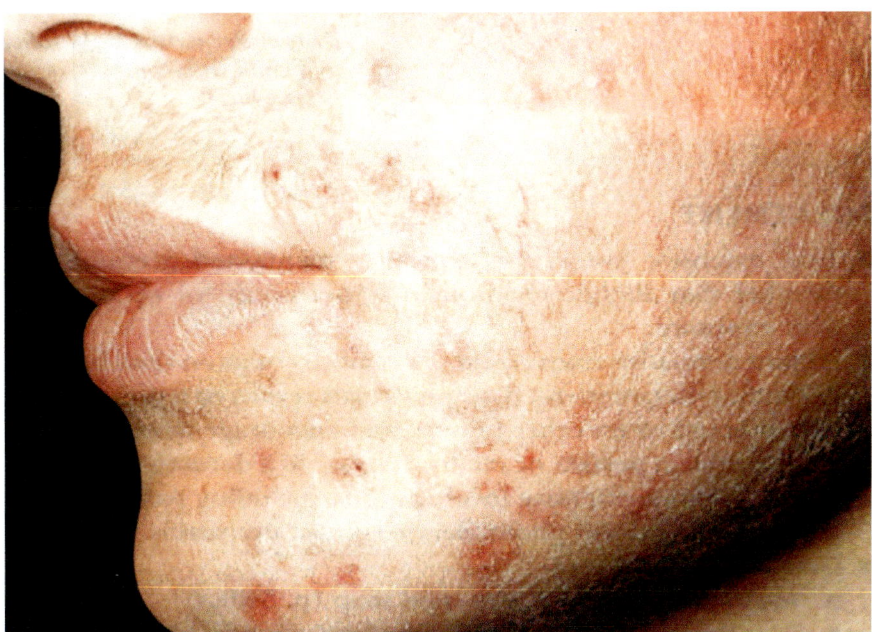

"Dishpan face," or irritant contact dermatitis, manifests as dry, irritated skin from excessive washing with an acne soap.

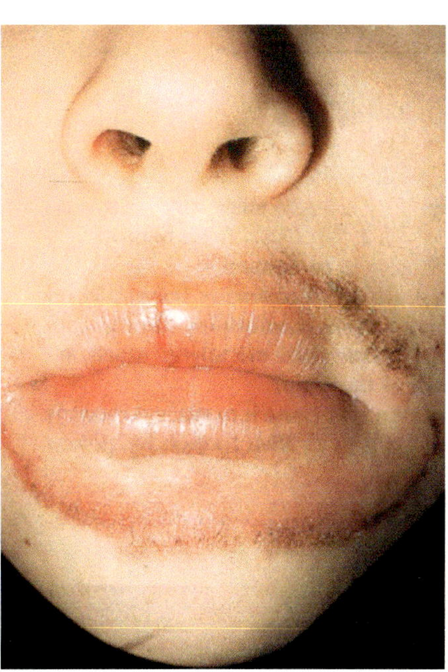

Irritant dermatitis from saliva in a child with compulsive licking habit.

TREATMENT

- Take extensive history for exposures mentioned previously. Remember that allergic reactions may not occur for up to a week after exposure.
- Irritant dermatitis from cosmetics is more common than is allergic dermatitis. Recommend that individuals return to a previously tolerated brand or try other brands, and encourage less use. Allergic contact dermatitis may not manifest for up to a week after exposure—in individuals previously sensitized.
- If the problem persists or recurs, referral to a dermatologist is necessary for more extensive investigations, including patch testing to rule out allergic and photoallergic contact dermatitis.
- General measures:
  - Wash less frequently, with mild soap (*See* page 242).
  - Stop the use of all possible offending agents. Use a simple lubricant, such as glycerin diluted in water.
- If inflammation and itching are significant, cool soaks (*See* page 241) or mild to potent topical corticosteroids are indicated (for a few days or weeks only, if potent).
- For severe allergic reaction, especially if also present elsewhere, systemic corticosteroid therapy is usually indicated.

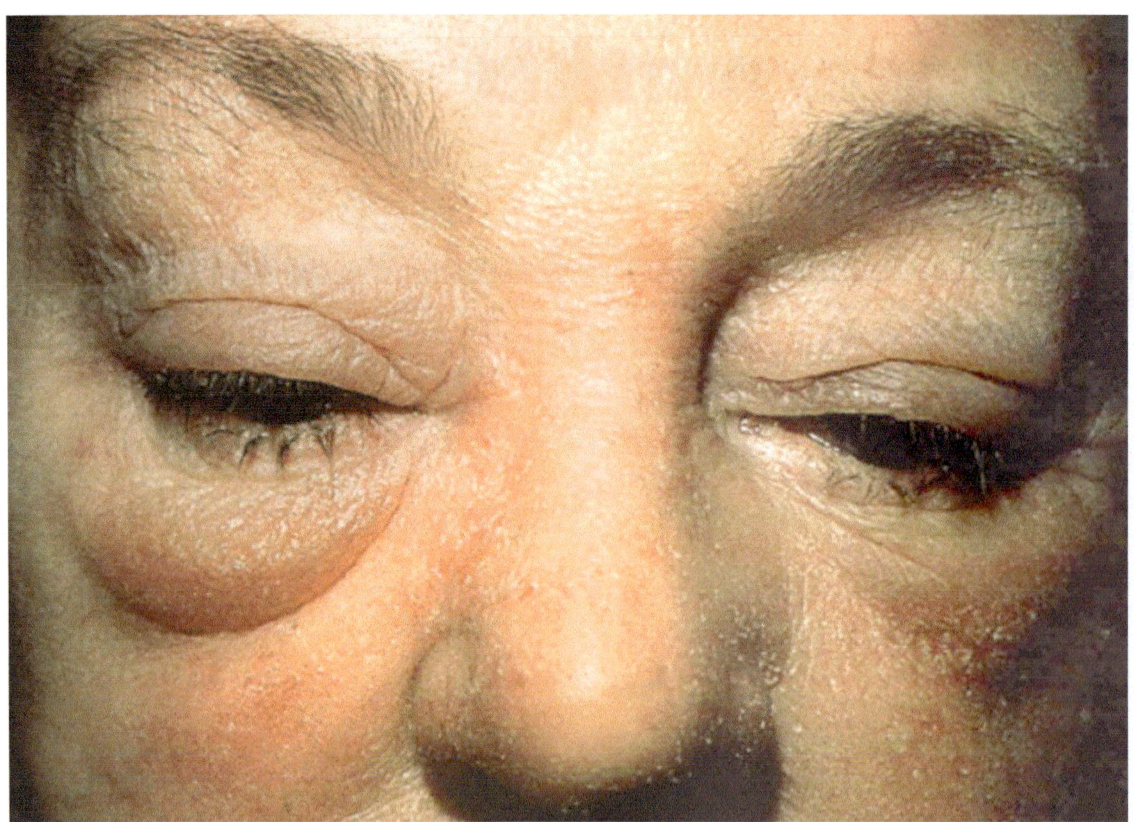

Allergic contact dermatitis from over-the-counter topical medication rubbed over congested sinuses.

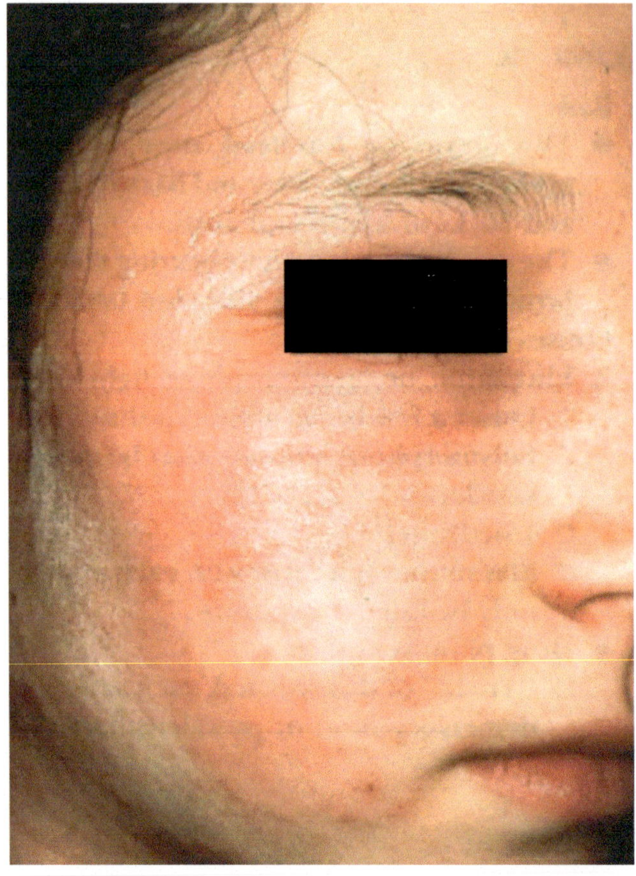

Allergic contact dermatitis from the poison oak plant.

Photodermatitis

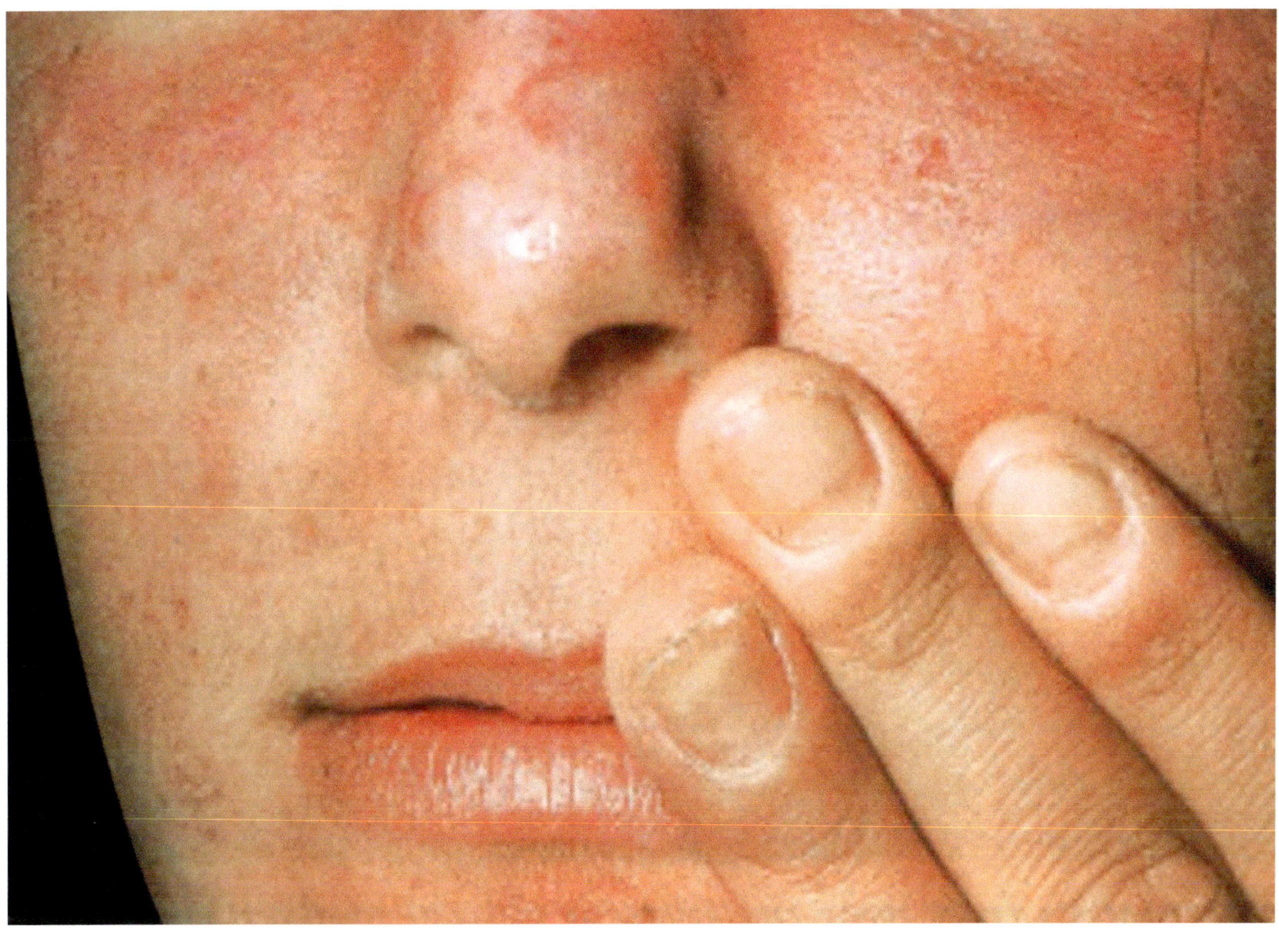

Phototoxic reaction in a patient taking tetracycline, with increased sunburn sensitivity and onycholysis (separation of nail plates from nail beds).

CLINICAL

- Rash
  - This occurs on forehead, nose, malar eminences, upper lip, point of chin, ears, sides and back of neck, V area of upper chest, and backs of hands and arms.
  - The condition spares hair-bearing scalp, eyelids, and area under brows, nose, lower lip, and chin (shaded).
- Causes
  - Idiopathic, or "polymorphous light eruption" ("sun allergy"):
    - Onset a few hours after exposure
    - Polymorphous lesions may be dermatitis, papules, plaques, and vesicles
    - Usually itchy
    - May or may not recur with each exposure or may be triggered only by intense exposure
  - Drug photosensitivity
    - "Toxic" or dose-related, such as with tetracyclines (especially demeclocycline) or psoralens; looks like severe sunburn
    - Allergic: Thiazides, thiazines, sulfa drugs, nitrofurantoin, and many others; itches, looks like dermatitis

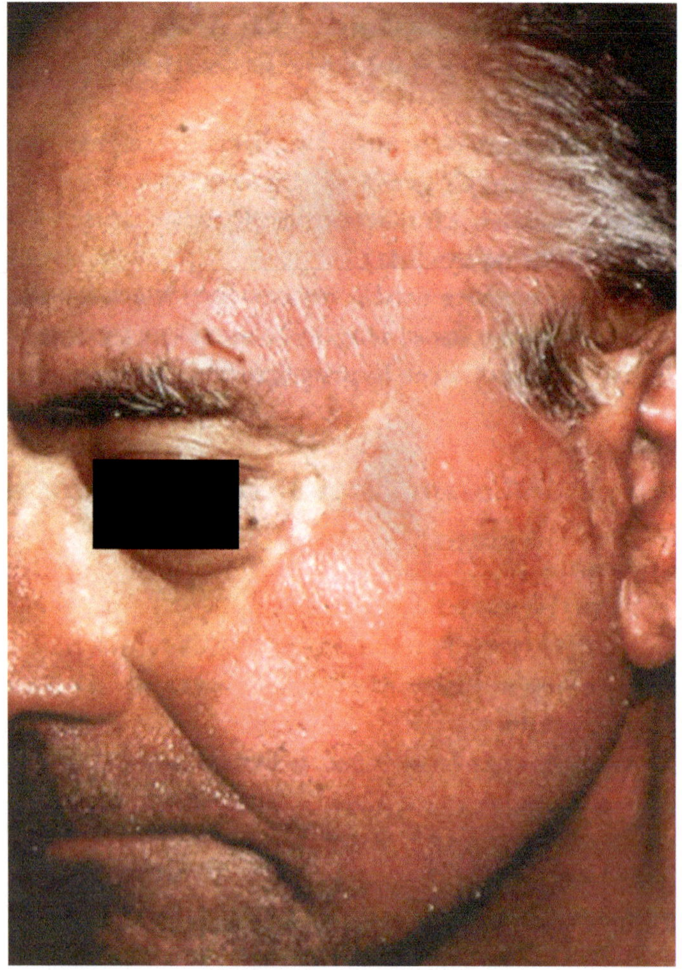

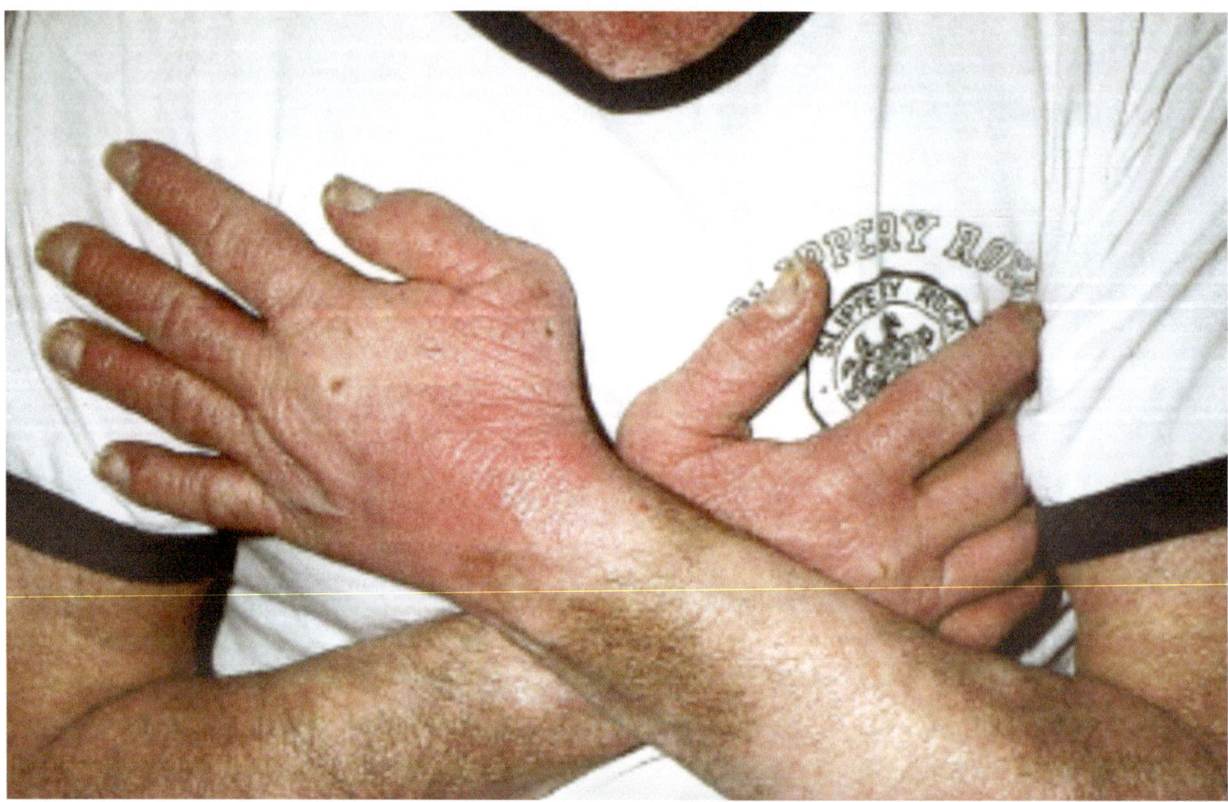

(Same patient) Long-standing, severe idiopathic photosensitivity of polymorphous light eruption of face and hands.

- Internal disease:
  - Lupus erythematosus: May be discoid (purely cutaneous) or systemic; varying degrees of redness, vasculitis, and scarring
  - Dermatomyositis: Characteristically also causes "heliotrope" (violet edema of eyelids)
  - Porphyria (cutanea tarda, especially): Leathery and hyperpigmented areas on face, fragile blisters on hands
  - Pellagra: Leathery and hyperpigmented areas

TREATMENT

- History and physical examination to detect drugs or internal disease. Treat accordingly.
- Reduce sun exposure:
  - Avoid potent 10 AM to 2 PM sun
  - Wear brimmed hats, long sleeves, and gloves
  - Use sun-blocking agents (*See* page 204), especially those with broad-spectrum protection.
- Topical corticosteroids (moderately potent) to reduce redness and symptoms
  - Sedating antihistamines may help to alleviate pruritus
  - Systemic steroids may be needed for severe, generalized eruptions
- Antimalarials (hydroxychloroquine) help polymorphous light eruption and the rash of lupus erythematosus. ***Caution:* Antimalarials in high doses are hepatotoxic to patients with porphyria. Moderate- to long-term use requires ophthalmologic follow-up to monitor for retinopathy.**
- Phlebotomy or cautious, low doses of antimalarials should be used for porphyria cutanea tarda.
- Refer puzzling and chronic cases to a dermatologist for phototesting and therapy.

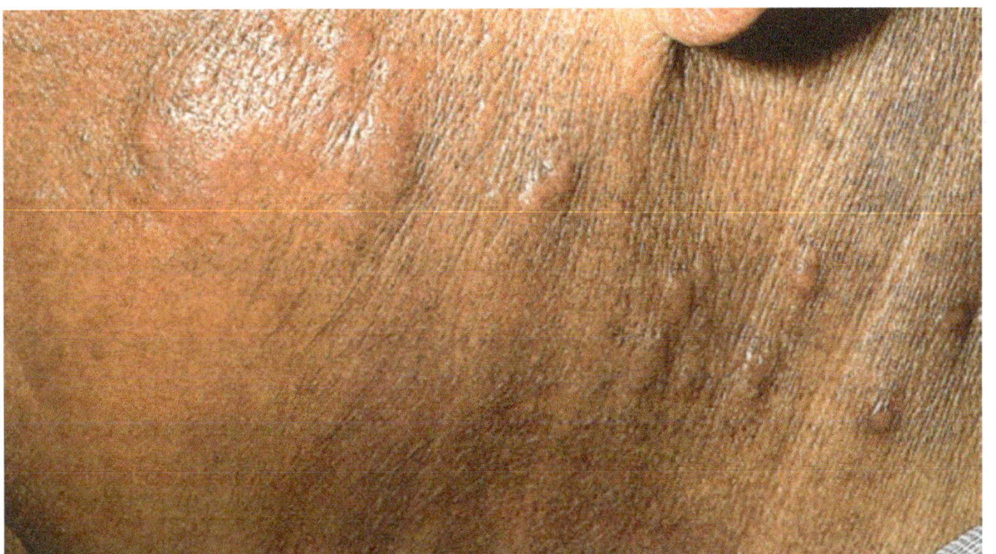

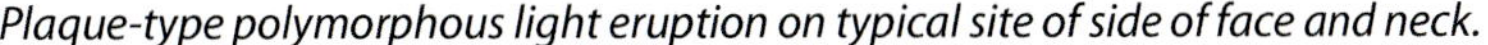

Plaque-type polymorphous light eruption on typical site of side of face and neck.

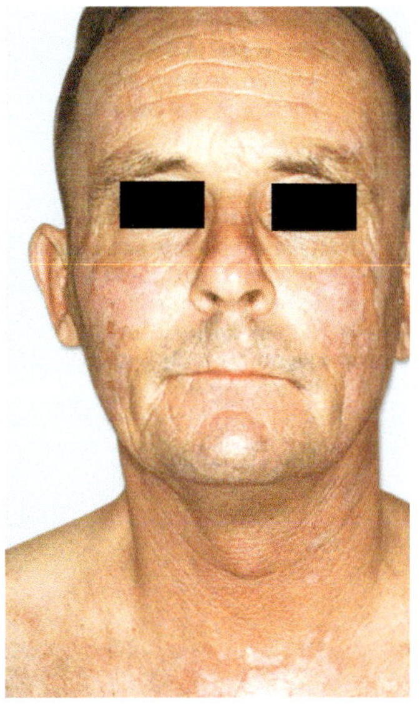

Inflamed and scarred lesions of discoid lupus erythematosus on sun-exposed sites. Note lesion in V of neck.

Tinea Faciei

CLINICAL

- In many patients, this is typical "ringworm" (expanding red and scaly border).
- Tinea faciei may present as an amorphous, asymptomatic, reddish patch, which **may be photosensitive**.
  - Scaling may be slight or absent because of oiliness and frequent washing.
  - This condition may be mistaken for polymorphous light eruption, lupus erythematosus, contact dermatitis, or others.
  - Topical corticosteroids decrease redness, but lesions do not resolve and may enlarge.

- When an amorphous facial eruption does not respond to conventional therapy, perform a potassium hydroxide (KOH) examination to rule out tinea faciei. **If KOH testing result is negative, repeat in 2 days after patient ceases washing** (to allow scale buildup), or apply adhesive patch for 12–24 hours and then collect scale that has accumulated under the nonadherent pad.

TREATMENT

- Use topical antifungal agents (*See* page 235) unless hair is involved. Apply an antifungal cream or lotion twice a day for 2–3 weeks or at least for several days past complete clearing of lesion.
- Use oral antifungal agent for the following:
  - Recurrent lesions
  - Hairline involvement
  - Extensive ear or eyelid involvement, where adequate topical therapy is difficult (*See* Treatment of Fungal Infections, page 235).

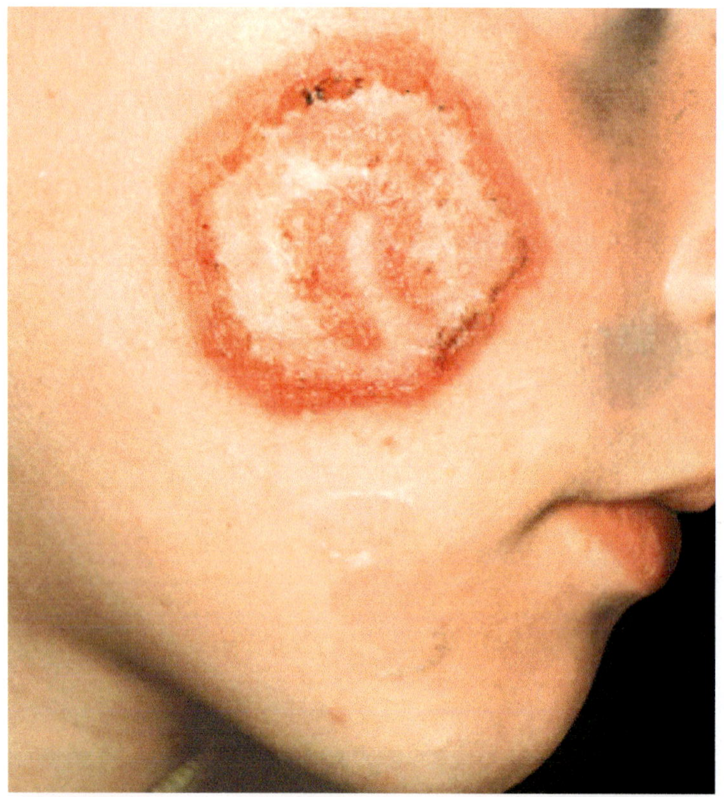

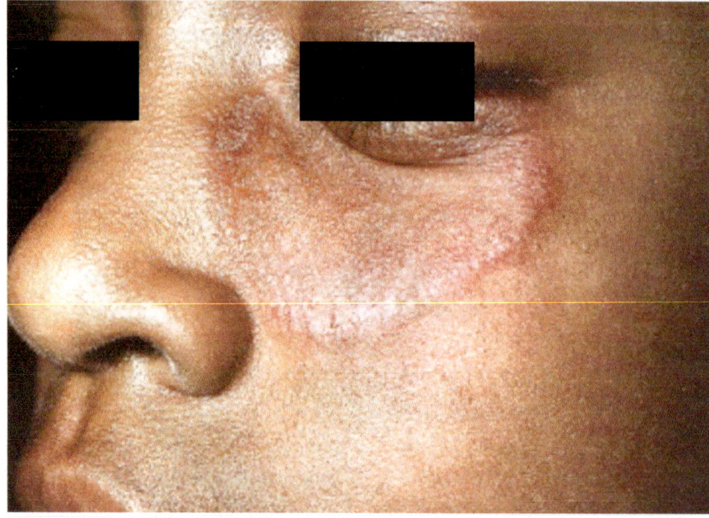

Classic ring-type "ringworm" on face.

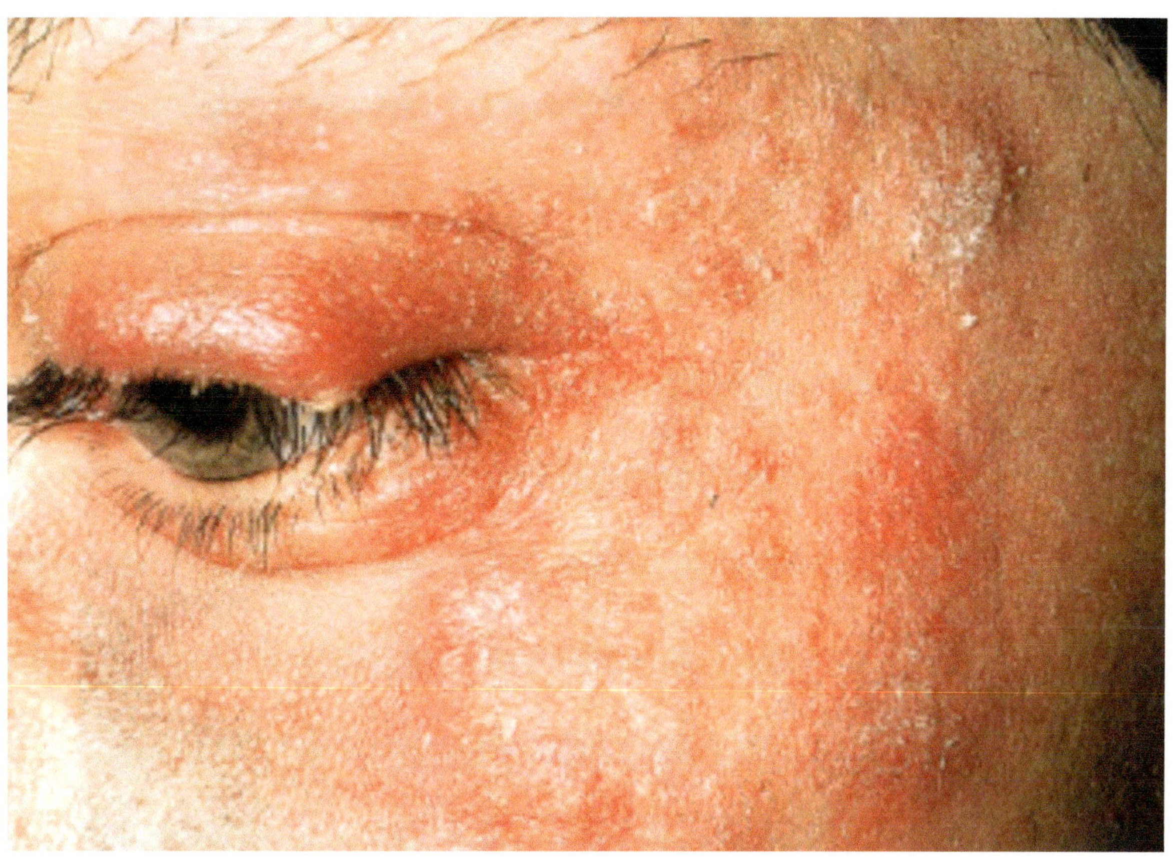

Somewhat accentuated "ring" border but less well defined. Note kerion of lash.

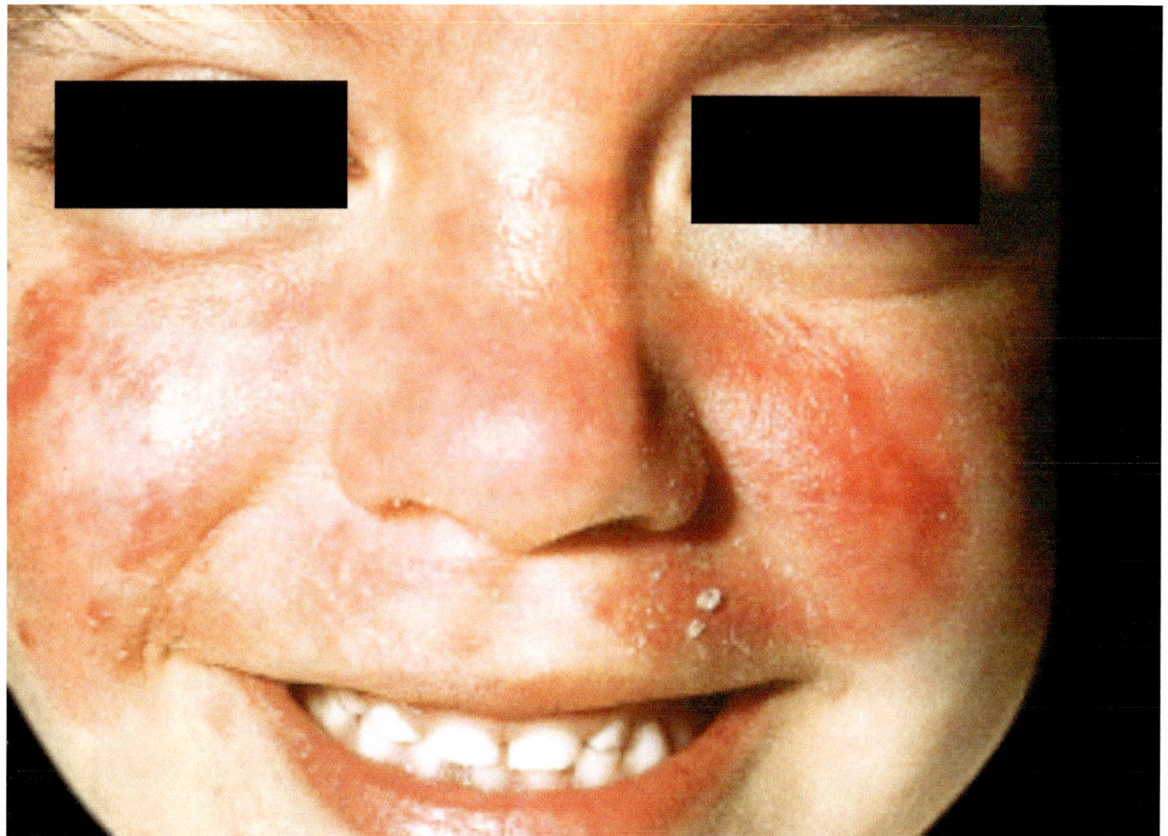

Diffuse butterfly rash of tinea faciei, partially resolved with treatment.

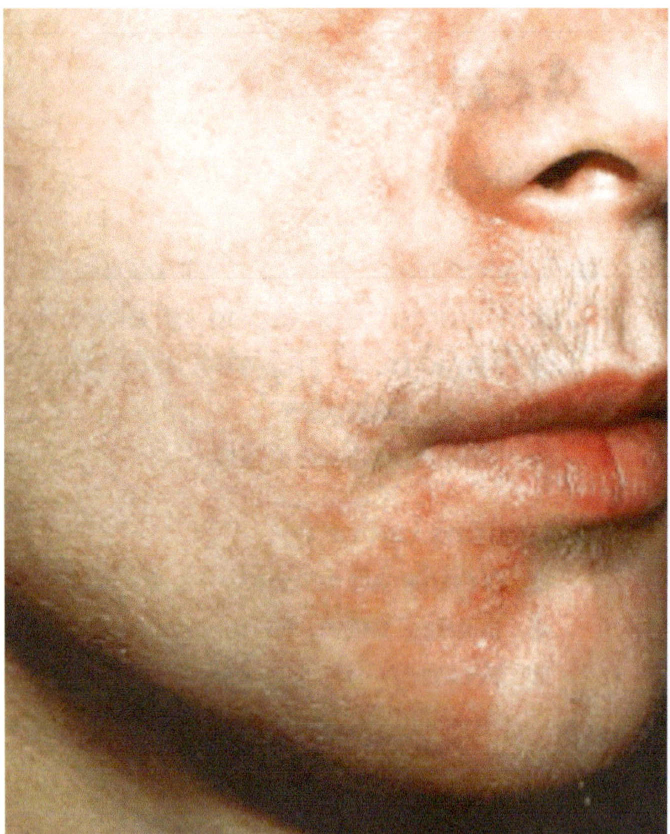

No ring pattern evident in this chronic tinea of the face.

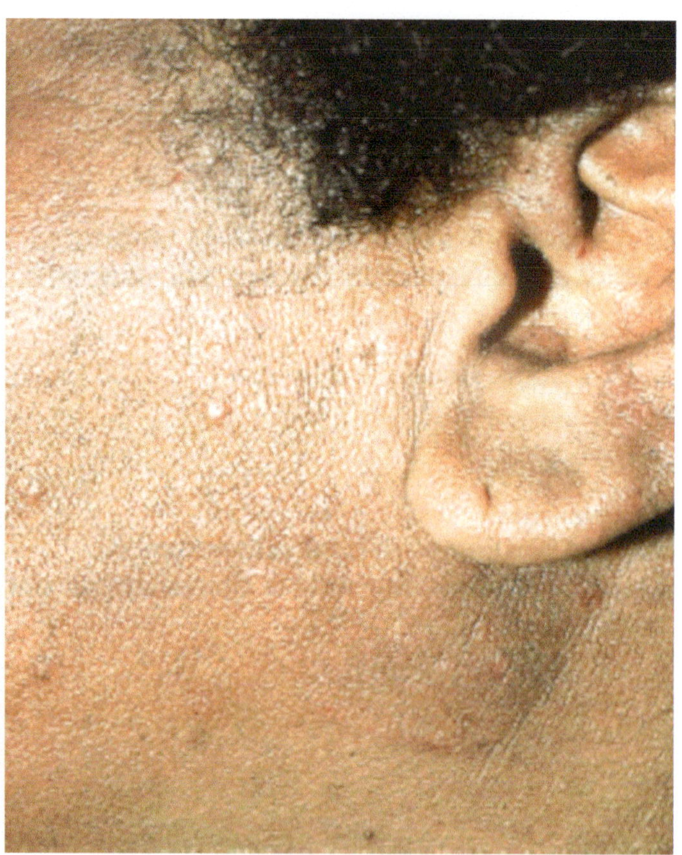

Very subtle tinea present and enlarging for >6 months, visible mostly as a coarsening of the texture of the skin.

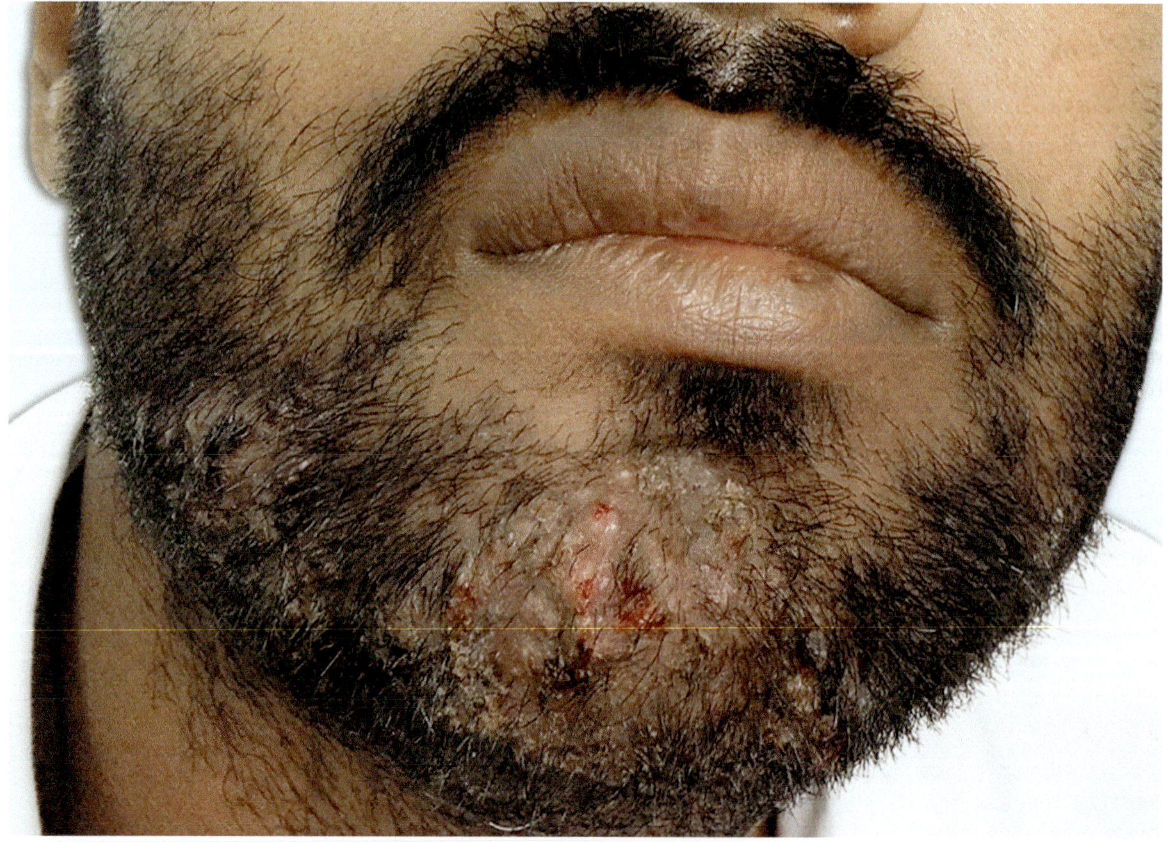

Tinea involving the beard.

Acne

CLINICAL

- Lesions may be one or more of the following:
  - Comedones: Open or closed
  - Superficial papules and pustules
  - Deep papules
  - Nodules and cysts
- Lesions occur in:
  - Nearly all teenagers, at least to a slight degree
  - Young men, when severe (nodular)
  - Women in the 20- to 35-year-old age group as chronic papules of the lower face, especially the chin
- Occurrence and severity are related to the following:
  - Inheritance (predominantly)
  - Sex hormones:
    - More frequent and worse in males
    - Better during pregnancy and high-estrogen oral contraceptive use
  - Chronic use of cosmetics, moisturizers, and pomades:
    - Certain ingredients are "comedogenic"
    - Not necessarily related to thickness or oiliness of cosmetic base
  - Stress in some individuals
  - Sunlight:
    - Improves acne in many individuals
    - Has no effect in some individuals but masks by tanning
    - Aggravates acne in a few (especially the very fair skinned)
- Exacerbations *not usually* related to:
  - Diet, junk foods, chocolate, vitamins, and minerals
  - Sexual activity
  - Cleanliness
- Scarring:
  - Is the natural result of healing of dermal inflammation
  - Is related to picking and squeezing only if that manipulation aggravates a specific lesion

TREATMENT

Patient education is paramount (*See* Patient Guides, page 246). Critical points that the patient must realize are the following:
- The occurrence of acne is preordained and is *not* due to something the patient did or did not do.
- Accordingly, the patient cannot control the disease by manipulating diet, behavior, or environment.
- Therapy usually helps. With the exception of intralesional or systemic corticosteroids, however, it prevents new lesions but does not accelerate healing of old ones, so it should be applied every day to the entire acne-prone area, **not just to individual pimples**.
- Often no improvement is seen for 3–6 weeks, so be patient.

- Washing with "acne" soap (including granulated soaps)
  - Has only minimal impact on superficial pustules
  - Does not prevent or remove comedones
  - Often irritates the skin, so that burning results from applying effective topical agents (*See* farther on), limiting or preventing their use
- Encourage a normal frequency of washing with a mild soap (*See* page 242)

Topical Agents

In general, topical agents should be applied thinly to the entire acne-prone area. They are less likely to be irritating if washing takes place infrequently, with mild soap, and if agents are applied to dry skin >15 minutes after washing. Effective topical agents include the following:

- Benzoyl peroxide (*See* page 234):
  - Effective against superficial papules and pustules

- Works by killing bacteria, possibly prevents pore-plugging, and possibly suppresses oil production
- Water-based gels less drying and irritating than alcohol or acetone-based products
- Concentrations of 2.5% and 5% sufficiently potent
- May bleach colored fabrics

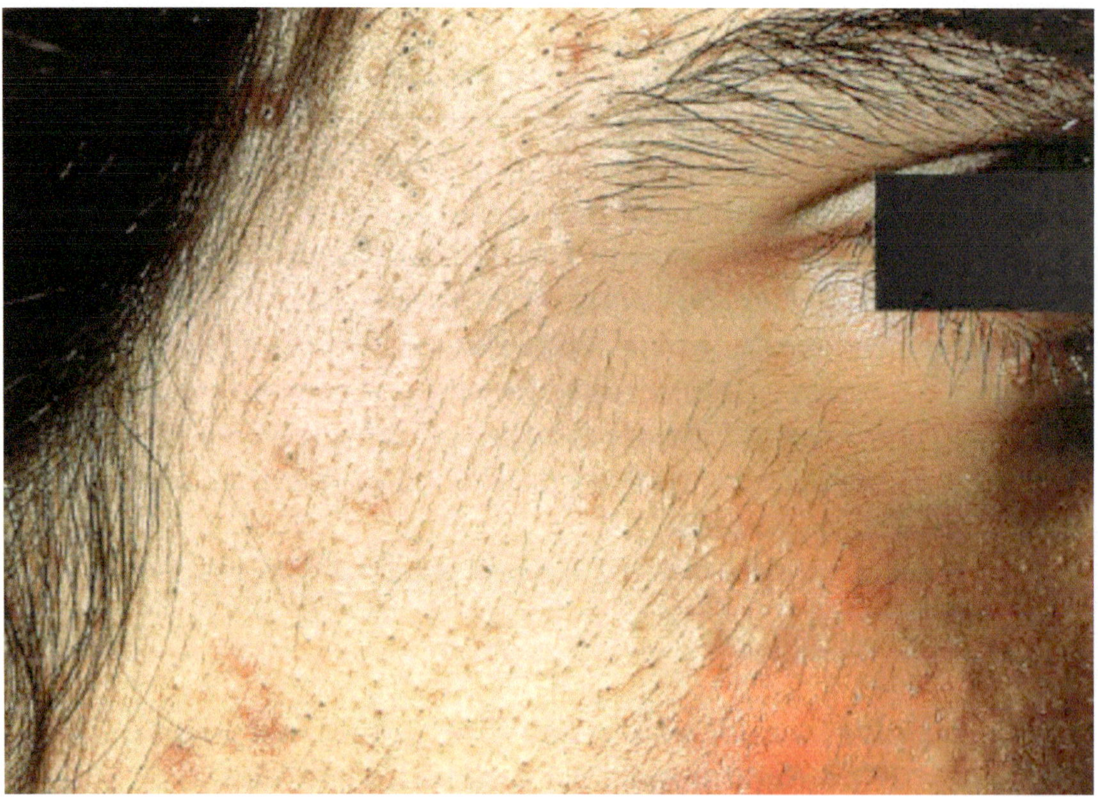

Almost pure open comedones (blackhead) acne, with only a few inflamed papules.

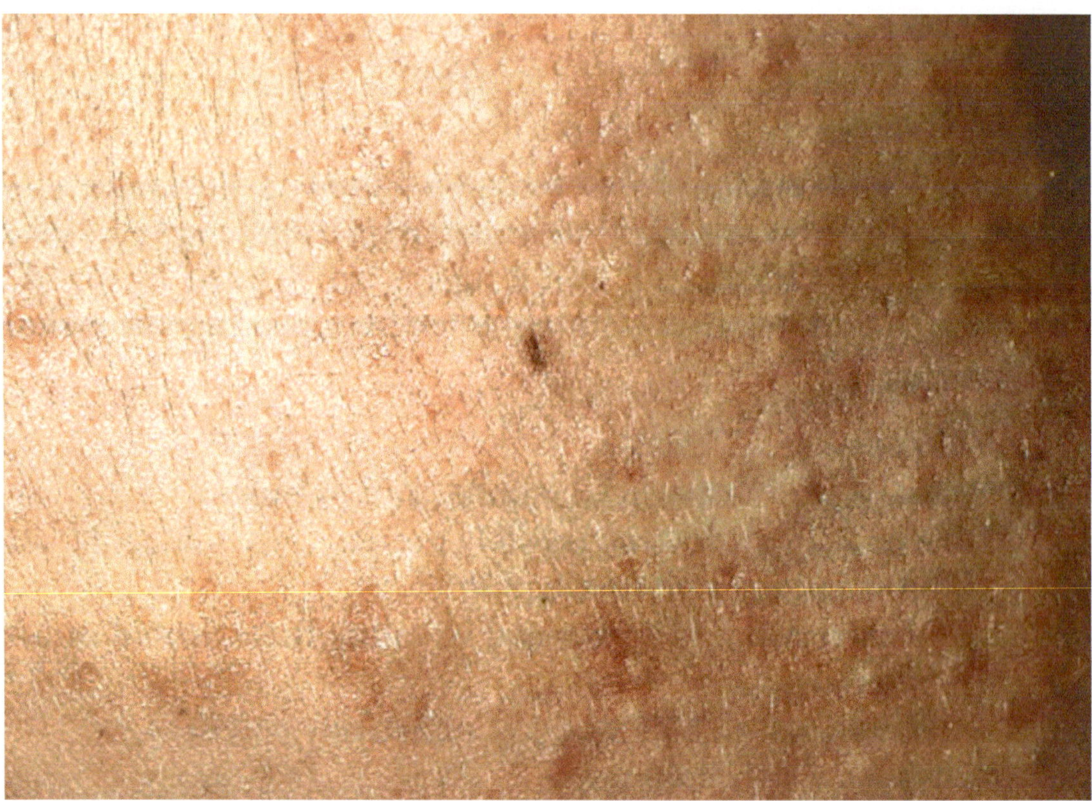

Closed comedones, or whiteheads. They are deep and tenacious.

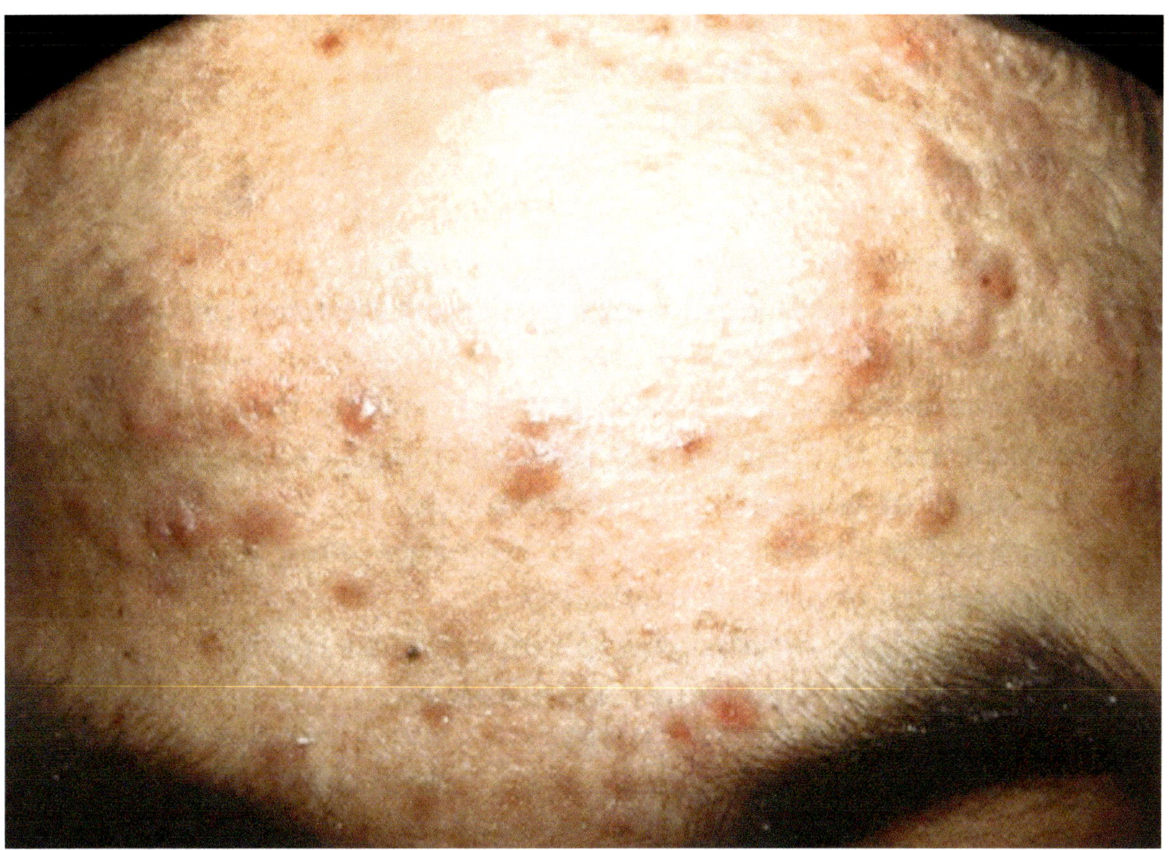

Typical papulopustular acne. No comedones are evident.

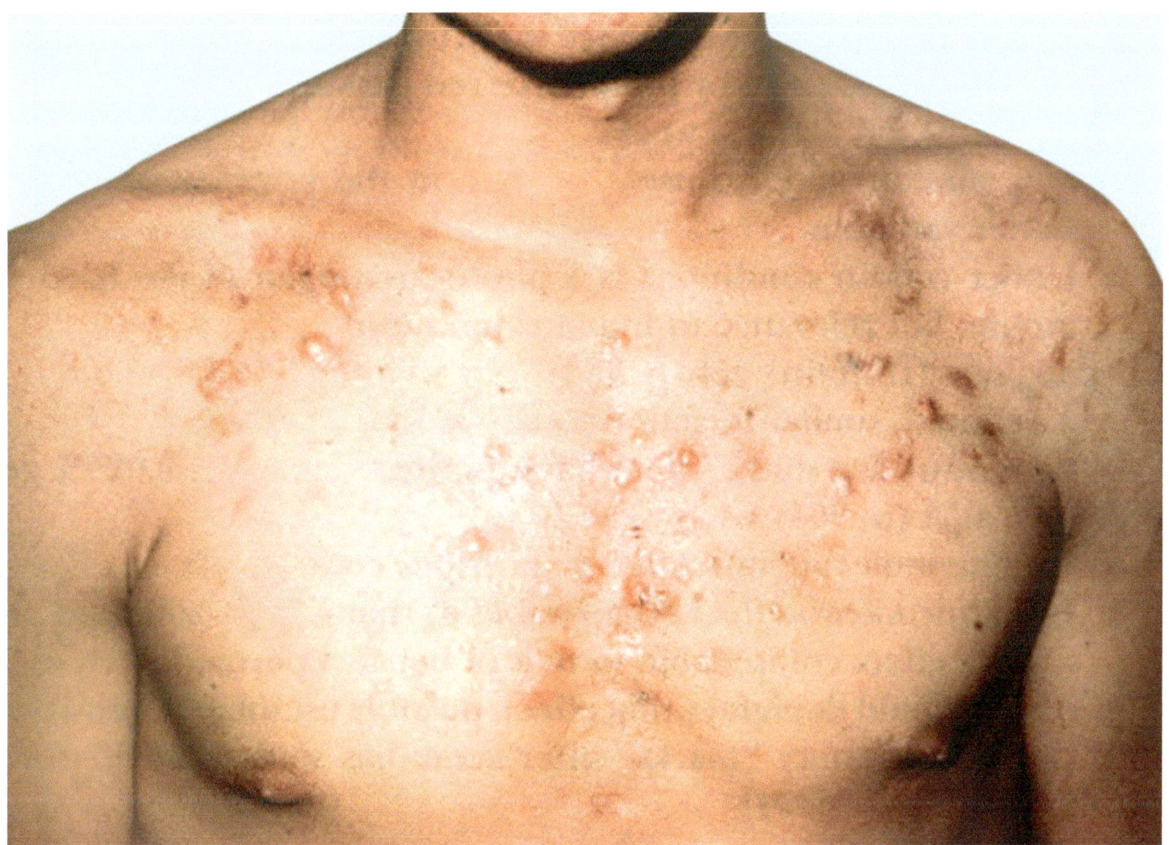

Nodular or nodulocystic acne.

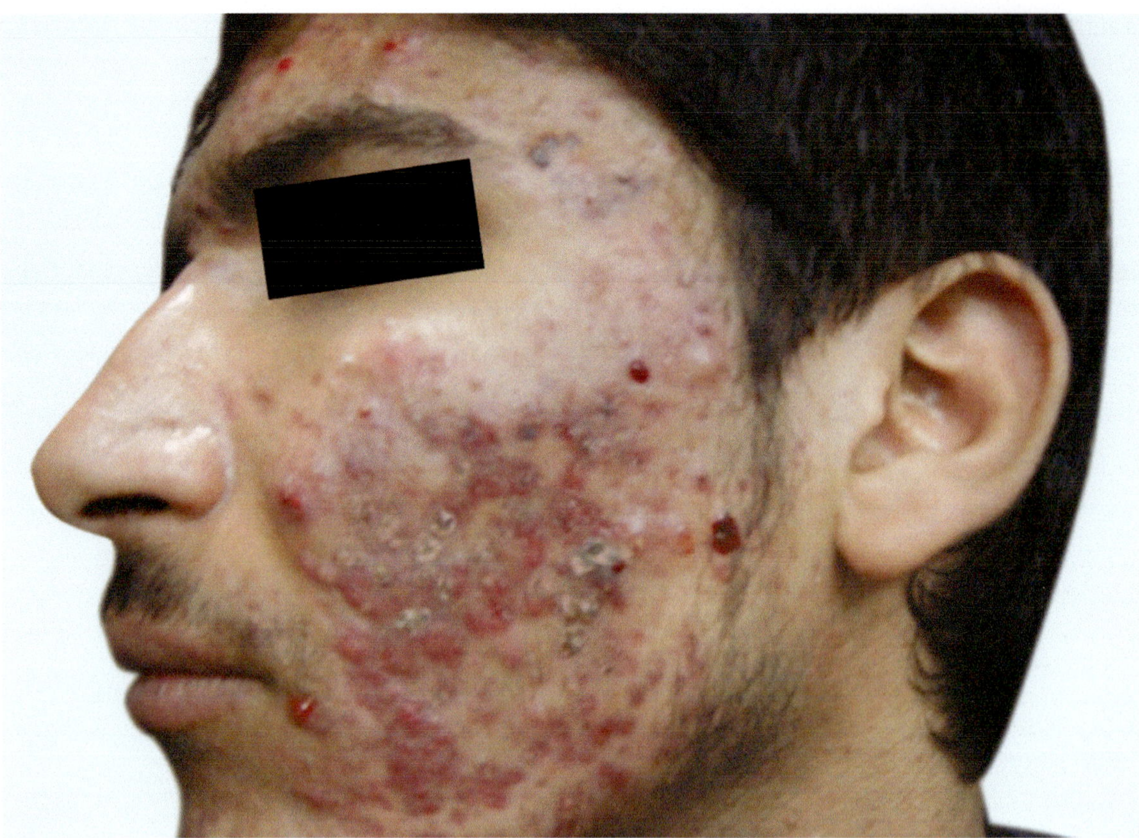

Severe nodulocystic acne.

- Occasionally causes allergic contact dermatitis
- Should be applied twice daily, if tolerated

- Topical antibiotics (*See* page 234):
  - Clindamycin, erythromycin, tetracycline, minocycline, and dapsone in penetrating vehicles kill bacteria in follicles and are effective against papulopustular lesions.
  - Effect is probably equivalent to that of benzoyl peroxides but without effect on comedones or sebum production.
  - Topical antibiotics are usually less irritating than benzoyl peroxides, but alcohol vehicle may be drying. Some are available in cream, foam, or moisturizing lotion vehicle.
  - Bacterial resistance frequently develops after months of use, making the treatment ineffective.
- Benzoyl peroxide-erythromycin and benzoyl peroxide-clindamycin combination (*See* page 234)
  - More effective than either agent alone
- Tretinoin (retinoic acid) (*See* page 234), tazarotene, and trifarotene:
  - Often effective against comedones and, eventually, papules and pustules
  - Work by loosening keratin pore plugs and preventing their development
  - May take 6–12 weeks to affect comedones
  - Lower concentrations (0.025% cream) less irritating than higher concentrations and as effective after 3 months of therapy; higher concentrations possibly reaching that benefit faster
  - Should be applied thinly once daily (usually at night)
  - May cause irritation or pimple-like red papules around plugged pores for the first few weeks
  - May photoirritate, so use is limited in the summer or during winter vacations
  - Under certain conditions is a photocarcinogen in the hairless mouse, but relevance to humans unknown
- Adapalene (Differin) gel (*See* page 235):
  - A retinoid, similar in action to tretinoin
  - Available over-the-counter as 0.1% and on prescription as 0.3%
  - In a controlled study, somewhat superior to tretinoin 0.025% gel
- Benzoyl peroxide-adapalene combination
- Azelaic acid (*See* page 235):
  - Unrelated to previous compounds

- Has anticomedo effect comparable to that of tretinoin and antibiotic effect comparable to that of benzoyl peroxide
- Also has mild depigmenting effect, possibly useful in minimizing postinflammatory "marks" after acne; has some benefit alone for melasma (*See* page 49)

▪ Clascoterone 1% cream is a novel topical androgen receptor inhibitor:
  - Should be applied twice daily

▪ Combination topical treatment:
  - The use of tretinoin or adapalene and benzoyl peroxide or topical antibiotic by the same individual is better than one drug alone in most cases of papulopustular acne.
  - Because of chemical incompatibility, drugs must not be applied at the same time. Usually, tretinoin is applied at bedtime and benzoyl peroxide, in the morning and at dinner time.
  - Irritation is common, so use only mild soap and add lubricant or a mild topical corticosteroid, if necessary.
  - Patient Guides (*See* page 246) encourages correct use.

Systemic Agents

Antibiotics

▪ Tetracycline or erythromycin in dosages of up to 1 g daily usually improves superficial and deep inflammatory acne after 3–4 weeks; dosages of up to 2 g daily may be needed for nodular acne. Maximum benefit occurs in 6–12 weeks.

▪ Doxycycline 100 mg daily or twice daily is easier to take than tetracycline because it can be taken with food, but it has a much higher chance of photosensitivity (3% if 100 mg/day and 40% if 200 mg/day).

▪ Minocycline may be effective in resistant cases (the organism does not develop resistance to it), it can be taken with food, and rarely causes gastrointestinal upset or vaginitis. However, it is very expensive, compared with the other drugs and may cause hyperpigmentation.

▪ Clindamycin or trimethoprim/sulfamethoxazole is alternative, possibly effective in resistant cases but with more potentially dangerous side effects (colitis and Stevens-Johnson syndrome).

Tetracycline and minocycline may reduce the effectiveness of oral contraceptives and (theoretically) allow pregnancy to occur, although the likelihood is thought to be very slight. Female patients should be informed of this possibility, and they may wish to use an additional or alternative form of contraception.

▪ Although not package-labeled, spironolactone at a lower dose is widely used as an antiandrogen in women

Isotretinoin (13-cis-retinoic acid):

▪ A derivative of vitamin A, this product reduces oil gland output by up to 90%.

▪ This product is taken by mouth for 3–5 months. Side effects occur early; improvement lags behind and may continue to increase for 1–2 months after stopping treatment. Side effects resolve in 1–2 months.

Unlike any other acne therapy, the benefit is prolonged long after the drug is stopped (months or even years).

▪ Side effects and their incidences are—cheilitis (90%), dry, chapped skin (90%), dry nose or eyes (80%), hair shedding (10%), peeling of palms and soles (5%), arthralgias or myalgias (15%), elevated liver transaminases (15%), and elevated serum triglycerides (25%). The serum abnormalities may return to normal during treatment.

▪ Serum testing is advisable before therapy and at 2- to 4-week intervals or until the results are normal.

Isotretinoin is a potent teratogen, especially if taken during the 1st weeks of pregnancy. To avoid pregnancy during administration of this drug, the manufacturer and the US Food and Drug Administration (FDA) recommend that all patients capable of becoming pregnant be:
- Started on oral contraceptives
- Tested for pregnancy initially and again in 1 month
- *Then* started on isotretinoin

▪ No supplemental vitamin A should be taken during treatment, as it may increase side effects.

▪ Skin dryness can be treated with moisturizers (*See* page 111). Ointments or lip balms may be used on the lips. Methylcellulose "artificial tears" may be used for dry eyes.

▪ Dose is 1–2 mg/kg. Give the lower dose for purely facial acne and the higher one for extensive truncal acne. Severe truncal acne may require a repeat 4-month course after a 2-month rest period.

▪ Drug cost is high.

Because of extensive known side effects and continuing investigation of additional side effects, the FDA recommends the use of isotretinoin only for severe cystic or nodular acne that is unresponsive to other medications.

In the United States, isotretinoin prescribing is controlled by the FDA—under iPLEDGE—See website for details.

- *See* Patient Guides, page 247, for isotretinoin.

Corticosteroids: Systemic corticosteroids are used occasionally in severe, painful flares of nodular acne for 1–2 weeks.

Intralesional injection of depot corticosteroids is an invaluable tool for individual nodules and large papules (*See* page 240 for technique). Physicians treating acne should acquire skill in administering this therapy.

Estrogens:

- Low-estrogen pills may have no effect on, and may even worsen, acne.
- High-estrogen oral contraceptives often improve acne in women, but benefits and risks must be considered and the patient monitored for side effects. Benefits may not be seen for 3 months.
- For the greatest benefit, estrogens should be given with replacement-dose corticosteroid (e.g., prednisone 5 mg daily) to suppress adrenal androgens.

Office Treatments

- Mild peeling induced by ultraviolet light, CO_2 slush, liquid nitrogen, or mild acid (trichloroacetic acid 20–30%, salicylic acid, and glycolic acid):
  - May cause mild improvement in superficial comedones and pustules
  - Used less often as self-administered topical agents and have become more effective
- Intralesional corticosteroids (*See* earlier)
- Liquid nitrogen cryotherapy to individual papules and nodules, which possibly enhances resolution
- "Acne surgery":
  - The removal of comedones, and possibly drainage of pustules, with a comedone extractor
  - Probably speeds resolution of pustules and prevents development of new ones
  - Made easier by the chronic use of topical tretinoin, which softens comedones

Treatment of Scars

Patients should be referred to a dermatologist or plastic surgeon for these specialized procedures.

- Dermabrasion, fractional erbium yttrium aluminum garnet (YAG) or CO_2 laser, or deep chemical peel:
  - Destroys superficial dermis and epidermis
  - *Causes scarring*, but it may be flat, not pitted and lumpy
  - Certain types of scars and certain areas of face respond best
  - Includes such possible complications as residual erythema, keloids, and permanent pigment changes
  - Often needs to be repeated for best results
- Excision of elevated or depressed scars:
  - Effective if only a few obvious scars are causing most cosmetic impact
  - May be combined with dermabrasion to eliminate deepest pits
  - Possible complications: Infection and scarring
- Injection of bovine collagen, hyaluronic acid, or calcium hydroxylapatite below depressed scars:
  - Adequately elevates large depressed areas and some furrows
  - Possibly makes more prominent "ice pick" pits
  - Possible hypersensitivity reaction
  - Benefits lasting 6–12 months, after which the scar reappears; procedure may be repeated

Practical Treatment of Acne

For all patients:
- Patient handouts, destroy myths, relieve guilt (*See* page 246)
- Discontinuation of excessive washing, abrasives, and irritants

Comedonal acne:
- Topical tretinoin, adapalene, tazarotene, and trifarotene
- Azelaic acid
- "Acne surgery"

Superficial papulopustular acne:
- Benzoyl peroxide alone
- Topical antibiotic alone
- Azelaic acid
- Benzoyl peroxide–topical antibiotic or benzoyl peroxide–adapalene mixture
- Addition of tretinoin often helpful
- Systemic antibiotic in widespread or resistant cases

Moderately deep papular acne:
- Topical antibiotic
- Benzoyl peroxide (possible irritant in women in their 20s)
- Azelaic acid
- Systemic antibiotic often required

Nodular acne:

Referral to a dermatologist for the required complex long-term care is recommended.

- Topical agents for superficial component
- High-dose systemic antibiotics
- Intralesional corticosteroids
- Possibly a brief dose of oral corticosteroids for flares
- Oral contraceptives and replacement corticosteroids in women
- Isotretinoin

Rosacea

CLINICAL

- Either or both clinical features of:
  - "Blushing erythema," "ruddy" complexion, or telangiectatic matting
  - Angry, red, pimple-like papules and pustules
- Possible sebaceous gland enlargement with enlargement of nose (rhinophyma) and coarsening of facial skin
- Location:
  - Central forehead
  - Nose, "butterfly" of cheeks
  - Central chin
- Occurs in:
  - Women more frequently than men
  - Middle-aged people
  - More common in the fair skinned (especially those of Celtic background)
- Idiopathic:
  - Worsened by heat, hot or spicy foods, and alcohol
  - Caused or worsened by *potent* topical corticosteroids

TREATMENT

- General:
  - Often moderately to poorly responsive to therapy
  - Often requires combination of topical and/or oral treatments
  - Slow to respond (several weeks) and may need treatment for weeks to months; may relapse
  - Avoidance of known aggravating factors such as heat, spicy and hot foods, sun, alcohol, and potent topical corticosteroids is helpful.
  - Avoidance of soaps and other irritants
- Topical therapy:
  - Topical metronidazole is effective in many cases. Benefit begins in 3–4 weeks, reaches a maximum in perhaps 6–8 weeks, with pustules and papules responding better than does erythema; available in the United States as a 0.75% and 1% cream and gel.
  - Azelaic acid 15% gel or 20% cream, sodium sulfacetamide lotion, cream, suspension, or cleanser; ivermectin cream, permethrin cream, brimonidine 0.33% topical gel, and oxymetazoline hydrochloride 1% cream are other treatment options.

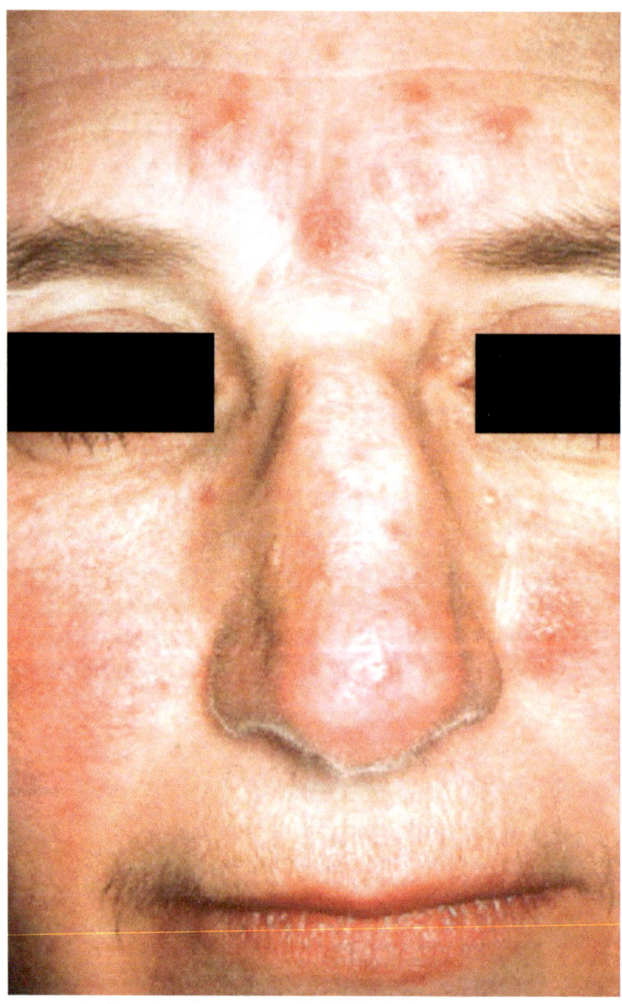

Almost exclusively papulopustular acne rosacea.

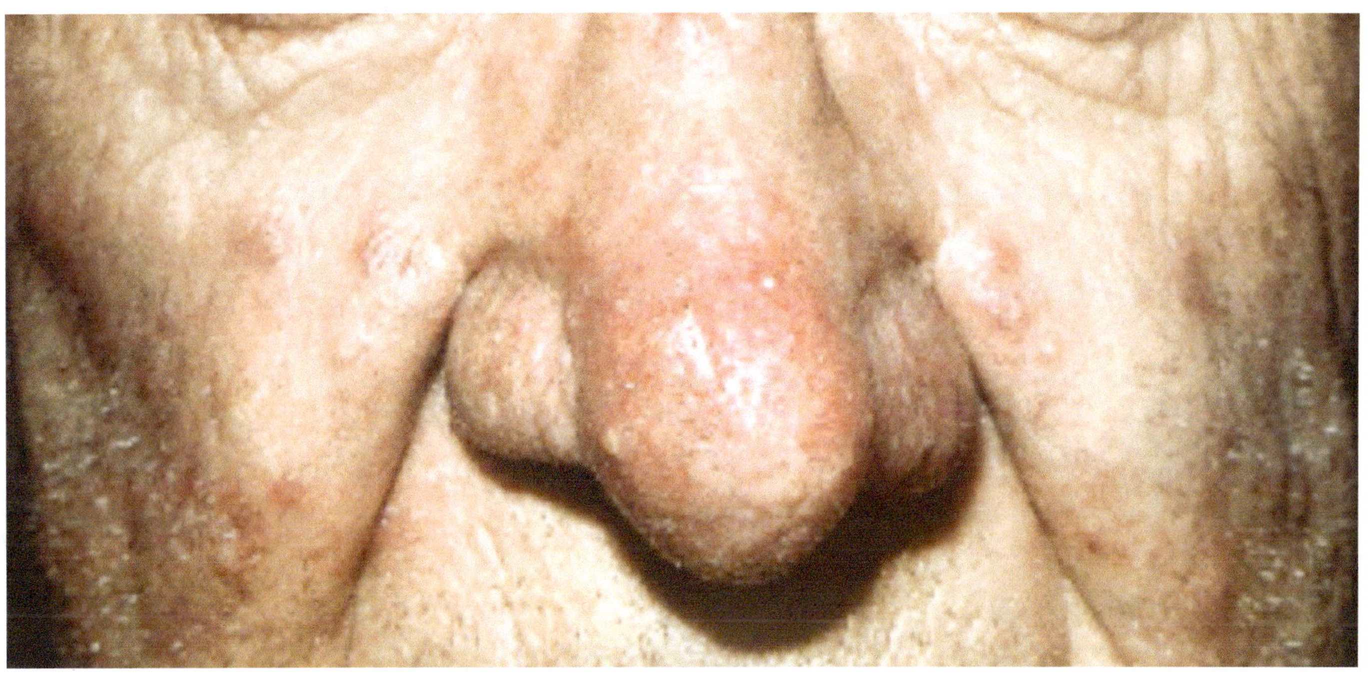

Rosacea with early thickening of the skin of the nose (rhinophyma).

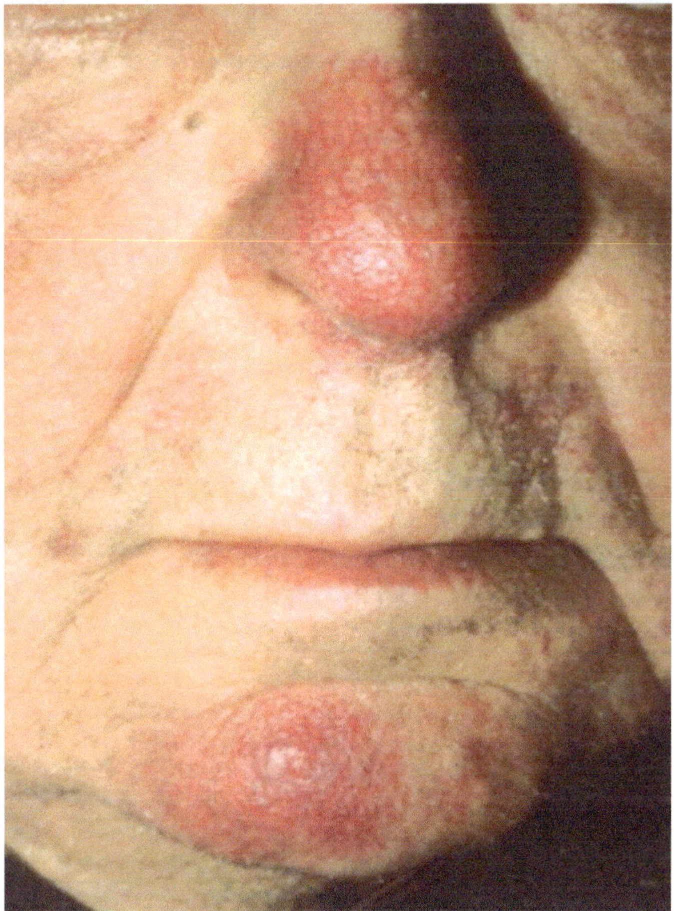

Almost exclusively telangiectatic rosacea.

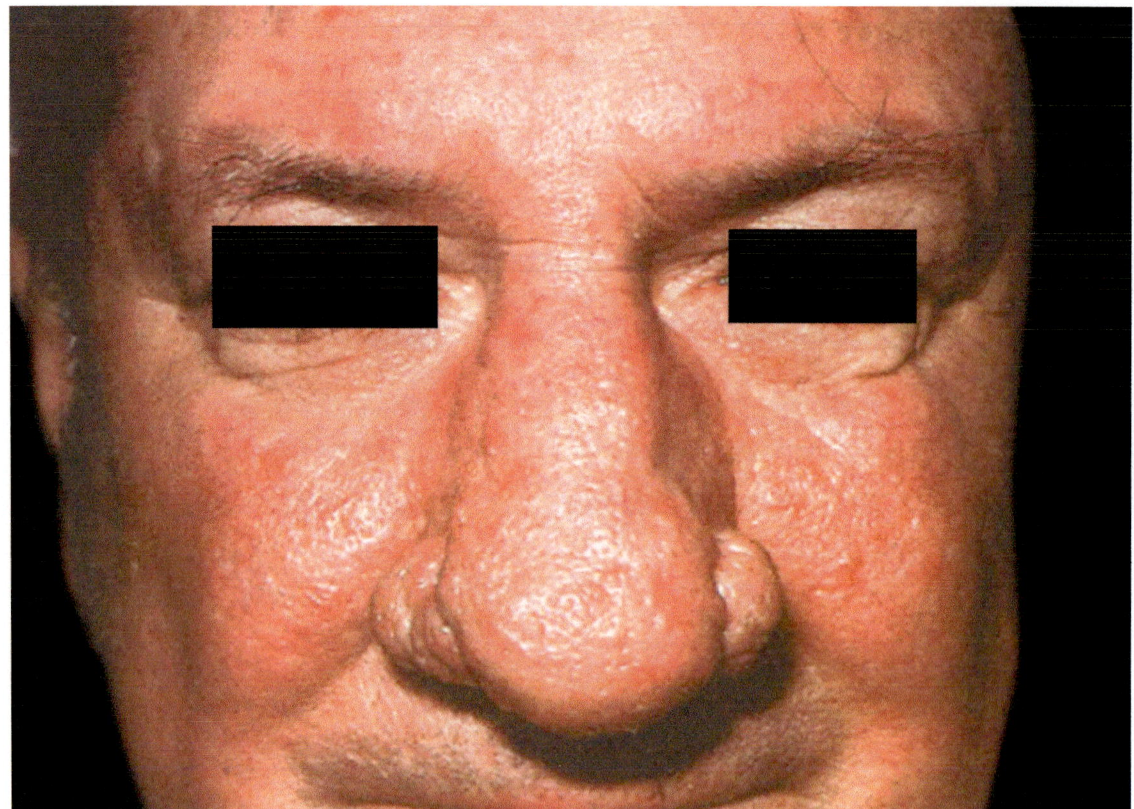

Rosacea and marked rhinophyma.

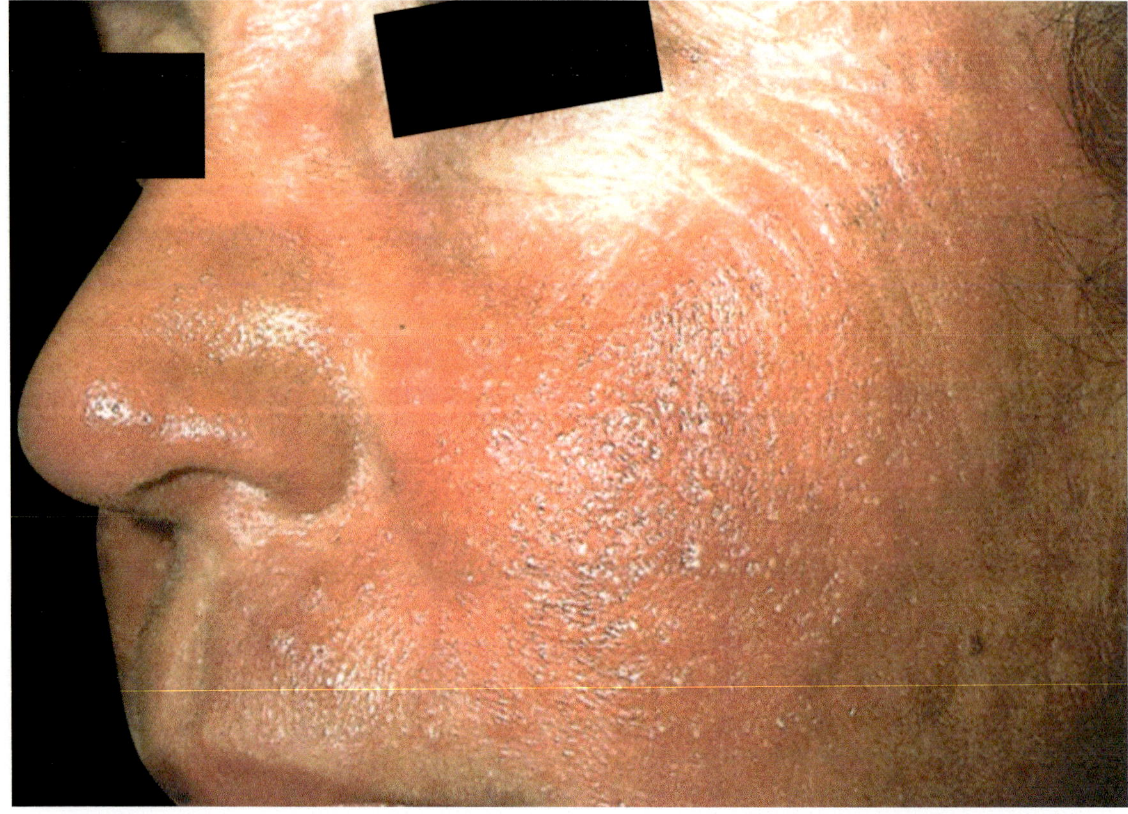

"Steroid rosacea." Marked vascular blush and pustulation from prolonged use of topical potent corticosteroid.

- Oral doxycycline or minocycline probably the drug of choice:
  - Doxycycline 50–100 mg twice daily or delayed release 40 mg daily or minocycline 50 mg at bedtime:
    - Marked benefits may be evident in 6–8 weeks, after which time treatment can be discontinued.
    - If relapse occurs weeks or months later, the course is repeated.
    - If relapse occurs immediately, maintenance on topical metronidazole or reduced daily or every other day doses of tetracycline or minocycline are advised.
- For rhinophyma, cold steel shave, surgical pairing, CO_2 or Nd:YAG laser.
- For resistant cases, low-dose intermittent dosing of the oral vitamin A derivative, isotretinoin, which may induce a prolonged remission; *See* page 247 for instructions on its use and the extensive side effects it often causes

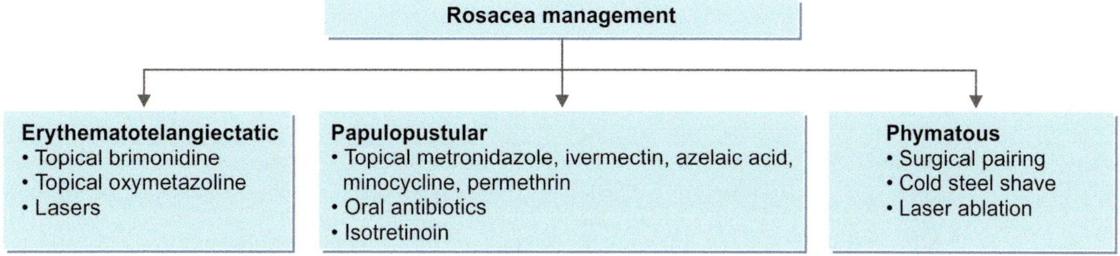

Perioral Dermatitis

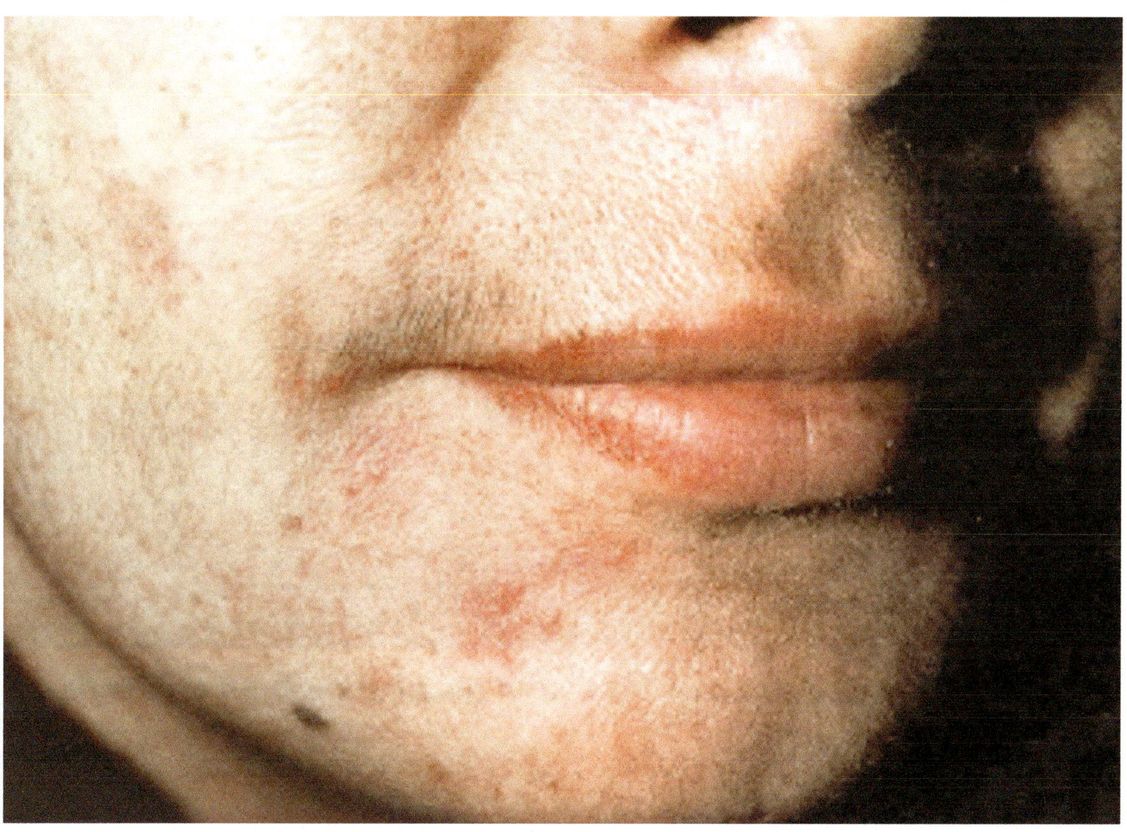

Typical mild perioral dermatitis in a young white woman. Faint, patchy erythema with a few pinhead-sized papules.

CLINICAL

- Faint, patchy pinkness, faint scaling, and/or tiny, pinhead-sized papules around the alae nasi, down the nasolabial folds, around the corners of the mouth, on the sides of the chin, below the lateral corners of the eye, or on the glabella; intermittently mildly itchy
- Occurs overwhelmingly in young white women; more recently noticed in older women (up to age 50), men (where it often is just below the lateral canthi, not around the mouth), and children; rare in dark-skinned individuals
- Outbreaks are often intermittent and recurrent but may be chronic for months.
- Cause unknown but may flare with stress; potent topical corticosteroids can induce this condition in susceptible individuals

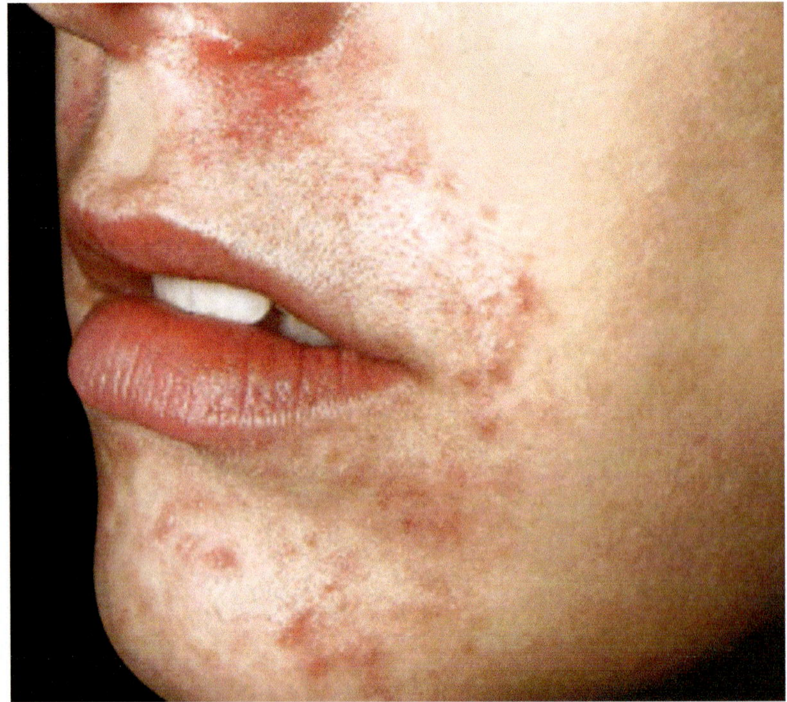

More severe perioral dermatitis extensively in the entire perioral area of a young woman.

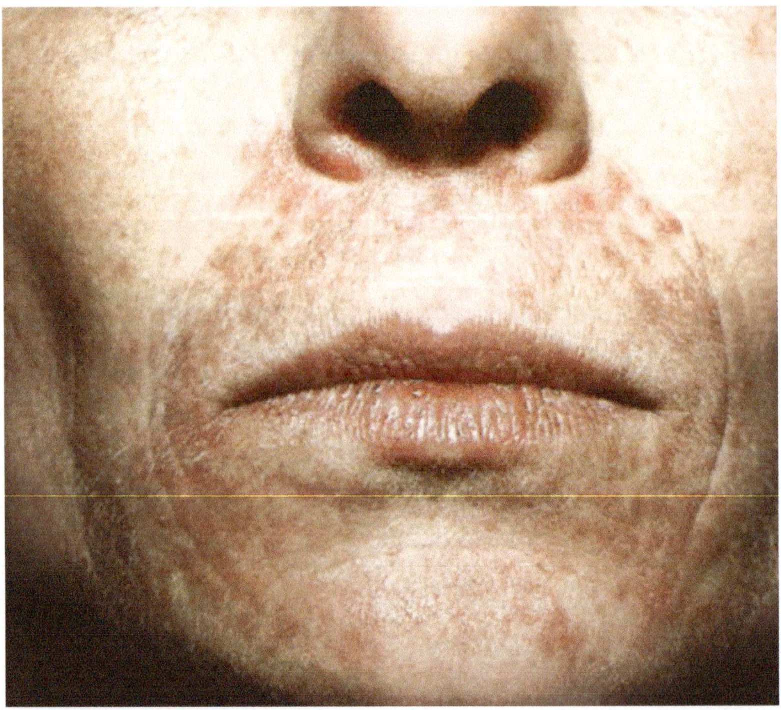

Dense, angry red perioral dermatitis induced by 3 months' use of a moderately potent topical corticosteroid cream (fluocinolone).

TREATMENT

Regard this as a variant of rosacea, but it occurs in a younger population and with a better long-term outcome. Rosacea treatments (*See* page 33) are even more dramatically effective in this population.

- Tetracycline 500 mg twice daily or doxycycline 100 mg twice daily, or minocycline 50–100 mg once daily usually causes complete resolution in 3–4 weeks and then may be discontinued. May be repeated intermittently as necessary.
- Topical metronidazole 0.75% or 1% cream or gel twice daily for 6–8 weeks is probably the most effective alternative and is safe in the occasional pediatric case. Topical erythromycin or clindamycin acne lotions may be effective but will also take up to 2 months to work.
- Topical azelaic acid, clindamycin, erythromycin, dapsone, and pimecrolimus are alternatives

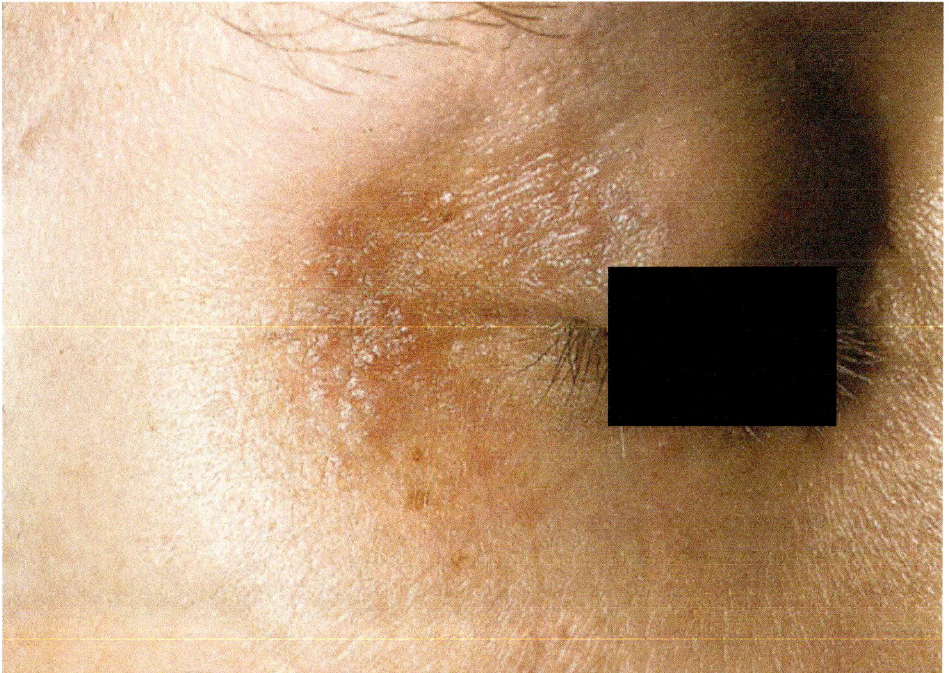

"Perioral" (periorificial) dermatitis of the lateral canthus.

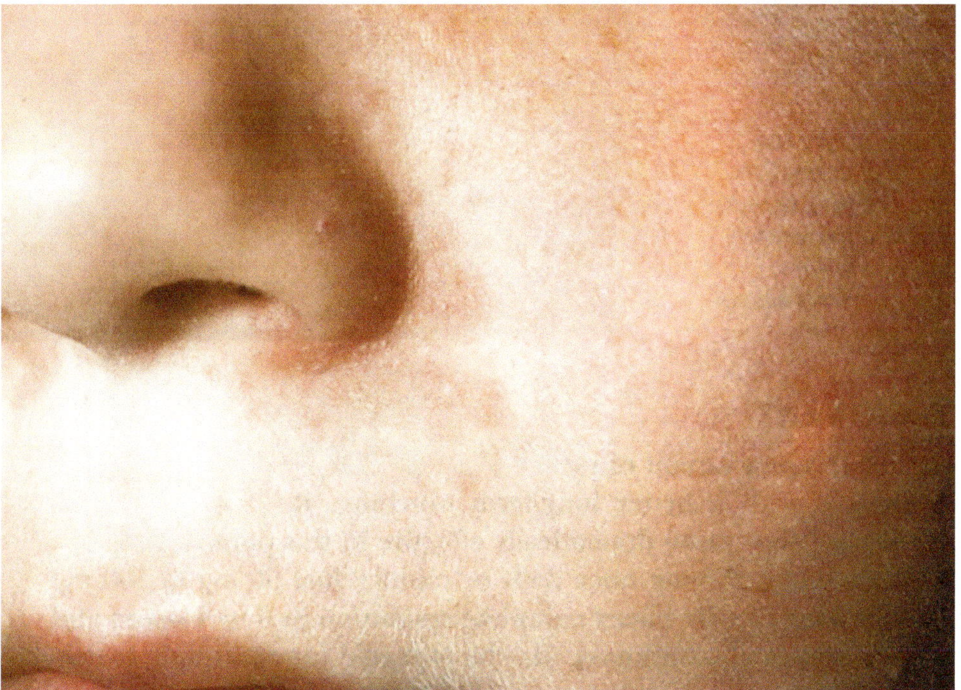

Perioral dermatitis in a localized area in a 7-year-old child. This is not seborrheic dermatitis because on palpation, one can feel tiny papules, and it will not clear with mild topical corticosteroid.

Pseudofolliculitis Barbae ("Beard Bumps")

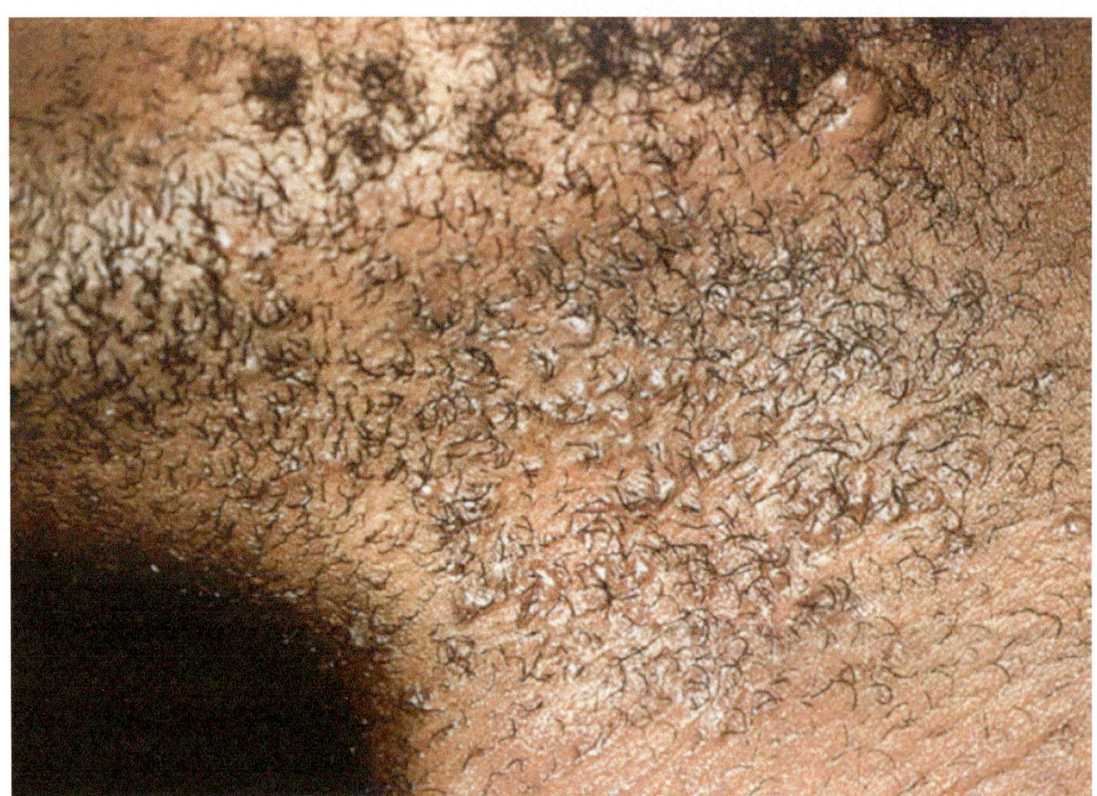

Slightly inflamed papules of pseudofolliculitis barbae confined to the area of beard growth.

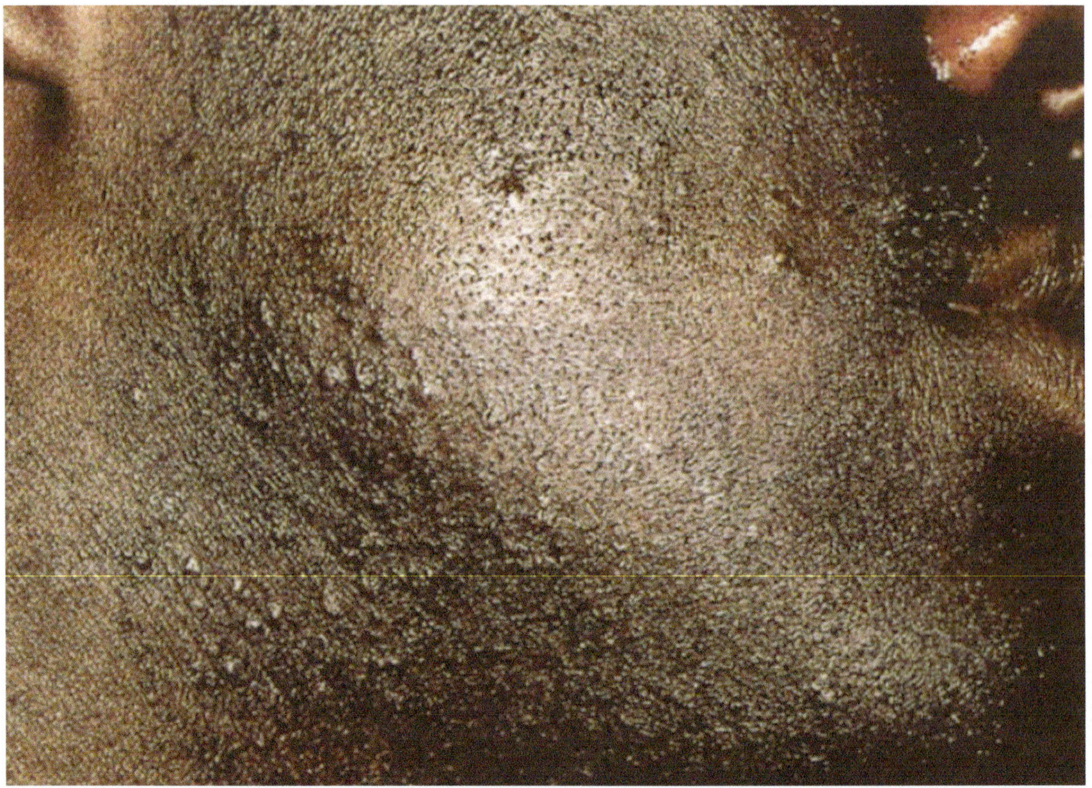

Chronic inflammation may lead to marked hyperpigmentation.

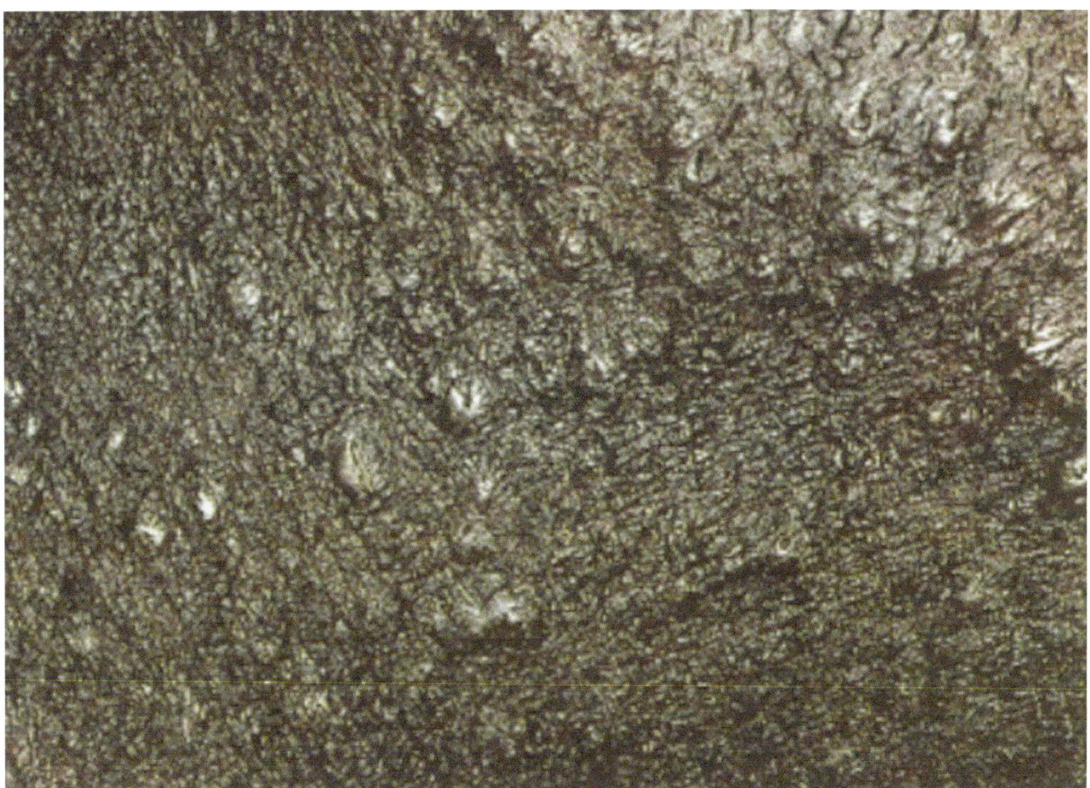

Close inspection shows hairs trapped in papules and pustules.

CLINICAL

- Ingrowing of tightly coiled beard hairs with resultant inflammation
  - This condition occurs mainly in dark-skinned individuals because of characteristically tightly coiled hairs.
  - After the beard hairs are shaved close to the skin, the pointed tips then catch on the edge of the pore and pierce the skin.
  - Inflammation is due to foreign body reaction and presence of skin flora in the dermis, as in acne.

TREATMENT

- The only sure prevention is not to shave.
- Lesions can be minimized by:
  - Shaving less often and less closely (with clippers rather than razor)
  - Using depilatory substances instead of shaving
    - "Dissolving" facial hair does not leave sharp tips that can pierce the skin.
    - These substances may be irritating in certain patients.
  - Patient or family member teasing out ingrown hairs with needle or pointed toothpick (wooden probe is less likely to injure tissue)
- Hydrocortisone 1% cream or lotion may reduce inflammation

Medications are likely to be only slightly beneficial.

- Doxycycline 100 mg once or twice daily, tetracycline or erythromycin 250–500 mg daily usually reduces inflammation (must be taken chronically).
- Benzoyl peroxide or topical antibiotic antiacne solution is usually of only slight benefit.
- Tretinoin (*See* page 234) thins keratin, releases some hairs, and prevents some ingrowing.
  - Must be used chronically
  - May be too irritating
  - Hair removal techniques such as laser and electrolysis may be beneficial.
  - Eflornithine hydrochloride cream 1% twice daily may be helpful.

Warts

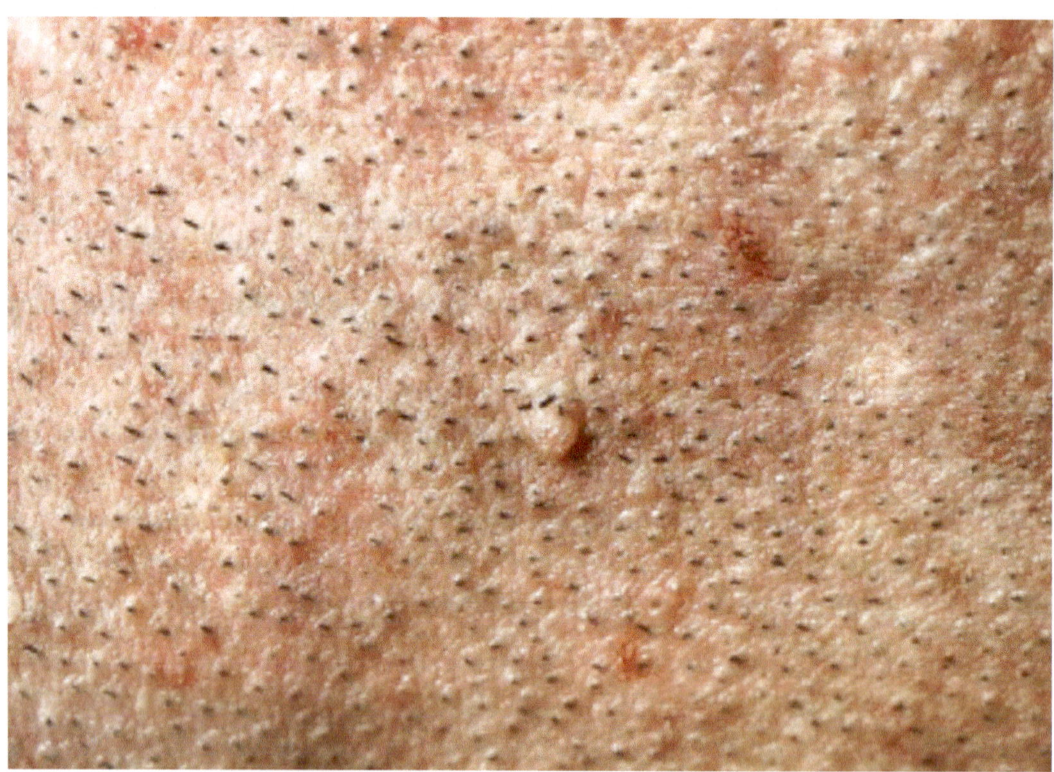

Typically subtle, tiny, slightly pink papule of wart in beard area. Examination with magnifying glass and tangential light helps to find them.

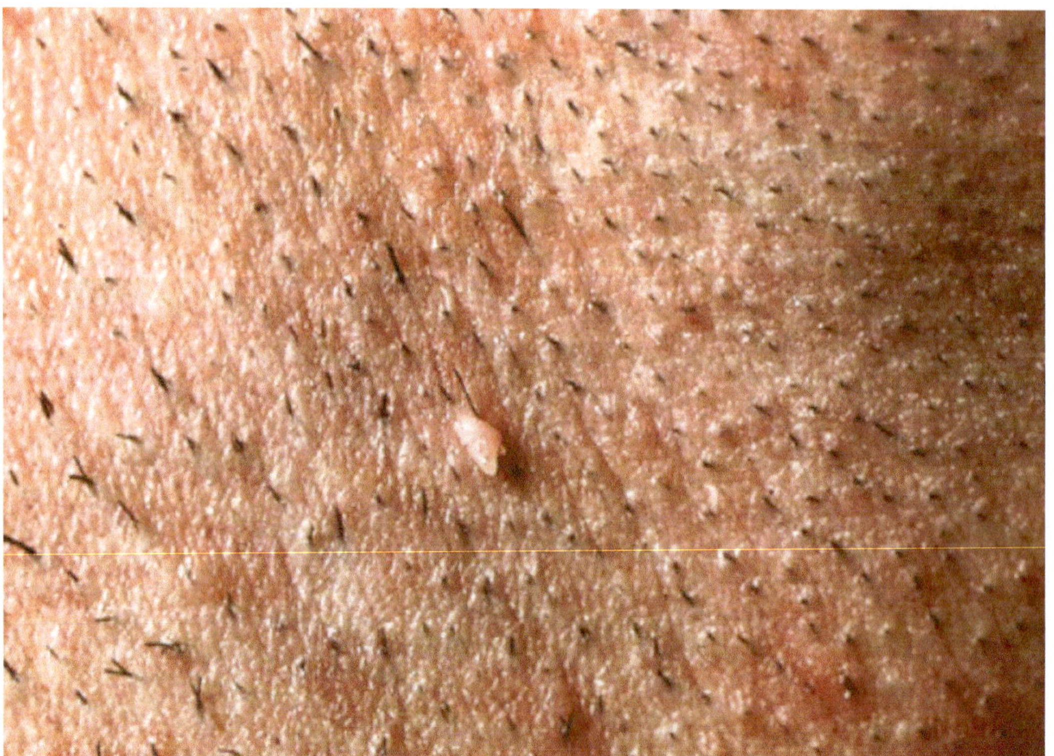

Warts may become elongated and fingerlike.

CLINICAL

- Tiny, pink, shiny papules in beard area of men:
  - Shaving spreads wart virus over entire beard area and causes lesions to bleed.
  - This condition is occasionally seen on other body areas after shaving.
- Caused by implantation of wart virus into skin:
  - Incubation period is several weeks to months.
    - New lesions keep cropping up after visible ones are destroyed.
  - Development of immunity after 6–24 months leads to spontaneous clearing.

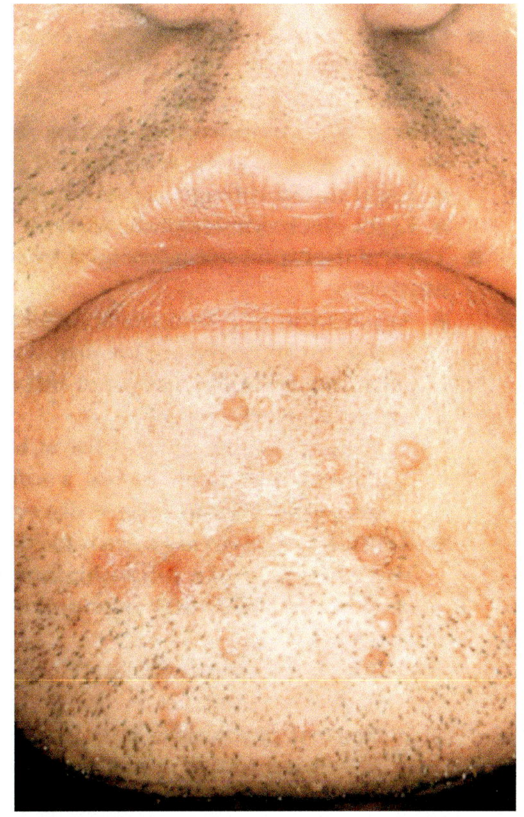

Large warts in beard area, spread by shaving.

TREATMENT

- One can wait for spontaneous resolution to occur, but shaving becomes difficult.
  - Allow hair to grow.
- Destruction of individual lesions is the most common management. Patient must be seen every 2–3 weeks to treat new lesions.
  - Light liquid nitrogen cryotherapy
  - Light electrodesiccation, without anesthesia
  - Vapor plume generated by electrodessication possibly contains viable wart virus, of uncertain danger to the operator and staff
- Topical therapies are advocated by some physicians, but efficacy is unproven.
  - Application of 5-fluorouracil (5-FU) cream or lotion twice daily to the entire beard area is postulated to work by killing growing cells, but it usually provokes inflammation, which may encourage involution.
    - Patient should use this for at least 3 weeks.
    - Patient may need to use a mild corticosteroid (e.g., hydrocortisone 1%) to relieve discomfort of inflammation.
- Keratolytics or drying agents used to "dry up" and peel off warts also often provoke inflammation. Because such drugs damage the keratin layer, they may encourage implantation of virus to new sites.
  - Whitfield's ointment twice daily
  - Benzoyl peroxide 5–10% twice daily
  - May need to use mild corticosteroid to relieve discomfort
- Over-the-counter 40% salicylic acid solution/plaster applied once daily and covered with strong adhesive tape can stay in place for 1–2 days.
- Imiquimod 5% cream applied three to five times per week for 6 weeks or longer until lesions disappear

Herpes Simplex

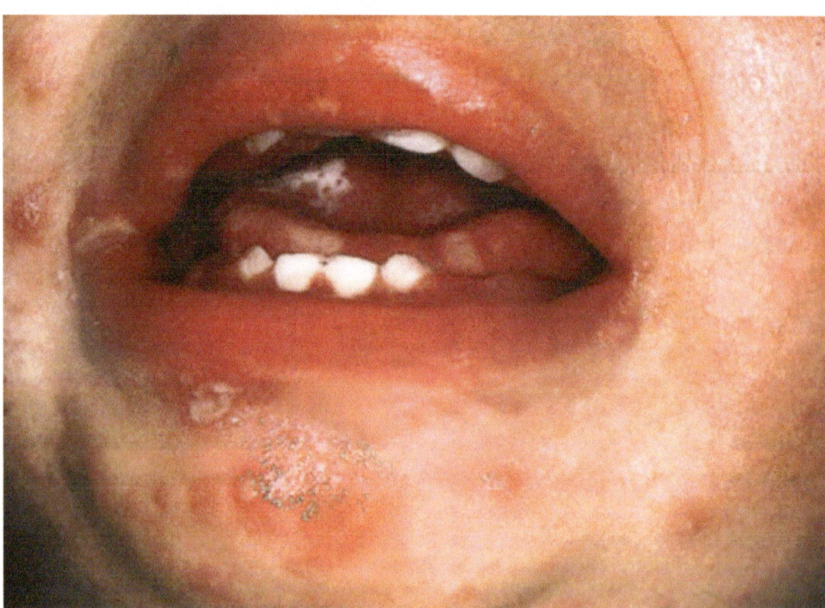

Primary herpes simplex infection of face and mouth in a child.

CLINICAL

- **Primary herpes (first attack) lesions:** Usually in a child or young adult, may present as—
  - Severe stomatitis, upper respiratory infection, lip and facial eruption, with fever and local adenopathy lasting 7–10 days
  - Very mild stomatitis or upper respiratory infection
  - Frequently completely asymptomatic
- **Secondary herpes (recurrent) lesions:**
  - Some individuals who have had a primary attack will have recurrent attacks, although the latent period may be years.
  - Lesions may occur on lips, occasionally on chin, cheeks, forehead, and eyelids, but always recur in same or contiguous sites.
  - "Fever blister," "cold sore": These are a few small vesicles or pustules on an erythematous base. In 2–4 days, these form crusts and heal in 5–7 days.

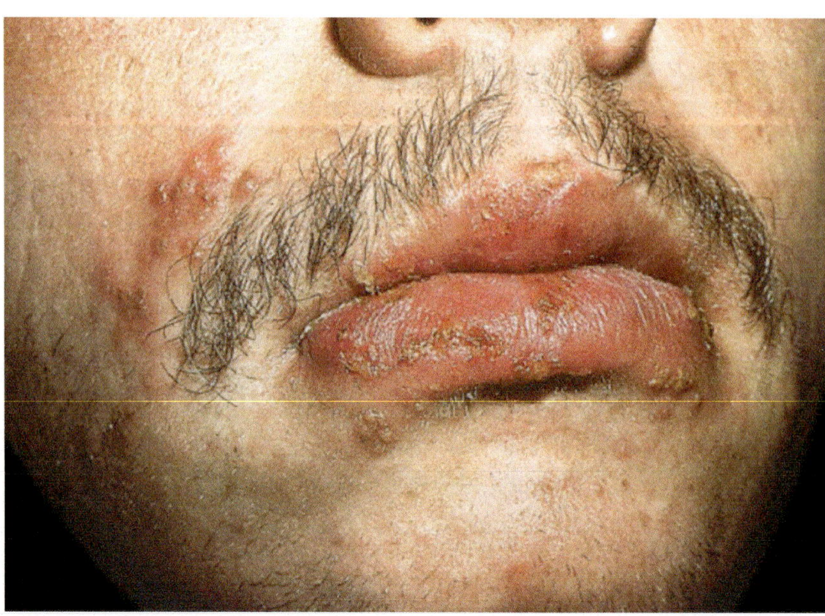

Primary infection in an adult; typical widespread distribution around mouth.

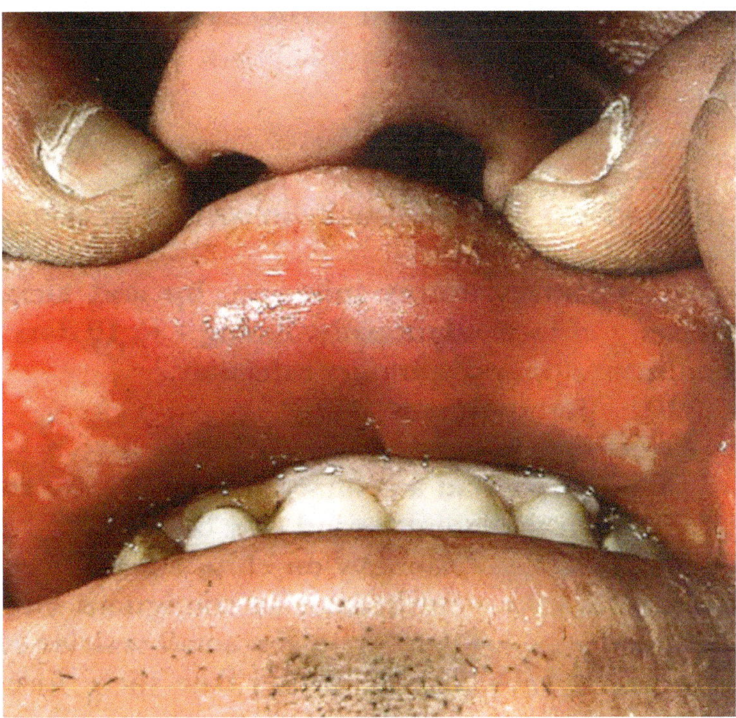

Typical clusters of punctate vesicles and erosions in primary infection.

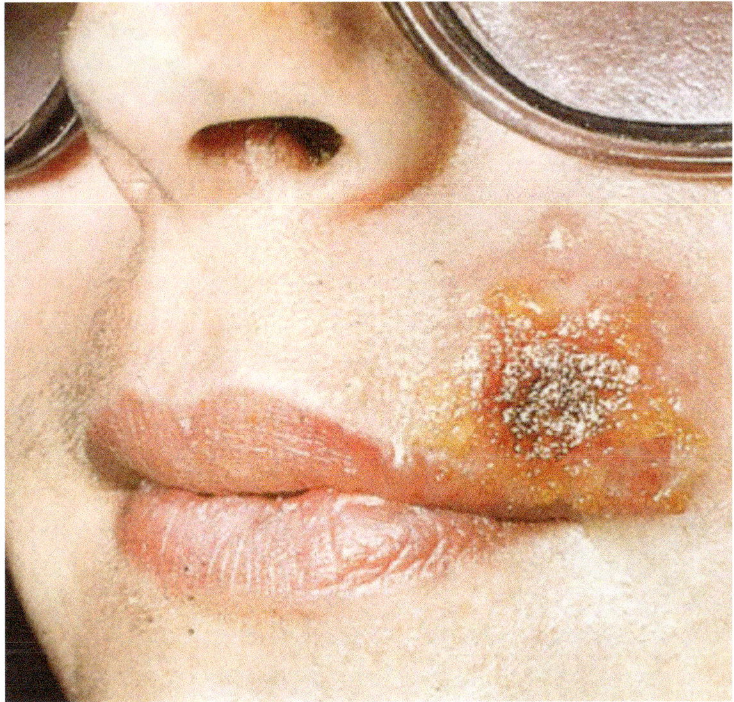

Primary infections are sometimes localized but severe.

- Secondary herpes may have a prodrome of burning at the site for a few hours before eruption. Lesion may burn or itch for 2–5 days.
- Pain, duration, number, and size of vesicles, and degree of crusting can vary considerably from attack to attack.
- Recurrences may be provoked by illness, fever, trauma, or sunburn, or may occur randomly.
- An individual may have only a few recurrences in his or her lifetime or many each year. This is unpredictable this early in the course. Often, frequent attacks may occur for a few years, followed by infrequent attacks.

▪ Primary and recurrent lesions may occur on the genitals (*See* page 54), sacral area, or hands and fingers.
  - Two viral strains occur usually type I above the waist, and type II, below.
  - Infection with one type of herpes may not confer immunity to the other type.

- Conjunctival, corneal, and ocular globe infections:
  - Encourage patients with oral or genital lesions not to rub their eyes during an attack to avoid inoculation.
  - If an eye infection is suspected, refer to an ophthalmologist for complete examination.
- Severe or chronic eruptions may occur in immunosuppressed patients.

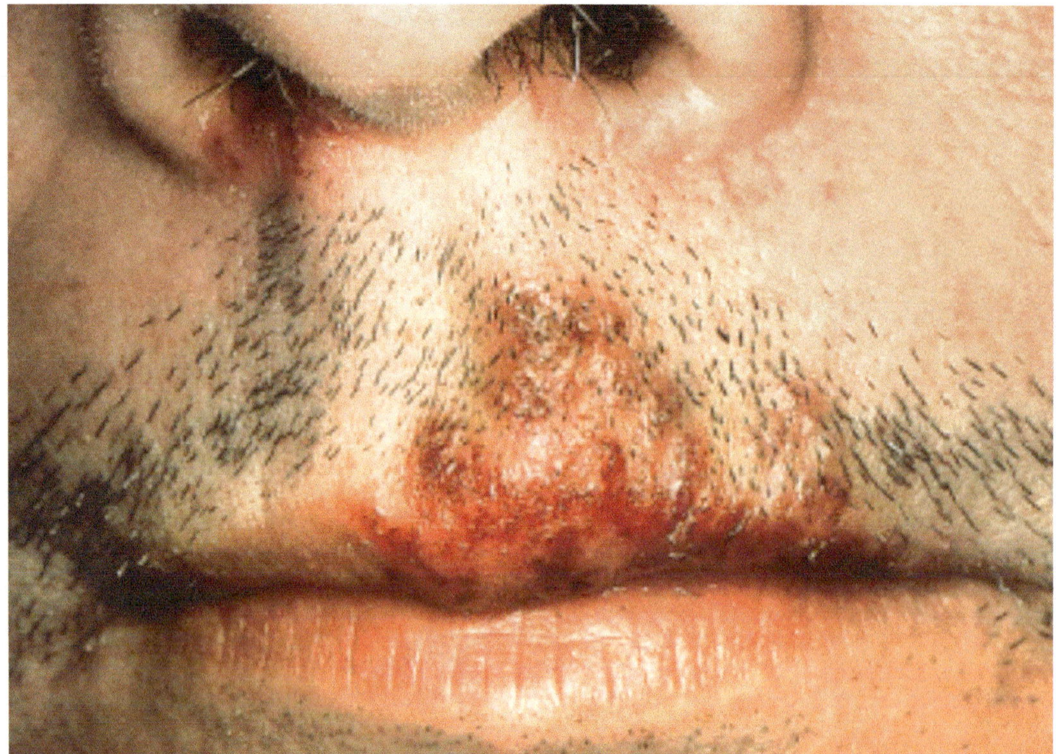

Typical recurrent herpes, in this case brought on by fever.

TREATMENT

A reservoir of viruses exists in nerve ganglia. No topical or systemic agent destroys this reservoir.

- General:
  - Patient education is paramount (*See* Patient Guides, page 248).
  - Avoid sunburn to face and lips by using hats and sunscreens, especially on lips.
- Penciclovir cream:
  - Approved for topical treatment of recurrent herpes. Applied every 2 hours for 4 days as soon as symptoms appear. Shortens outbreak by ½ day, compared with placebo.
- Acyclovir (*See* page 237):
  - Topical ointment:
    - May accelerate healing of primary lesion, but short course of oral acyclovir is more effective
    - Of no benefit in recurrent attacks
- Oral tablets:
  - These accelerate healing of primary lesions
  - Oral acyclovir prevents recurrent attacks if taken prophylactically. Usual dose is 400 mg three times daily, for 5–10 days. When the drug is discontinued, attacks usually resume, and first recurrent attack may be especially severe. Acyclovir

400 mg twice daily is recommended for those having six or more attacks per year. Regimen has been continued up to 5 years with safety and efficacy. If attacks occur at predictable times (e.g., with sun exposure), oral acyclovir may be taken intermittently in advance of and during those times.
  - If taken 400 mg three times daily as soon as prodrome starts for recurrent attack, may shorten long attacks but will not affect short ones. Effect, in general, in these situations is modest.
  - This regimen is strongly indicated for severe primary or long-lasting recurrent lesions in the immunosuppressed.
- Famciclovir:
  - Oral analog of acyclovir
  - Indicated for herpes zoster but also effective against herpes simplex virus
  - 500 mg twice daily for 7 to 10 days is used for primary lesions and 1.5 g as a single dose may be given for recurrent attacks
- Valacyclovir:
  - Oral agent for herpes zoster, but effective also against herpes simplex
  - More completely and more rapidly absorbed than acyclovir and famciclovir and may work faster than those agents
  - Approved in United States at dose of 1 g twice daily for 7–10 days for the initial infection or 2 g twice daily for 1 day when outbreaks occur
- Acyclovir-resistant herpes simplex:
  - This disease is becoming a frequent problem in HIV-infected persons; organism also resistant to famciclovir and valacyclovir.
  - Foscarnet is the next drug of choice but must be administered intravenously.
  - Refer patient to infectious disease specialist for evaluation and management.

Erysipelas

CLINICAL

- Superficial streptococcal cellulitis
- Typical symptoms include:
  - Sudden-onset, painful, rapidly spreading, vivid red macule on face
  - Chills, fever, and malaise
- Most often found in older adults
- Before the advent of antibiotics, often fatal
- Sometimes, a wound, fissure, or nasal folliculitis is portal of entry, but usually none evident.

TREATMENT

This is an emergency.

- If erysipelas is suspected, immediately initiate systemic antibiotic therapy (penicillin, unless the patient is allergic to it).
- Consider admitting the patient to hospital overnight to ensure compliance and monitor response.
  - Temperature drops dramatically in 12 hours.
- Cultures grown from wound, fissure, or nasal antrum are only occasionally positive.

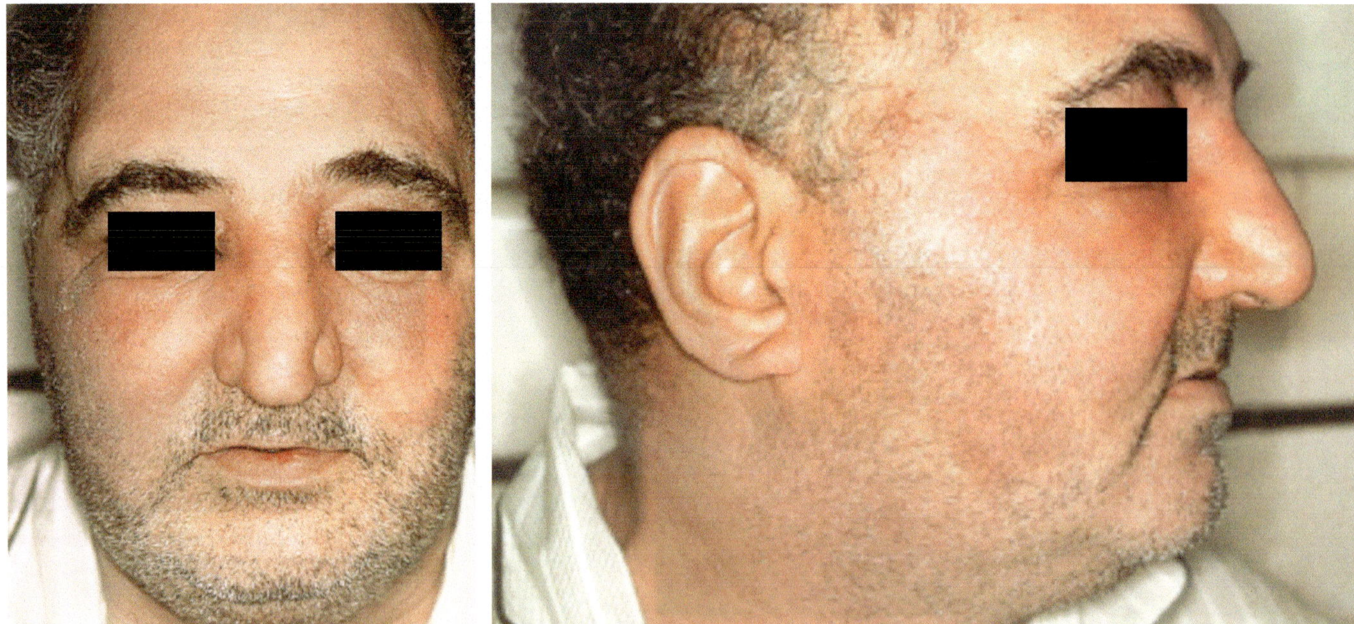

Front and side views of face show sharply demarcated, bright erythema, and swelling of nose and cheeks.

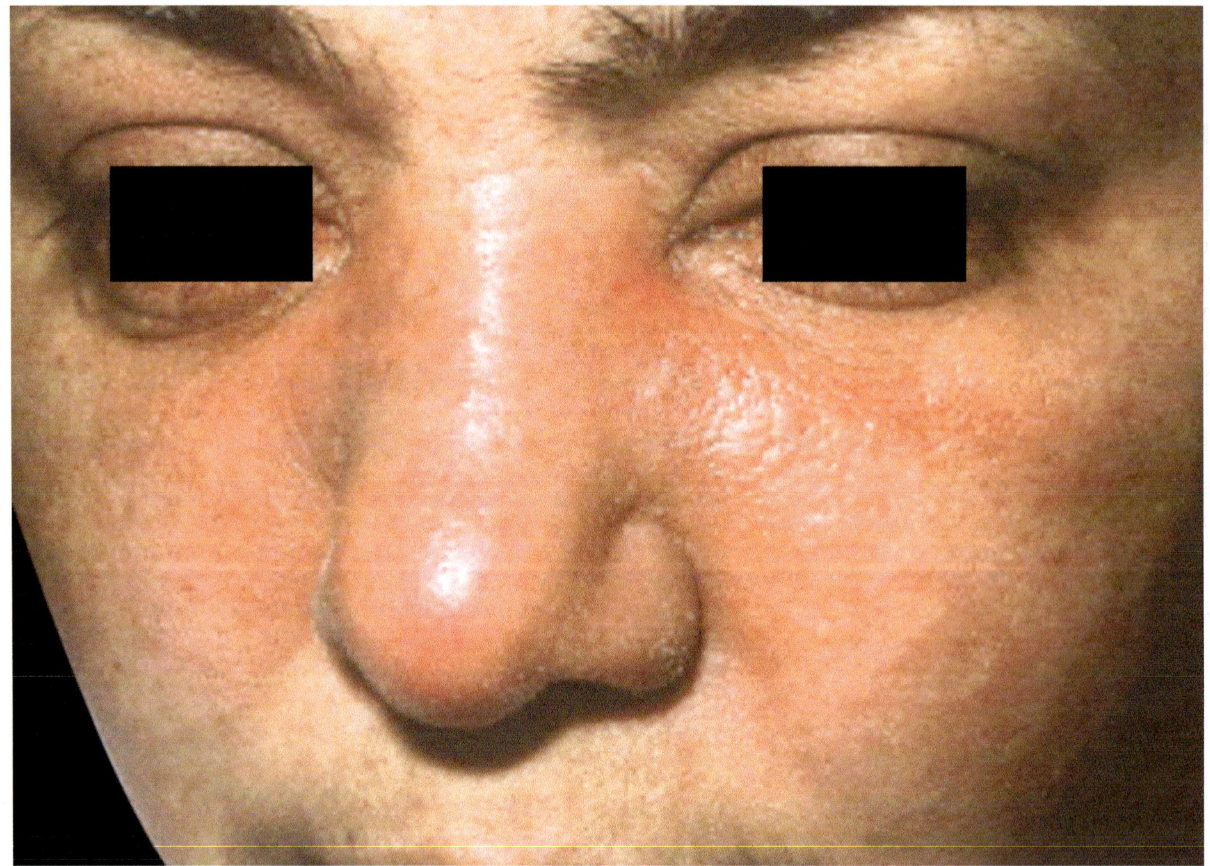

Similar classic facial erythema of erysipelas with involvement of eyelids as well. Temperature was 39.8°C.

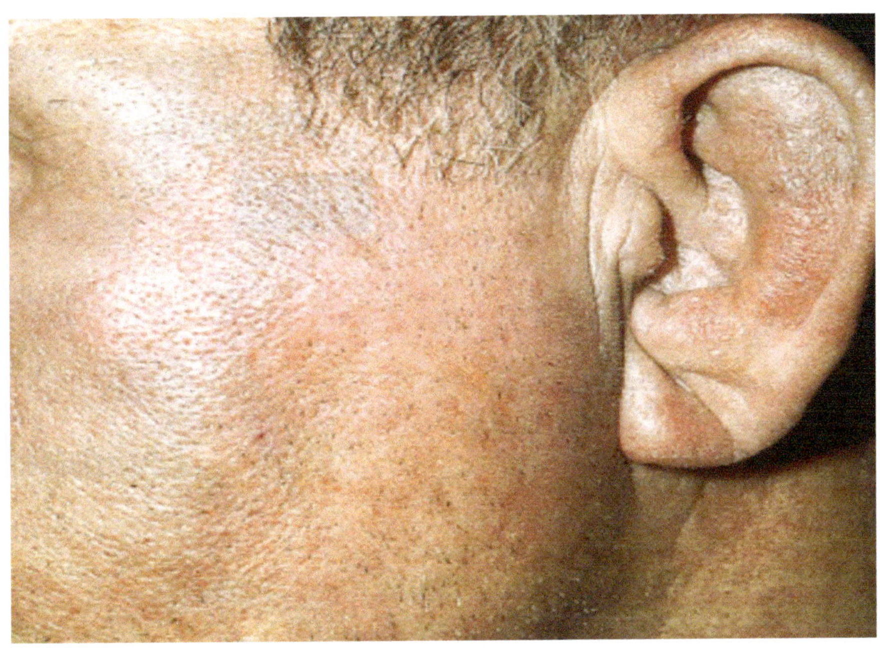

Redness and swelling started on the ear and rapidly spread across cheek in this patient with erysipelas.

Melasma (Chloasma)

CLINICAL

- Macular hyperpigmentation, sharply defined but with irregular borders
- Forehead, malar eminences, and upper lip
- Becomes evident or darkens dramatically with sun exposure
- Commonly occurs in women during pregnancy or during use of oral contraceptives or estrogens but may occur at other times and occasionally occurs in men; often improves in months or years
- Idiopathic; represents increased melanocyte activity; pigment solely in epidermis
- May be mimicked by postinflammatory pigmentation from photoirritation or contact dermatitis

TREATMENT

- Discontinue estrogens; condition may then slowly resolve, or it may persist.
- Minimize sun exposure:
  - Shading with a hat
  - Use of broad-spectrum sunscreens (*See* page 204)
- Hydroquinone:
  - Topical hydroquinone suppresses melanocyte activity.
  - Was available over-the-counter
  - Hydroquinone will lighten pigment, if epidermal (will not affect postinflammatory hyperpigmentation, which is dermal).
  - Sun must be avoided and broad-spectrum sunscreen must be used during treatment.
  - Treatment may completely clear melasma in persons with fair skin, but there may be a relapse. Only occasionally clears melasma completely in darker-skinned individuals, and relapse is common.
  - It is prescribed in 4–10% concentrations in creams or lotions (*See* page 241). These may be irritating and occasionally cause a contact allergy.
    - Apply thinly once daily to dark areas.
    - If effective, this treatment usually bleaches melasma without much effect on surrounding normal skin.
    - Ochronosis (noted as skin darkening) may occur.
    - If melasma clears, use hydroquinone only as needed for recurrences.
    - Effect is seen in weeks in the fair skinned but may require months of use in the dark skinned.

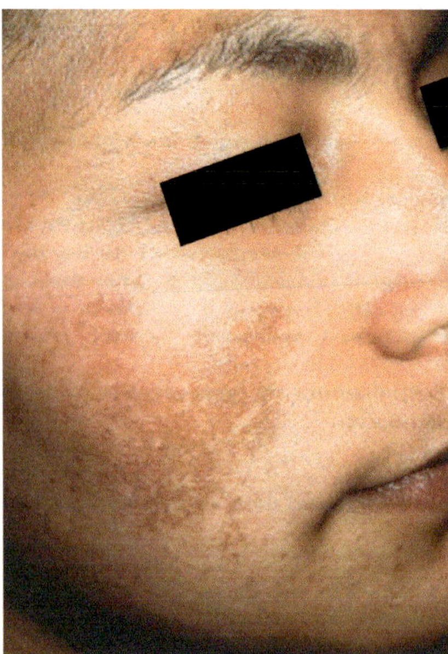

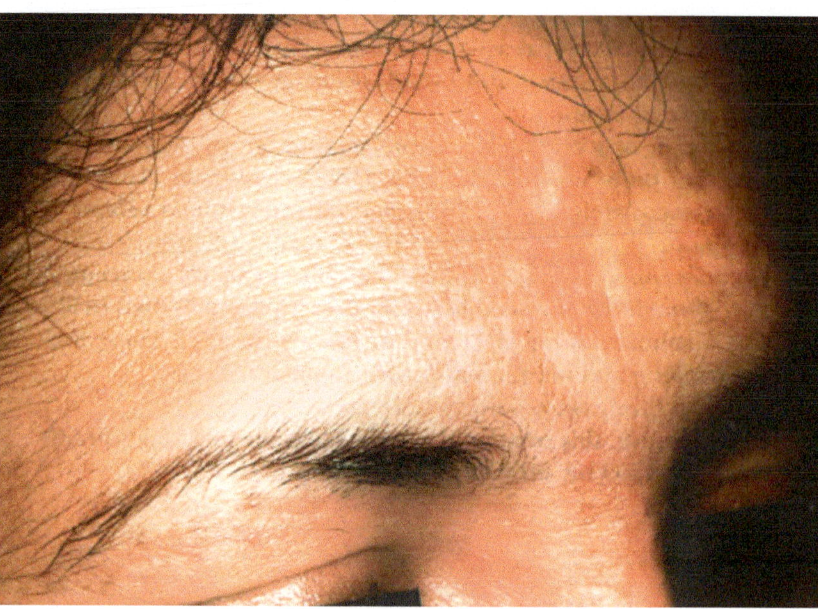

Melasma: Blotchy hyperpigmentation with irregular borders, usually seen on forehead, cheeks, and upper lip.

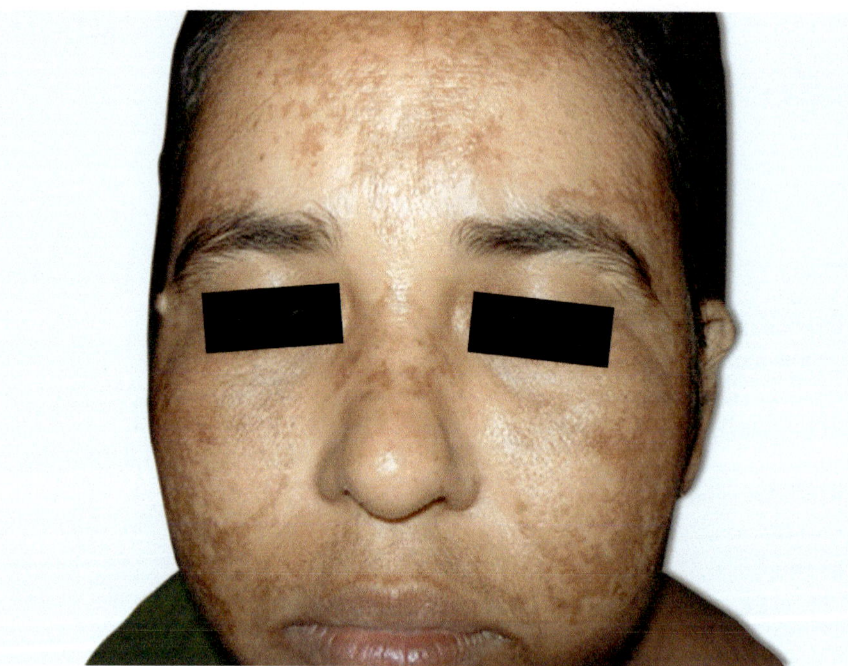

Patient showing brownish nonhomogeneous pigmented patches over forehead, nose, malar areas, and upper lip.

More effective and reliable (better penetration) if used with tretinoin cream or gel (*See* page 234). This makes irritation more likely, so topical corticosteroid is often added to reduce irritation; it also enhances the bleaching action.
These materials may be applied sequentially, usually using tretinoin only once a day, hydroquinone once daily, and corticosteroid as necessary.

- Azelaic acid:
  - Topical 15% foam or gel and 20% cream applied twice daily suppresses melanocyte activity similarly to hydroquinone. A 10% cream is available over the counter.
  - This treatment is about equal to 4% hydroquinone.
  - Azelaic acid is occasionally slightly irritating.
  - This treatment takes several months for favorable benefits to be seen.
  - Benefit is enhanced, if azelaic acid is applied once a day and tretinoin cream is applied at another time during the day.
  - Kojic acid 4% (as a cosmetic formulation) may be used

Lichen Simplex Chronicus

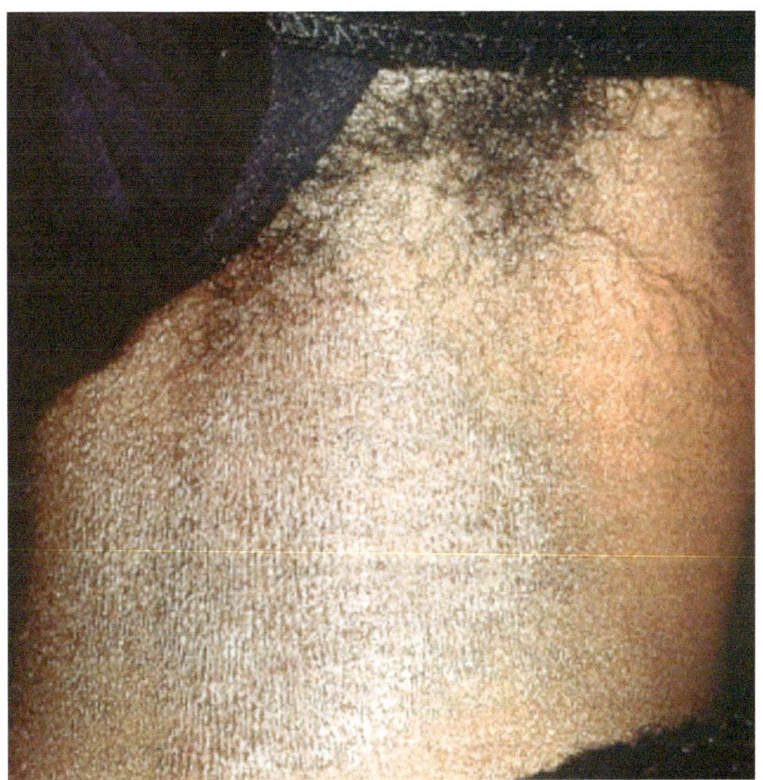

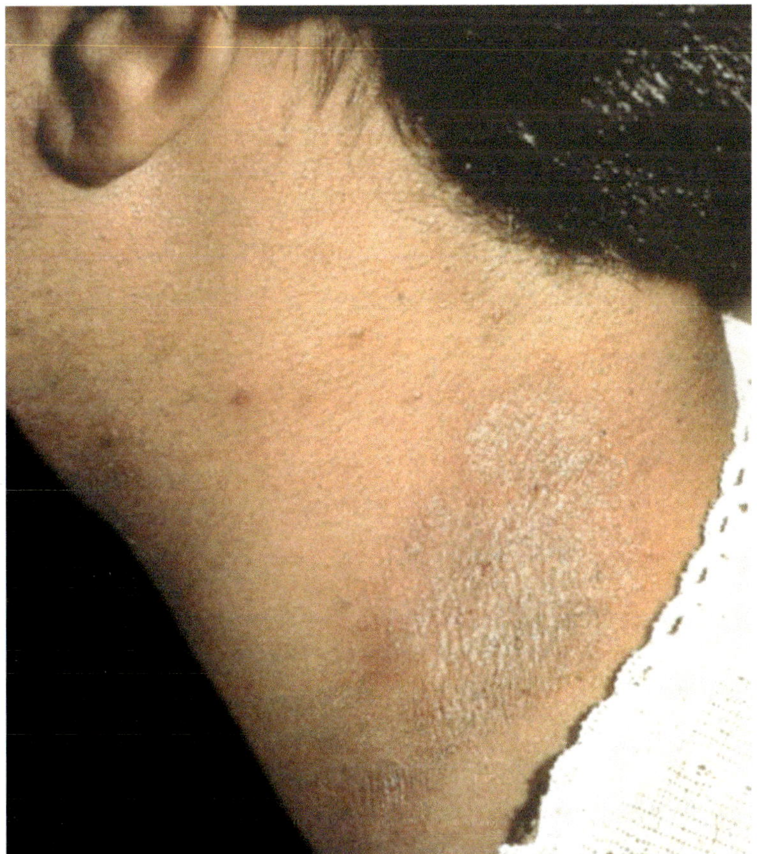

Typical well-circumscribed lichenified plaques of lichen simplex chronicus on the neck in women.

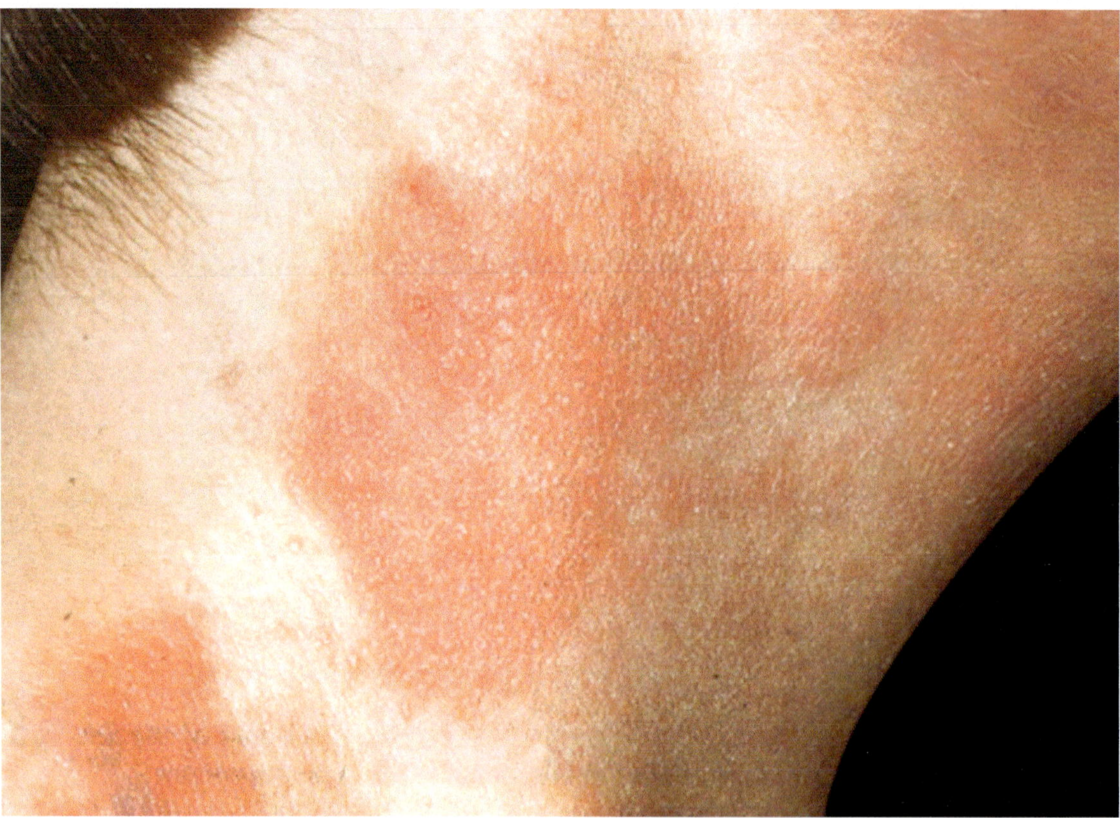

Early (3 weeks) patchy dermatitis on the side of the neck. Patient rubs more when tense.

CLINICAL

- Large (5–20 cm), fairly well circumscribed plaque of lichenification (skin thickened, scaly, hyperpigmented with accentuation of normal skin marking lines)
- Location:
  - Rare on the face but common on nape and sides of neck in women
  - In men, common on ankles (*See* page 99)
  - Perineum in both sexes (*See* page 74)
- Atopic history is common.
- Often develops or worsens during stress but rubbing becomes a chronic habit.

TREATMENT

- Instruct patient that:
  - It is not dangerous, contagious, or likely to spread.
  - It may have been caused by insect bite, contact irritation, or other skin problem but now rubbing has become a habit and tension-releasing mechanism (like biting fingernails).
- Treatment of choice is external or intralesional corticosteroids.
  - Tacrolimus 0.1% ointment and pimecrolimus 1% cream are nonsteroidal alternatives that may be helpful.
  - Very potent corticosteroid ointment (because lesion is usually dry) or cream is necessary.
    - Apply as often as necessary for itching *instead of scratching* for a few days, then two or three times a day.
    - Occlusion with plastic film or steroid-impregnated tape (*See* page 238) is very helpful if the preceding method fails, because it greatly enhances the effect of the corticosteroid and blocks scratching.
    - Discontinue potent corticosteroid when lesion is flat. Use milder preparation, if itching continues.
  - Intralesional injection of corticosteroid (*See* technique, page 240) is temporarily painful but often helpful, especially if topical therapy fails.
  - May tell patients that they must not rub area now that medication is in the skin.

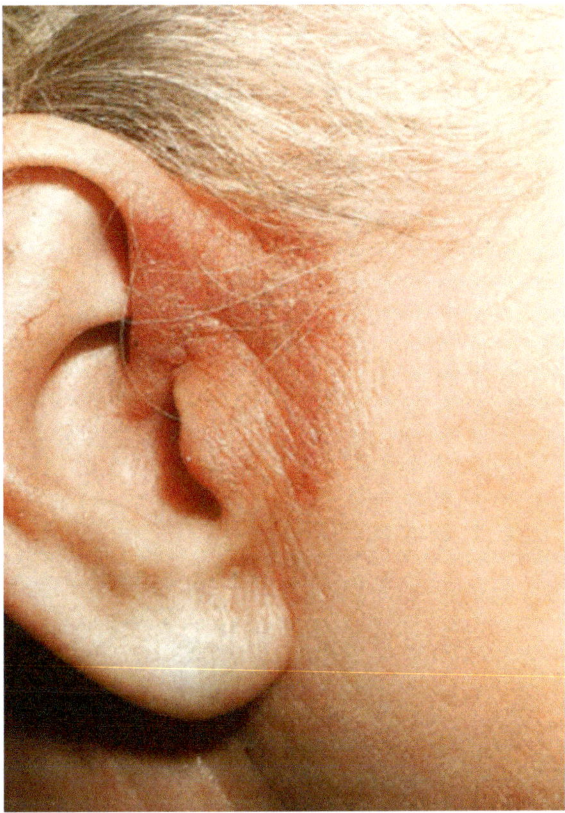

The side of the face is a less common site.

- Alternate or concomitant treatment with topical coal tar preparations (*See* page 244), especially in chronic cases. Beware of irritant folliculitis at nape of neck.
- Antihistamine as a sedative (*See* page 243) or a mild tranquilizer may be helpful in tense individuals, but **is not a substitute for topical medication.**

3 CHAPTER Genitals, Groin, and Axillae

Herpes Simplex

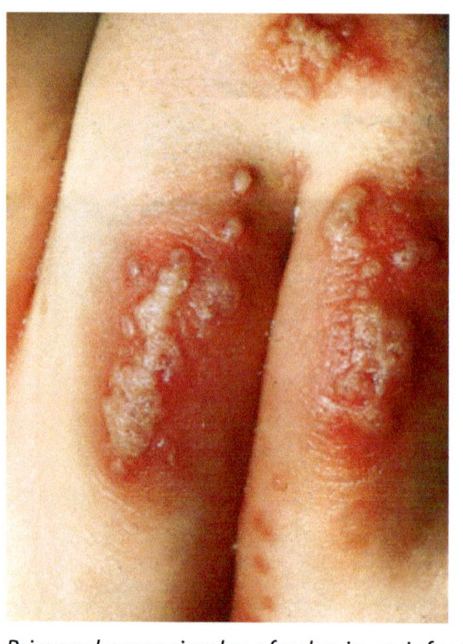

Primary herpes simplex of vulva in an infant. Organism probably came from parent's hand during diaper change.

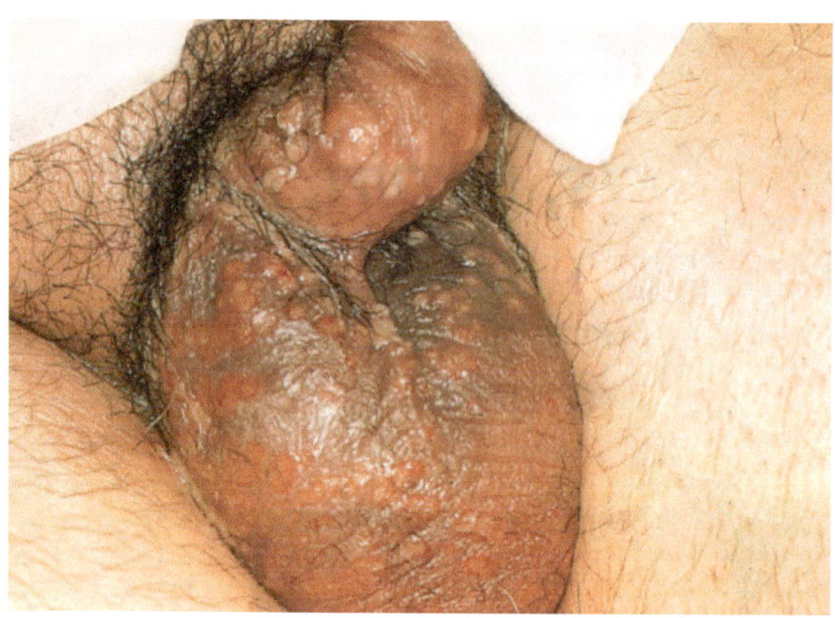

Widespread primary herpes genitalis in an adult.

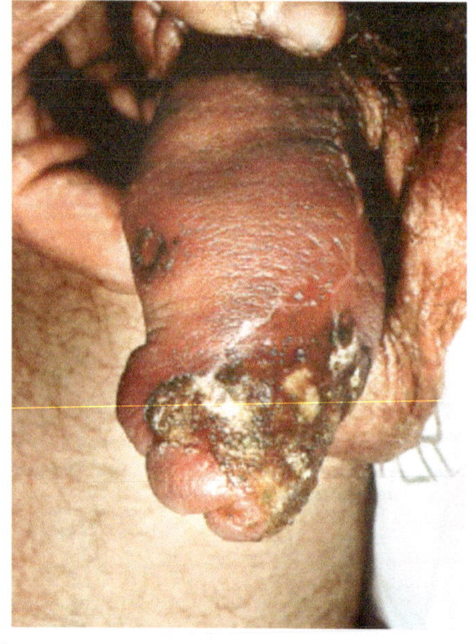

Severe, necrotic primary herpes simplex infection.

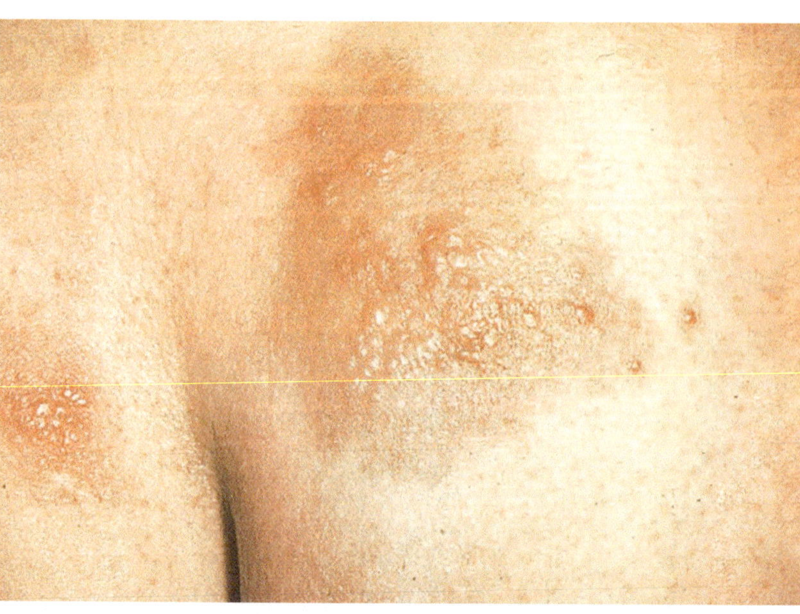

Primary herpes simplex of sacral area; often bilateral.

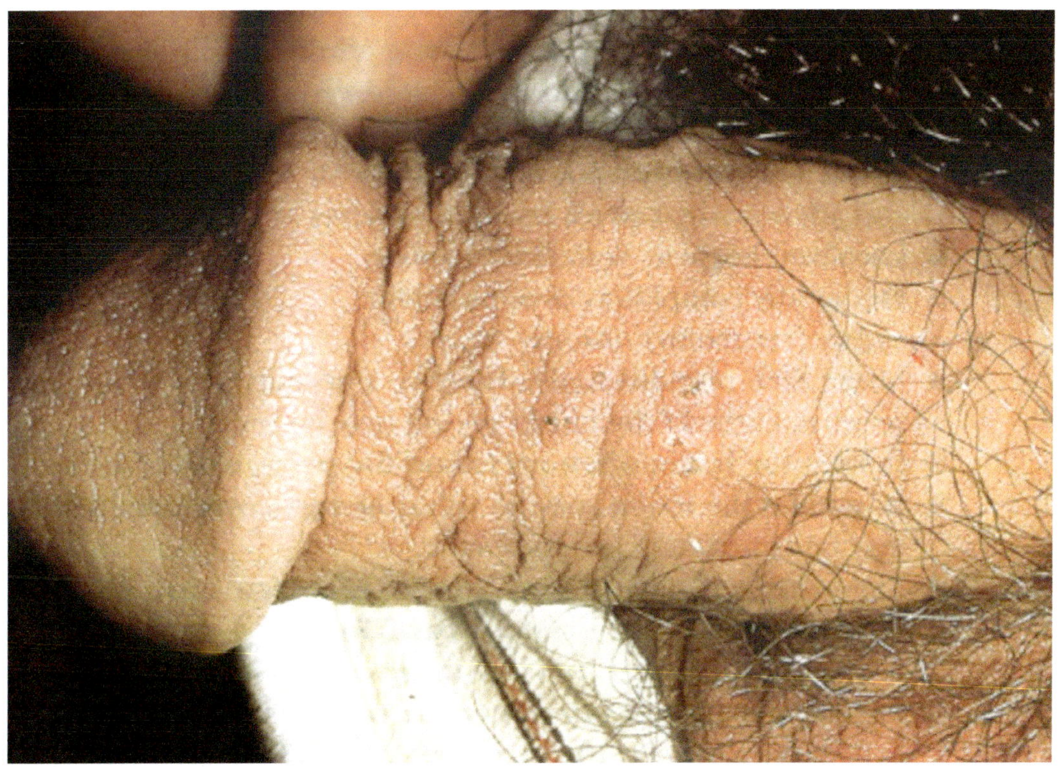

Typical mild eruption of small cluster of vesicles in recurrent herpes on penis.

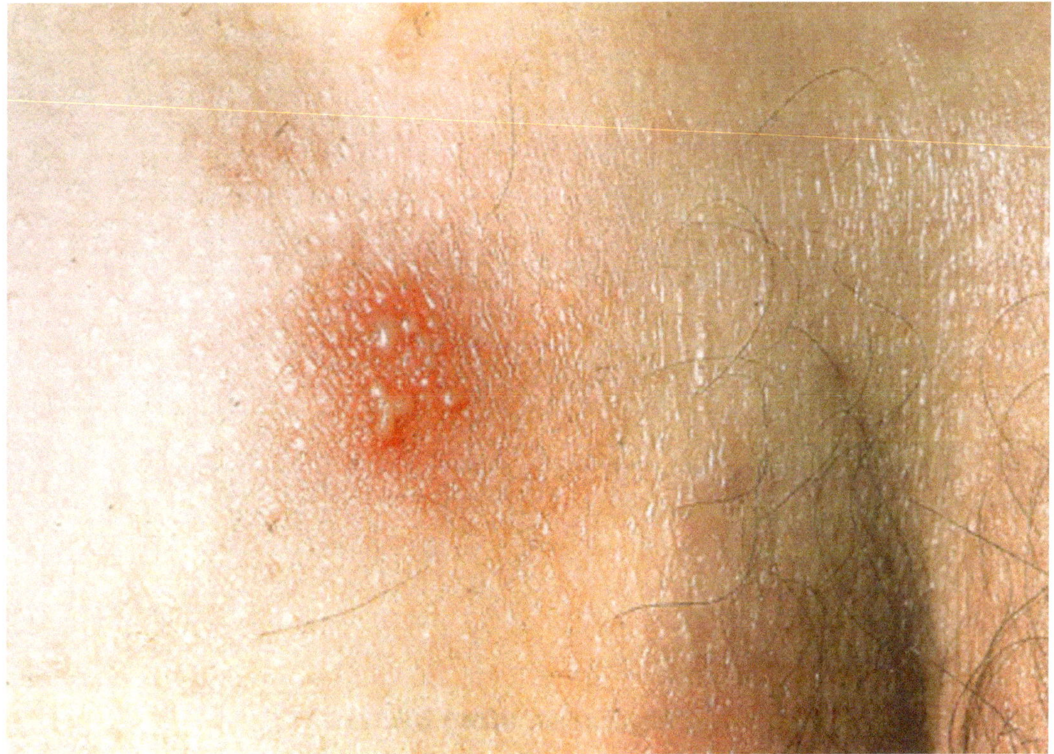

Recurrent herpes of buttocks. Also present are scars from previous eruptions.

CLINICAL

- *Primary* attack usually occurs in young adults (as opposed to oral herpes, which often first occurs in children). It presumably is sexually transmitted and may present as:
  - Severe balanitis, vulvitis, or vaginitis with vesicles, edema, pain, and adenopathy (rare); lasts 7–10 days

  - Localized herpetic vesicular eruption
  - Frequently completely asymptomatic
- *Secondary* (recurrent) lesions:
  - Some individuals who have a primary attack will have a recurrent attack; the latent period may be years.
  - In men, the lesion often occurs on the penis, usually distal.
  - In women, the lesion may be vulvar or cervicovaginal; the latter may be completely asymptomatic.
  - "Fever blister," "cold sore": These are a few small vesicles or pustules on an erythematous base. In 2–4 days, sores form crusts, and they heal in 5–7 days.
  - Patient may have prodrome of burning at site for a few hours before eruption. Lesion may burn or itch for 2–5 days.
  - Pain, duration, number, and size of vesicles and degree of crusting can vary considerably from attack to attack.
  - Recurrences are often provoked by intercourse but may occur with fever, illness, or at random.
  - An individual may have only a few recurrences in his or her lifetime or many each year. This cannot be predicted early in the course. Often, there are frequent attacks for a few years, followed by infrequent attacks.
  - Lesions are contagious for 2–4 days, before dry crusts form.
- Transmission of herpes from women to men is frequently from *asymptomatic shedding*. Even though the woman may have had clinically evident lesions only a few times a year, several times a month she may shed small numbers of live virus, which are contagious. Because this shedding is undetectable, there is no "safe" period for intercourse; thus, continual use of condoms is recommended. Asymptomatic shedding by men is much harder to document but is known to occur, probably less often than in women.
- When herpes simplex is present in the newborn, it often becomes disseminated and frequently is fatal. In more than half of cases, there is no prior sign of herpes in the mother. It is thought that the infection is acquired from the father by intercourse with the mother near term. If herpes is known to exist in a pregnant woman, her obstetrician should be apprised of it so that careful examinations can be performed as birth approaches. Previously, cesarean section was always performed if herpes was detected during labor, but this practice is now being questioned.
- Primary and recurrent lesions may occur on the face (*See* page 44), sacral area, or hands and fingers.
  - Two viral strains occur—usually type I above the waist and type II, below.
  - Infection with one type of herpes may not confer immunity to the other type.
- Severe or chronic eruptions may occur in immunosuppressed patients (*See* page 172).

TREATMENT

Because the viral reservoir is *in* spinal ganglia, topical treatments cannot be expected to prevent recurrences. No systemic therapy is available to eradicate the reservoir, so "cure" is not possible. Only patient immunity will ultimately control the infection.

- General:
  - Patient education is paramount (*See* Patient Guides, page 248).
  - Condoms and spermicidal jellies and foams probably prevent transmission of the virus.
- Acyclovir *(See* page 237*):*
  - Topical ointment:
    - May accelerate healing of primary lesion, but oral acyclovir is superior
    - No benefit in recurring attacks
  - Oral antivirals: *See* page 237 for details
- Penciclovir cream
  - Topical treatment of recurrent herpes.

Anogenital Warts (Condylomata Acuminata)

CLINICAL

- Soft, fleshy papules, tags, or plaques:
  - In this moist environment often not keratotic
  - May be pink, whitish, or pigmented
- Found on:
  - Penis:
    - Especially under the foreskin and in the coronal sulcus
    - Occasionally around urethral meatus and in urethra
  - Vulva and vagina:
    - Vaginal examination of all female patients necessary
  - Perianal skin and anus:
    - Anoscopy of all patients necessary

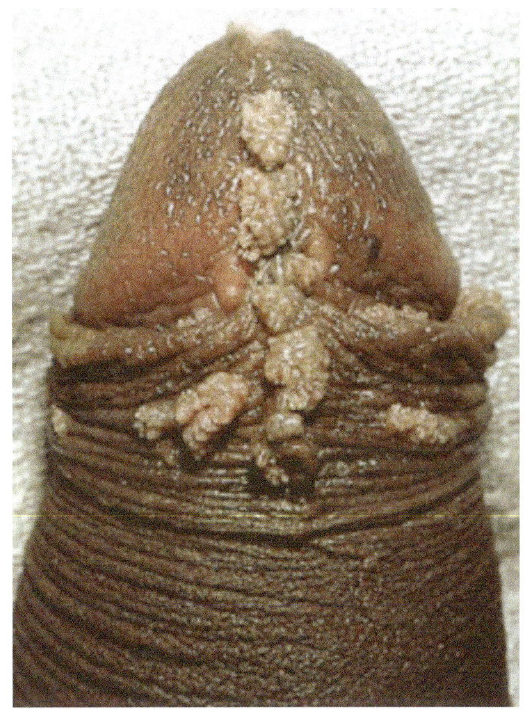

Exuberant growth of penile warts.

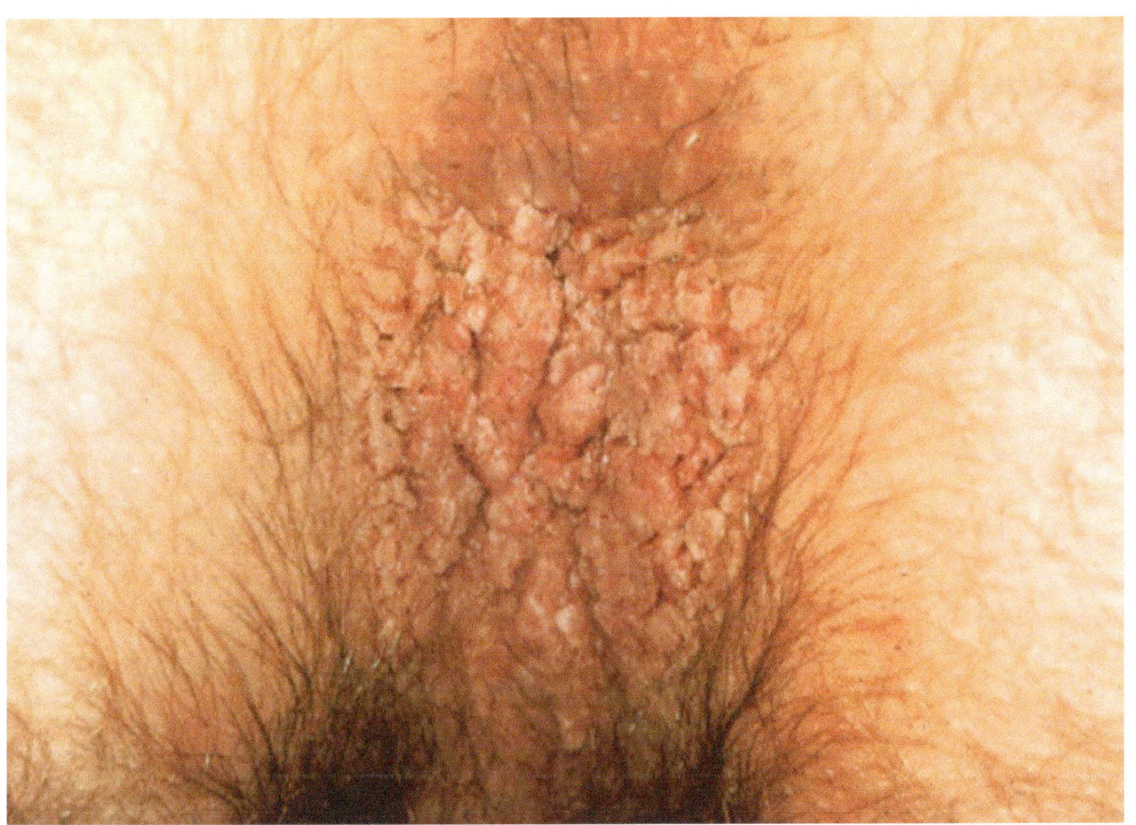

Profuse growth of perianal warts.

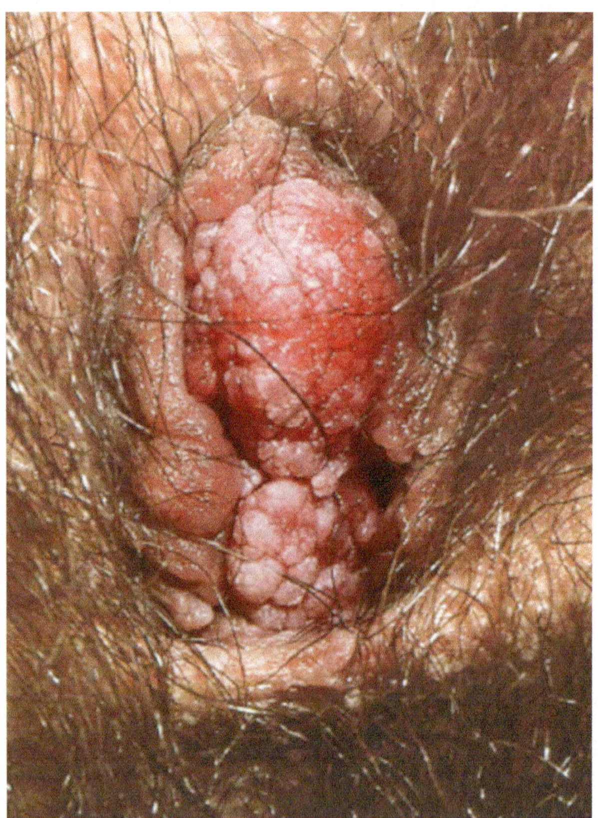
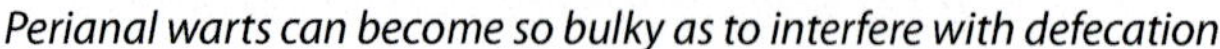

Perianal warts can become so bulky as to interfere with defecation.

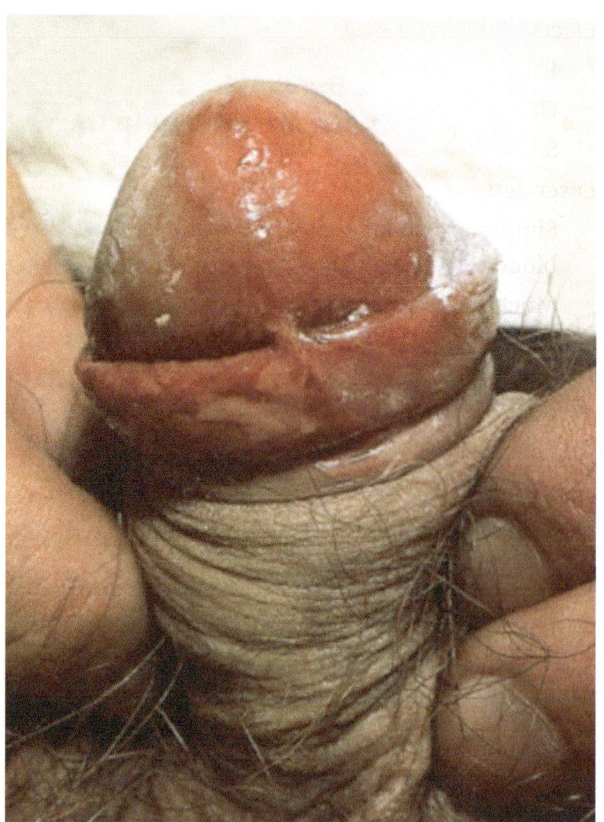

Severe irritant contact dermatitis from podophyllin left on for 48 hours.

Subtle or latent lesions may be detected by soaking the affected area for 3–5 minutes with 5% acetic acid solution, causing white patches to appear. White vinegar diluted half and half with water makes an acceptable solution. Compressing the area with moistened gauzes is a practical technique. In men, a majority of positive results may not contain wart virus—a fact that has led to decreased use of the test.

- Viral-induced benign tumor:
  - Virus probably slightly different from those causing nongenital warts
  - Transmitted by sexual contact
  - Incubation period of several months; makes determination of source of infection uncertain
  - Reduces confidence in "cure" because newly seeded viruses may not produce lesions for months
  - Resolves spontaneously in months or years when immunity develops
  - Associated with the development of laryngeal polyps in infants when vaginal warts are present in the mother at childbirth

Certain viral strains are implicated in the pathogenesis of cervical dysplasia and cancer in women. Sexual partners must be examined to eradicate sources of reinfection. Close monitoring of infected women with Pap smears is recommended for early diagnosis of dysplastic and neoplastic changes.

TREATMENT

Cytotoxic: Podophyllotoxin

- Apply twice daily for 3 days, then withhold use for 4 days, for up to four cycles.
- Side effects are minimal.

Destruction of Wart Tissue (If Podophyllotoxin Fails)

- Liquid nitrogen cryotherapy:
  - Mildly to severely painful
  - Effective
  - Follow-up in 2–4 weeks to check for regrowth of new lesions

- Electrocautery:
  - Painful local anesthesia required
  - Often leaves mild scar
  - Sometimes, the therapy of last resort in huge perianal warts; close follow-up and repeat treatments are necessary
- Laser destruction:
  - Similar to electrocautery but easier to distinguish wart from normal tissue during destruction, so cure rate is higher; bloodless, so much tidier when removing very large perianal warts
  - Much more expensive than electrocautery
  - Vapor plume generated by electrocautery or laser possibly contains viable wart virus, of uncertain danger to the operator and staff

Keratolytics (salicylic and lactic acid), though safe when used elsewhere, are often highly irritating to genital and perineal skin. They are not effective at this site.

- Imiquimod (3.75% or 5% cream)—apply 5% cream three times a week at bedtime until clearance or up to 16 weeks. Alternatively, apply 3.75% cream nightly at bedtime for up to 8 weeks.
- Sinecatechin (extract of green tea) 15% ointment three times daily and cidofovir 1% gel once daily are alternative treatment options
- The 9-valent HPV vaccine gardasil-9 protects against types 6, 11, 16, 18, 31, 33, 45, 52, and 58. Types 6 and 11 cause most anogenital warts. The vaccine is not effective as treatment of existing lesions, but it can prevent infection if administered prior to the first sexual intercourse.

Syphilis

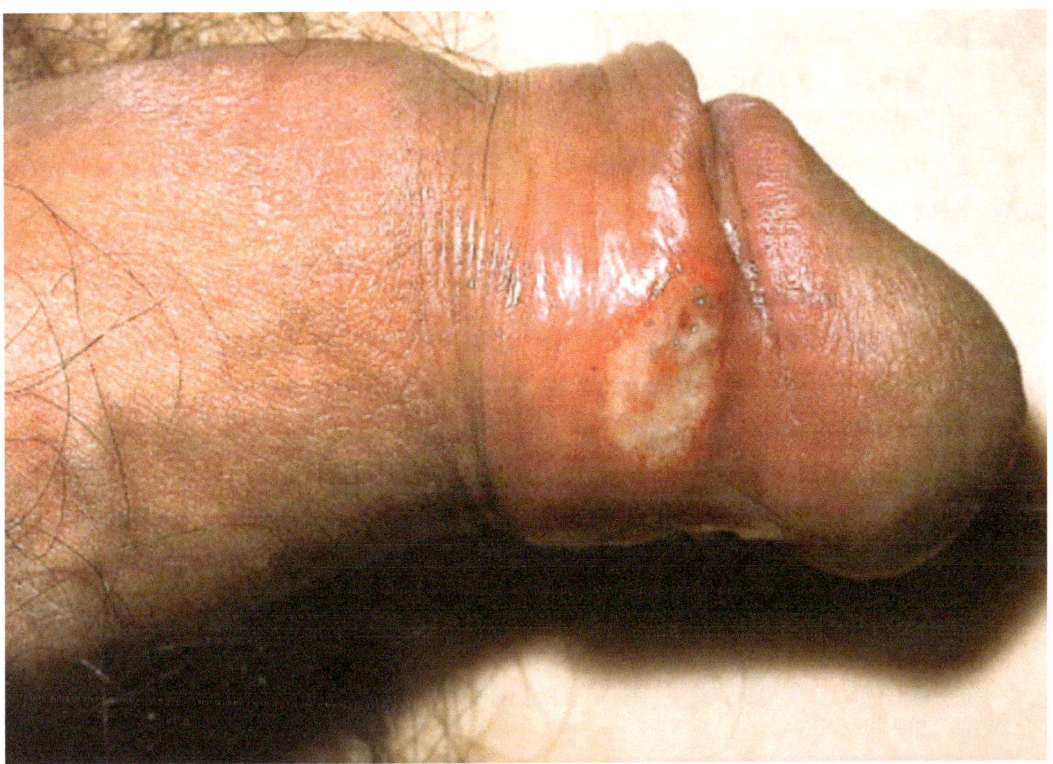

Typical single punched-out ulcer of primary syphilis.

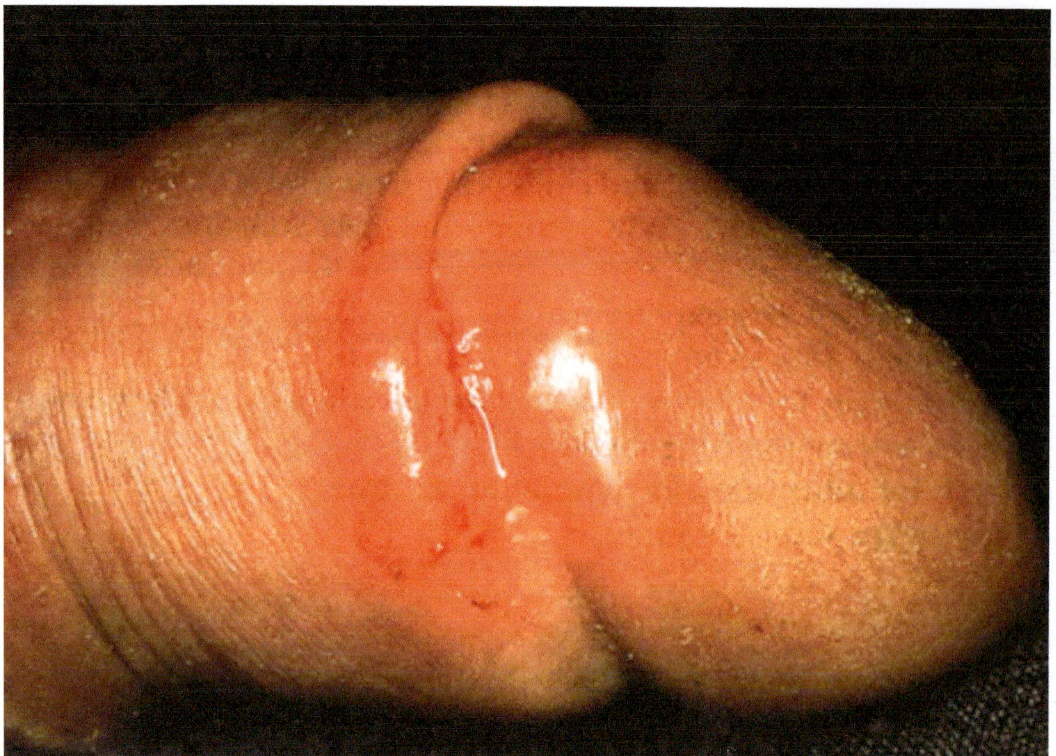

Commonly, the chancre is not ulcerated but is only an area of induration.

CLINICAL

- The primary chancre is typically a single, firm, painless, buttonlike induration with an eroded, oozing surface.
  - Infrequently noticed on female genitalia
  - May be multiple
  - May be painful, especially when secondarily infected
  - May be deeply ulcerated
  - Usually accompanied by painless, unilateral, rubbery node ("bubo"):
    - May be tender
    - May be bilateral
- Secondary syphilis of the genitals may occur in two forms:
  1. The rash of secondary syphilis (*See* page 143) usually involves the penis and scrotum.
  2. *Condylomata lata* are soft, whitish, flat-topped velvety plaques in genital and perianal creases.

In both forms, the lesions, teeming with organisms, are highly contagious, including to the examiner. Gloves must be worn.

- Serologic tests: Nonspecific serologic test for syphilis (STS) and fluorescent treponemal antibody (FTA)—
  - In *primary* syphilis, test results may or may not be positive.
    - FTA often becomes positive before the STS does.
    - Positive results are more likely the longer the lesion has been present.
    - STS results are often of low titer (up to 1:16).
  - In *secondary* syphilis, both test results should be positive.
    - Titer is high (above 1:8) in STS.

The STS result may be negative because of the *prozone* phenomenon. The titer is so high that it will not precipitate in test plates at the low dilutions used in the screening tests. If secondary syphilis is strongly suspected, send another blood sample and ask for a "prozone test" or examination of higher dilutions.

- Results of dark-field examination are positive for primary and secondary lesions.
  - **Training and skill are required for successful examination.**

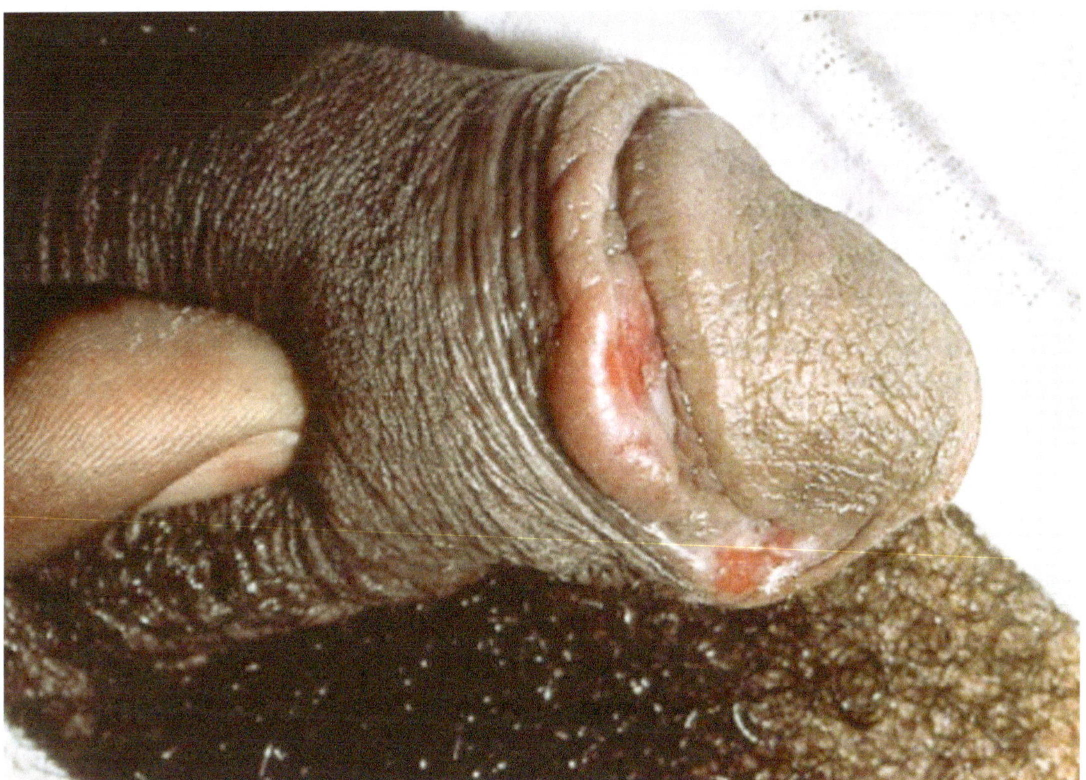

Lesions of primary syphilis may be multiple. Location is commonly in coronal sulcus.

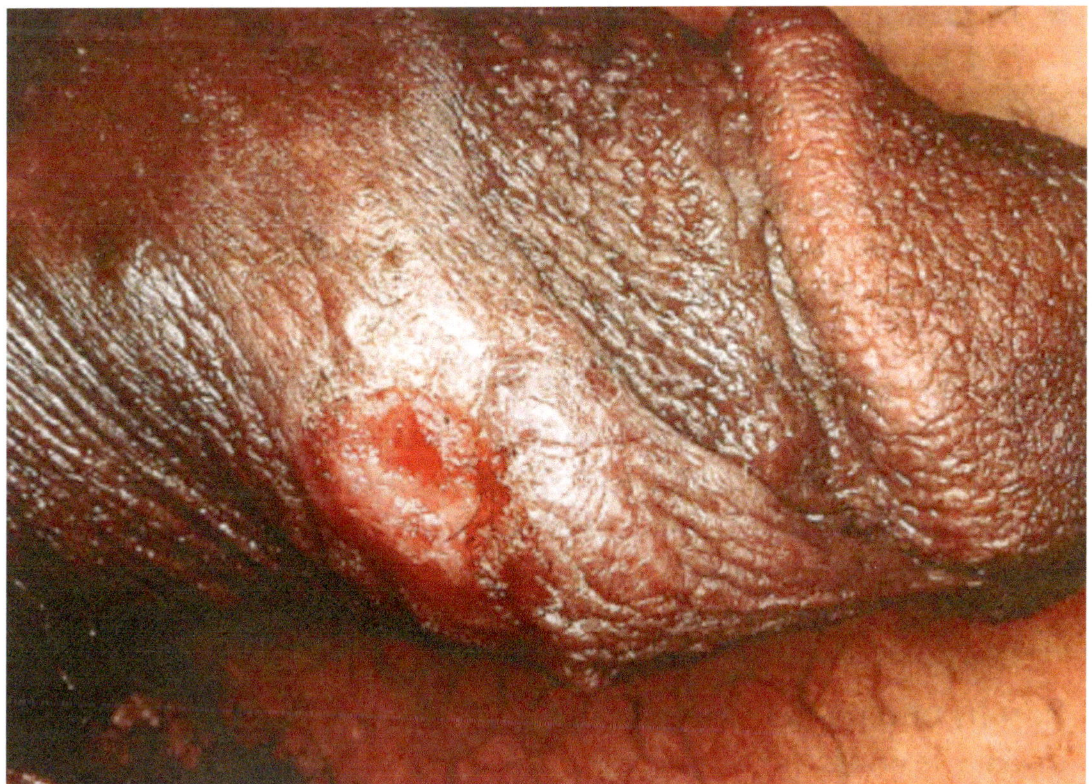

Chancre may become secondarily infected, then exudative and painful.

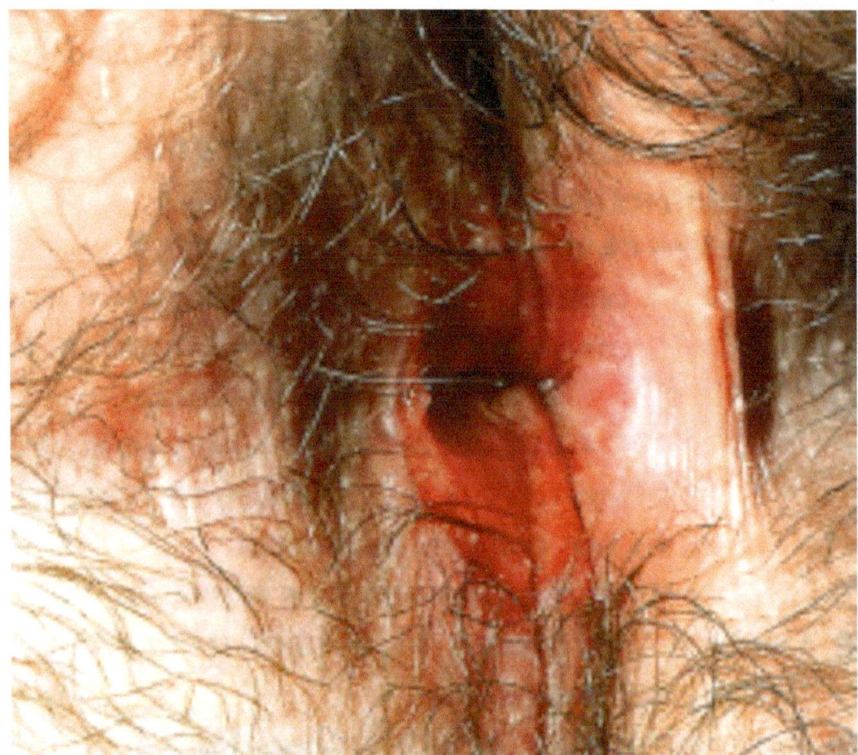

Perianal erosion due to chancre, which usually goes unnoticed by patient and physician.

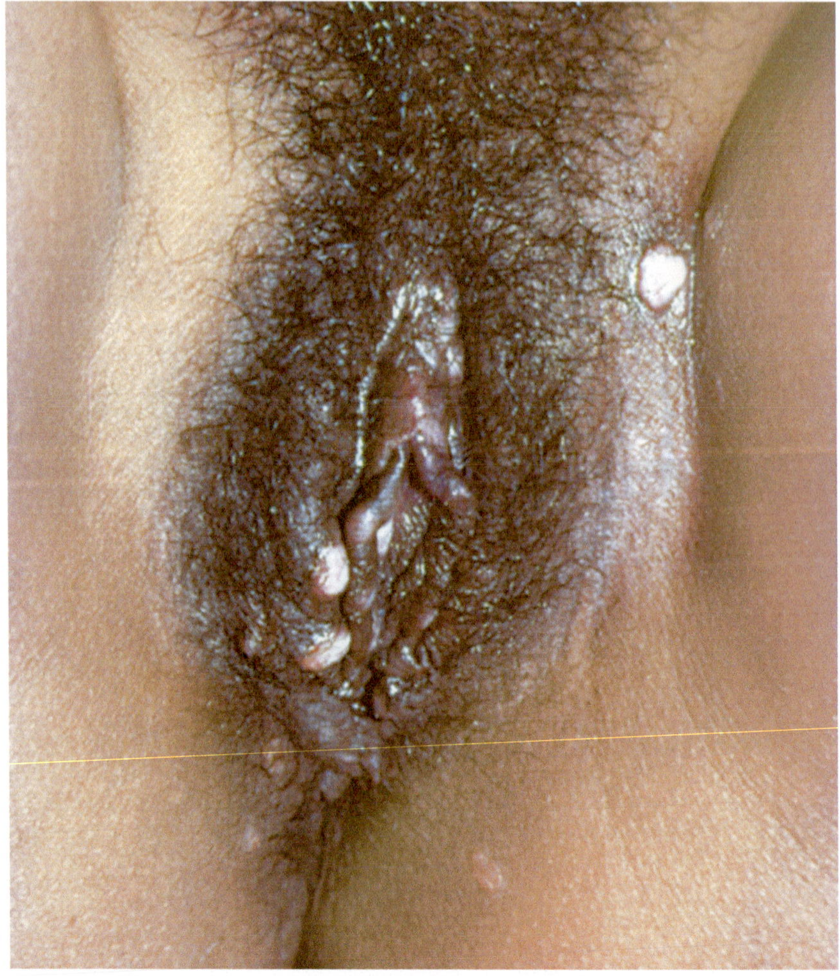

Syphilis: *Secondary syphilis. Condyloma lata. Moist plaques with smooth well-defined margins on labia.*

- Squeeze fluid from lesions with firm pressure, even using the jaws of a hemostat.
- Keep the organisms motile in a saline drop on the microscope slide; do not allow to dry out.
- Examine immediately under a well-calibrated dark-field microscope.

TREATMENT

- Be aware of updated national and local treatment recommendations. Current US Public Health Service recommendations for *primary* and *secondary* syphilis are:
  - Benzathine penicillin 2.4 million units intramuscularly once
  - If the patient is unable to take penicillin, then give doxycycline 100 mg twice daily or tetracycline 500 mg four times daily for 14 days.
  - Pregnant patients allergic to penicillin should undergo desensitization
- Local soaks or compresses (*See* page 241) may be applied for a few days if ulcer is painful, infected, or oozing copiously.
- Follow-up serologic testing:
  - FTA result remains positive indefinitely; do not retest.
  - Nonspecific STS.
    - Check titers every 6 months for 2 years.
    - STS result usually becomes negative in 6–12 months after treatment for primary syphilis and in 12–18 months after treatment for secondary syphilis.
    - STS result may fall to low titer (e.g., 1:2) and remain so indefinitely. This is a "persistent reactor," or "serofast," and does not require treatment.
    - If titers rise, assume new infection and treat again.
- Caution the patient to abstain from intimate contacts until 24 hours after treatment.
- Report to public health authorities.

Pubic Lice (Crabs)

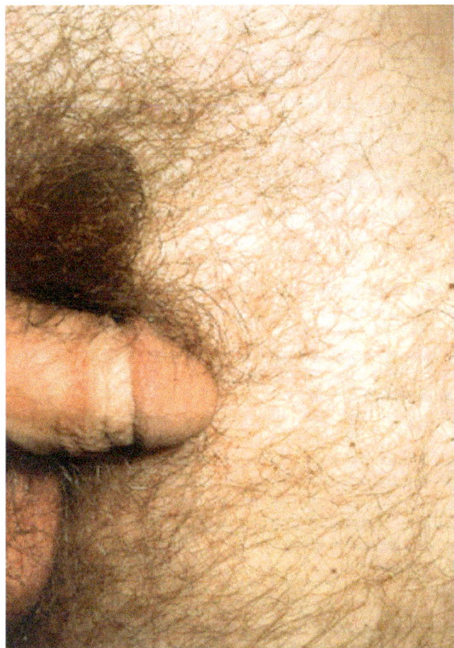

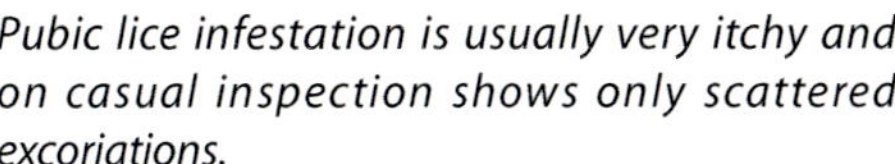

Pubic lice infestation is usually very itchy and on casual inspection shows only scattered excoriations.

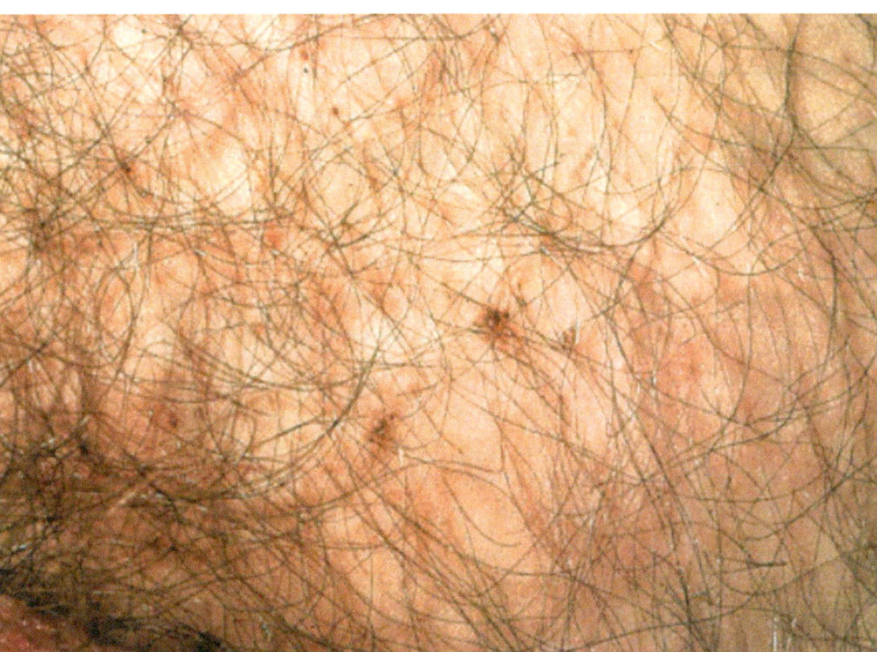

Closer inspection shows some blood-colored "scabs" to be flat, flakelike organisms.

CLINICAL

- *Pthirus pubis* is a 2 mm, flat, crab-like creature that holds onto the base of a hair shaft with one pincer, periodically bites its host, and attaches eggs (nits) to the hairs.
  - Passed by skin contact, usually during intercourse
  - Survives for 1–2 days off the host
- Physical examination:
  - Organism is gray, flakelike, slow-moving, and possibly difficult to see.
  - Gray, oval, 1-mm nits may be found on scattered hairs.
  - Mild-to-severe itching may be present.
  - Location
    - Pubis, lower abdomen, and upper thighs
    - Axillae, occasionally chest
    - Rarely, eyelashes

TREATMENT

- Patient instruction (*See* page 248) is important to destroy myths, ensure adequate treatment, and discourage overtreatment.
- Pthirocides:
  - These products kill adults and eggs, but dead nits remain attached to hairs.
  - Apply lotion, cream, or shampoo from waist to knees (or other affected areas **except eyes**); wash off in 10 minutes.

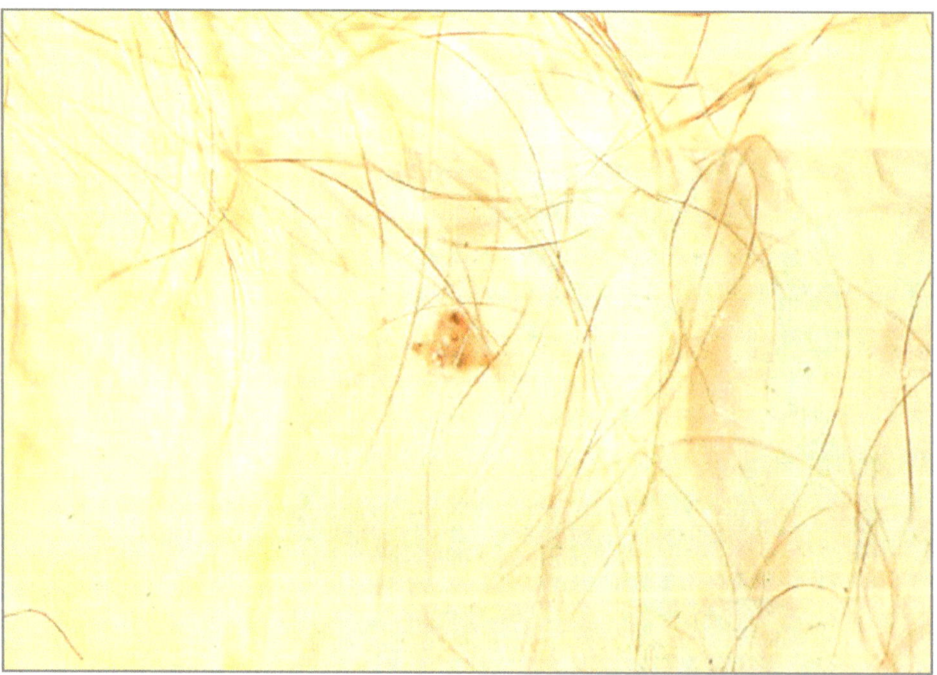

Slight magnification reveals the crablike organism, in this case headed downward.

  - Permethrin 1% cream rinse (*See* page 237) or a mousse containing pyrethrins and piperonyl butoxide are the treatment of choice: safe, effective, and available over the counter in the United States.
  - Treat bedmates simultaneously
- For lash infestation:
  - Apply ophthalmic-grade petrolatum ointment (only available by prescription) two to four times daily for 10 days, with cotton-tipped applicator.
  - Apply yellow oxide of mercury or other thick ointment or paste (to smother organisms) twice daily for 1 week.
  - Remove organisms gently, with fine-toothed tweezers.
- Environmental treatment:
  - Wash clothes, bed linen, and pajamas from previous day.
  - Don clean clothes after treatment.
  - It is not necessary to clean entire wardrobe, bed, and rooms because of short life span and relative inertia of organism.

Erythrasma

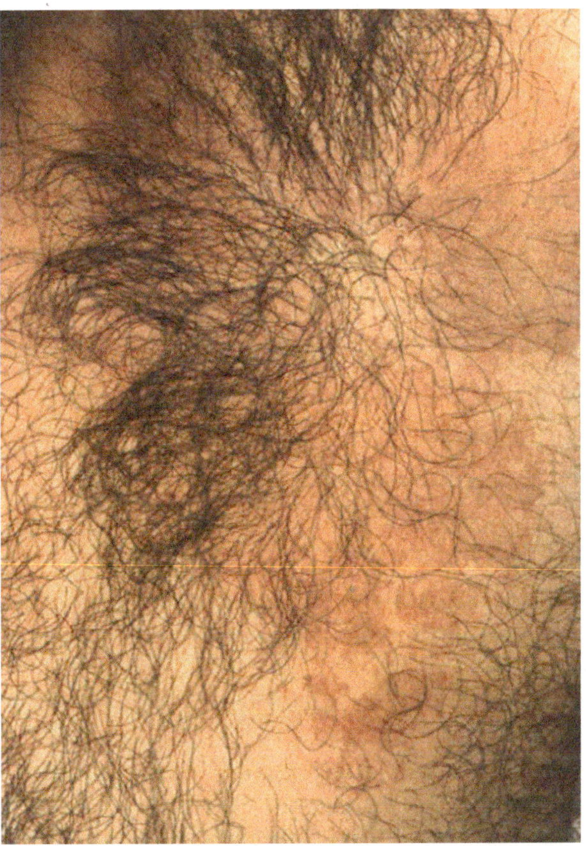

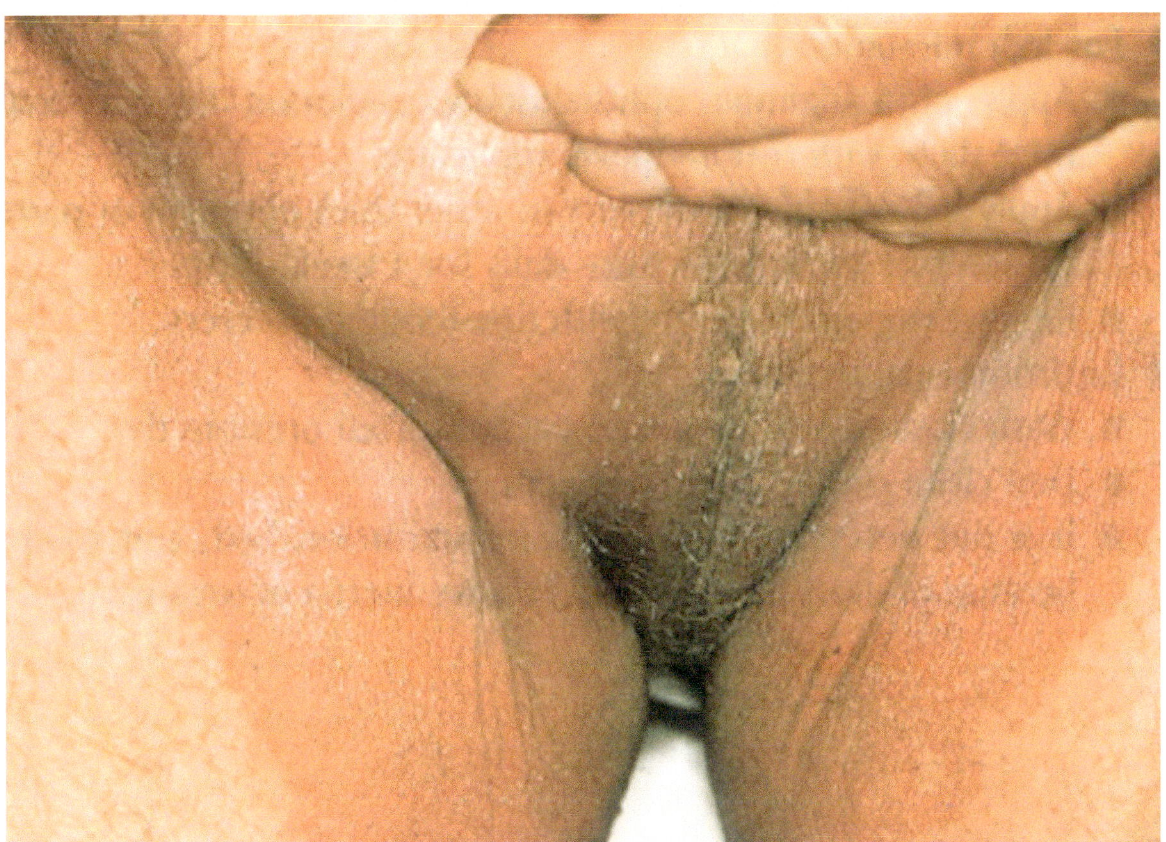

In light-skinned individuals, erythrasma is beefy red.

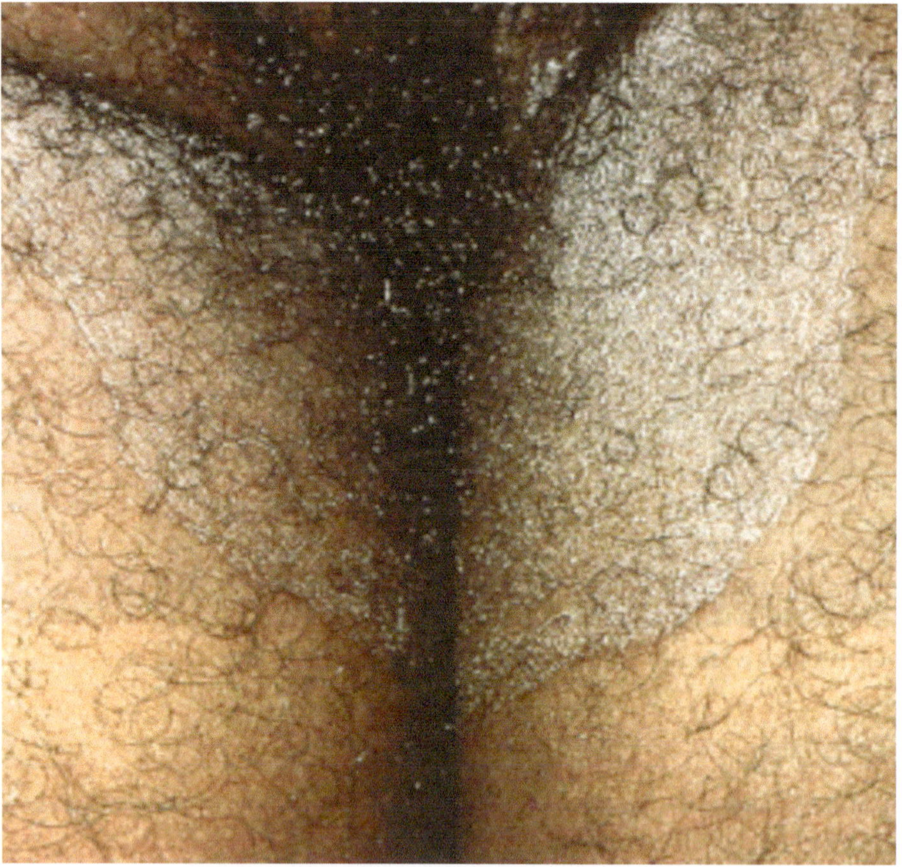

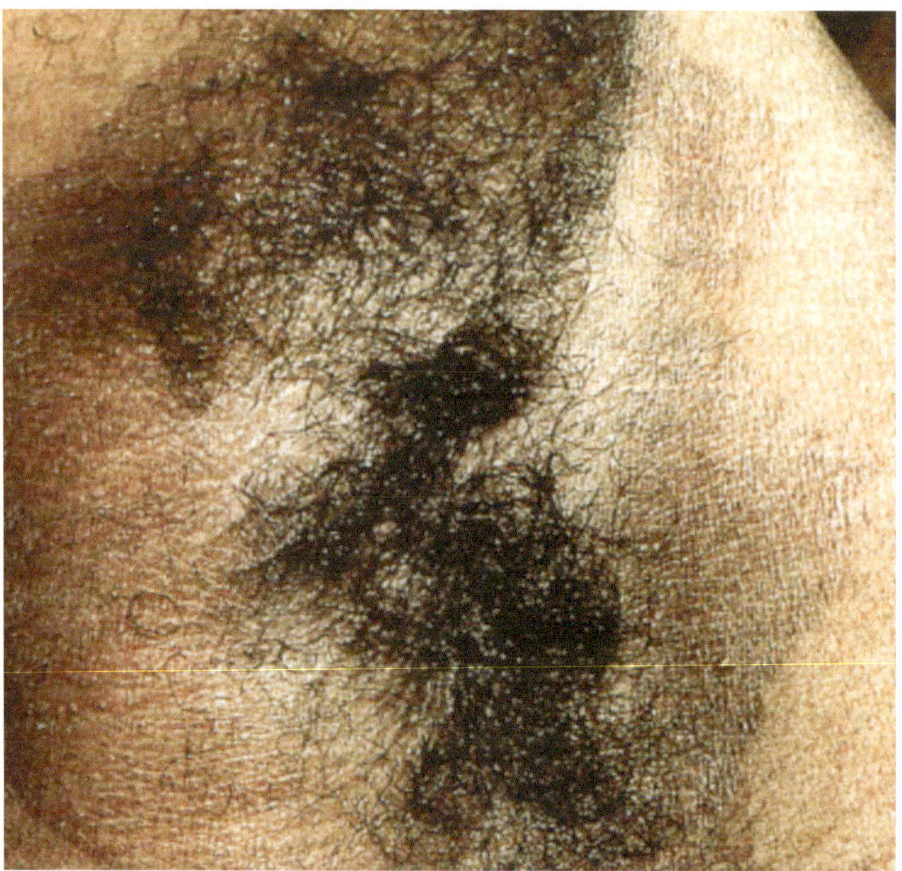

In dark-skinned individuals, the slightly scaly, circumscribed patches are pigmented.

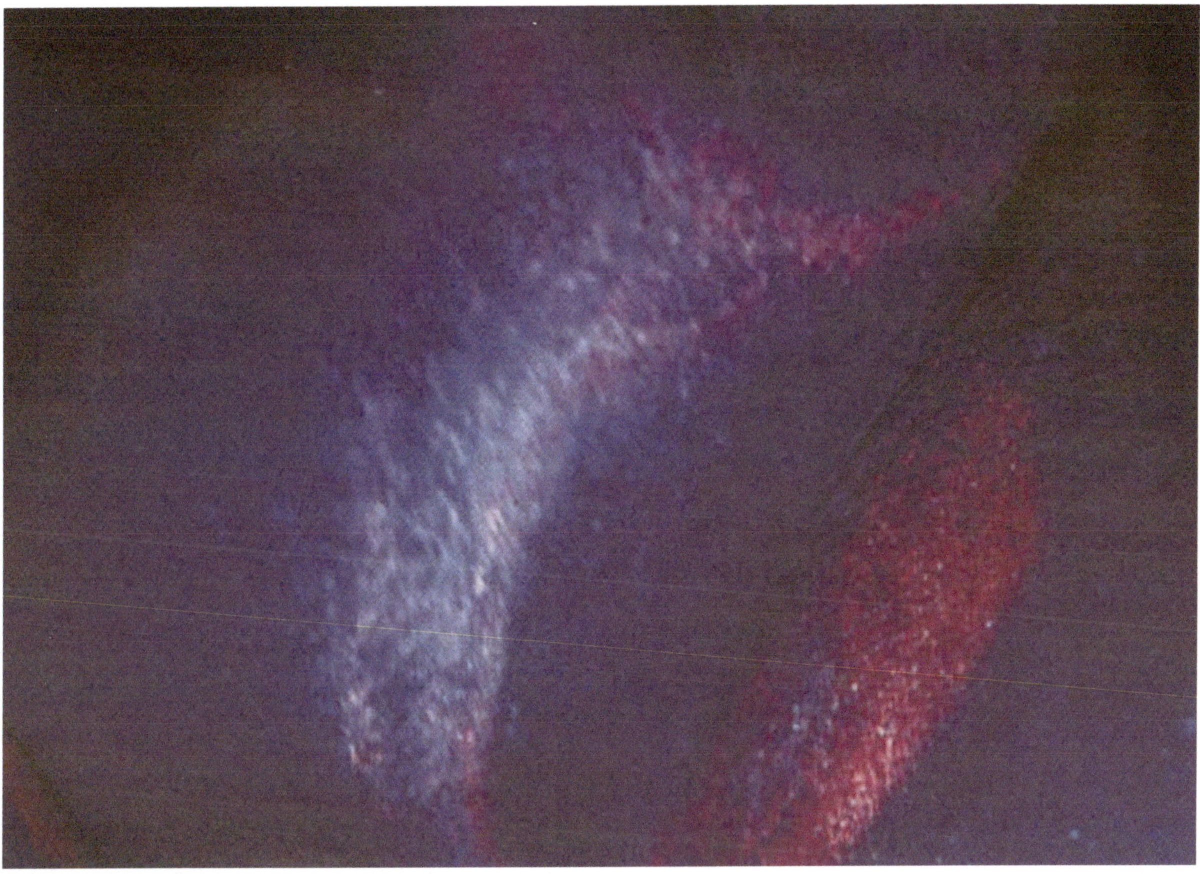

Wood's light reveals the diagnostic coral-red fluorescence.

CLINICAL

- Pinkish-tan to brownish-red confluent maculae in axillae or groin folds, radiating down thighs or chest wall:
    - Sharply marginated but irregular border
    - Mildly scaling or tight and shiny surface
    - Asymptomatic
- Wood's light examination shows coral-red fluorescence.
    - Negative for a few hours after bathing
- Potassium hydroxide (KOH) examination results negative:
    - Causative organism is *Corynebacterium minutissimum*

TREATMENT

- Topical antimicrobial drugs are effective, but few have been scientifically studied. Use twice daily for 1 week.
    - Clindamycin or erythromycin in thin solution, as used for acne (*See* page 234)
    - Miconazole or clotrimazole cream (*See* page 236)
- Systemic antibiotics are effective.
    - Erythromycin 500 mg twice daily for 2 weeks

Tinea Cruris (Jock Itch)

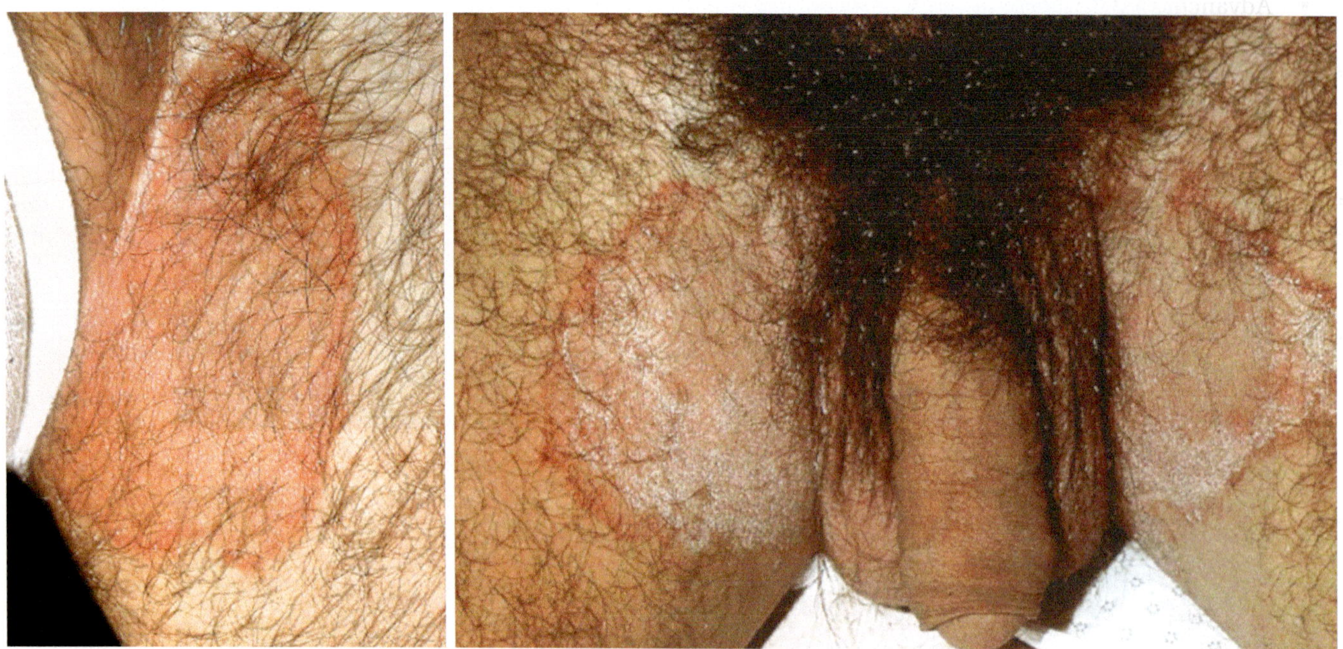

The inner thigh is the typical location for tinea cruris, or "jock itch." The border is pronounced and scaly.

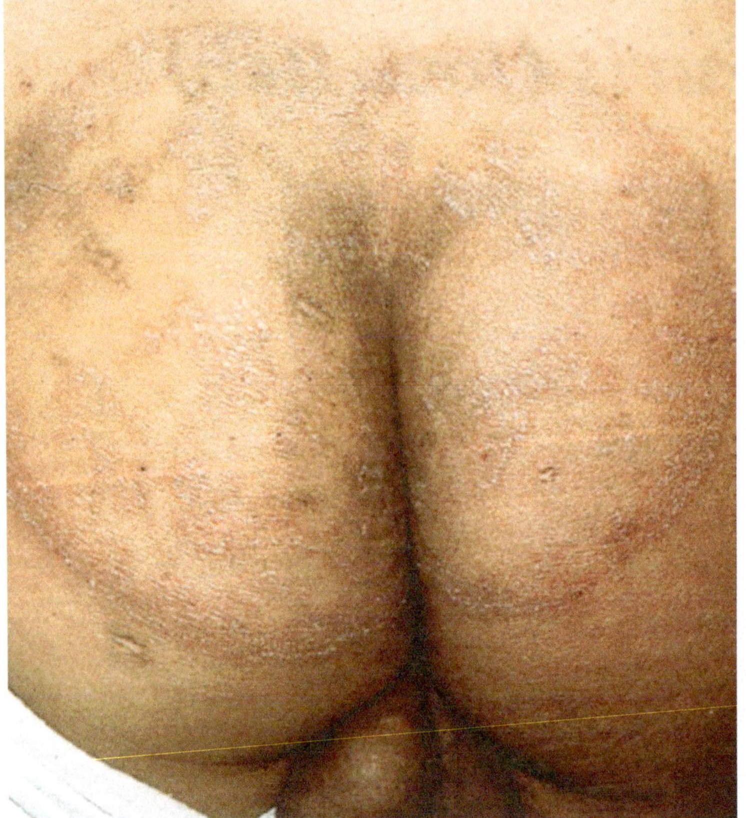

Tinea may thrive in the moist environment of the intergluteal fold.

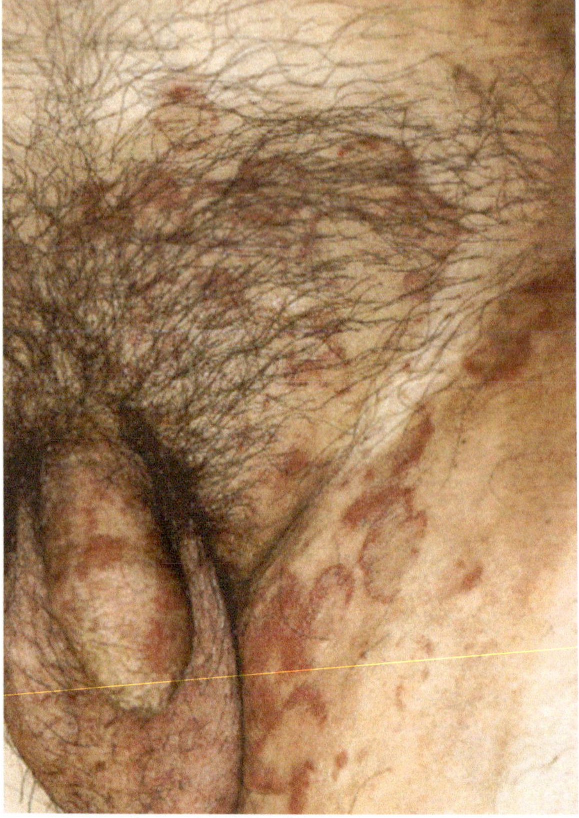

Topical corticosteroid applications activated tinea colonies in this chronic indolent infection.

CLINICAL

- Brick-red rash enlarging from inguinal folds down inner thighs and into pubic area
  - Advancing red, scaly border, clearing in center; sharply demarcated
  - Commonly, the penis and scrotum appear uninvolved but close examination and potassium hydroxide (KOH) preparation may reveal subclinical infection
  - Itching absent or mild to severe
- Often occurs in people who perspire freely or are obese
- Positive KOH examination (*See* page 226) result is usually easy to obtain.

TREATMENT

- General measures:
  - Wear loose, cool clothing
  - Reduce physical activity to reduce sweating and chafing
- Topical antifungal agents (*See* page 235) may be applied thinly to the rash and to normal skin a few centimeters beyond borders twice daily for 2–3 weeks or for several days past complete clearing.
  - Alcohol/propylene glycol solutions are usually superior to creams but may burn.
    - Penetrate to skin surface through hair
    - Drying to the skin
    - Little unpleasant residue
  - Medicated powders poor in delivery of active ingredient to the skin
- Fluconazole 150–200 mg once weekly for 2–4 weeks may be administered, if the rash is widespread
  - Resistant to topical therapy:
    - A problem in hairy areas where the fungus might grow down into follicles
- An alternative oral agent (unapproved for this indication) is itraconazole 100 mg daily for 1 week (*See* page 236)
- Topical corticosteroids:
  - Relieve itching quickly:
    - An antifungal agent alone may take many days to reduce inflammation and itching.
  - Mild preparation (hydrocortisone) adequate
    - Good penetration in thin, moist skin
    - Atrophy and striae may occur after just a few weeks' use of *potent* corticosteroid
  - Lotion or solution vehicle most pleasant to use
  - Combination of corticosteroid and antifungal agents:
    - Iodoquinol (Vytone) is moderately effective against dermatophytes.
      - Slight yellow staining of underclothes
      - May rarely cause allergic contact dermatitis

Candidiasis

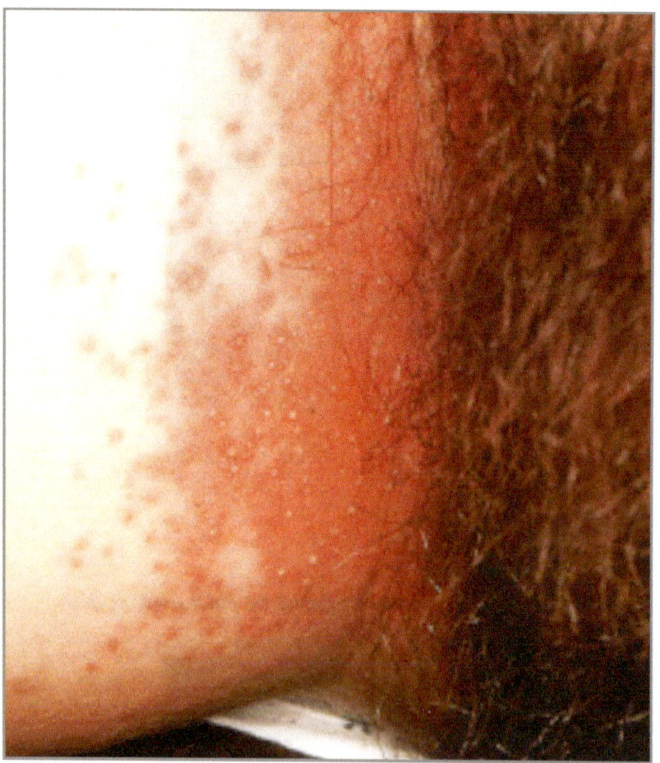

Bright erythema and satellite papules or pustules typify an acute intertriginous Candida infection.

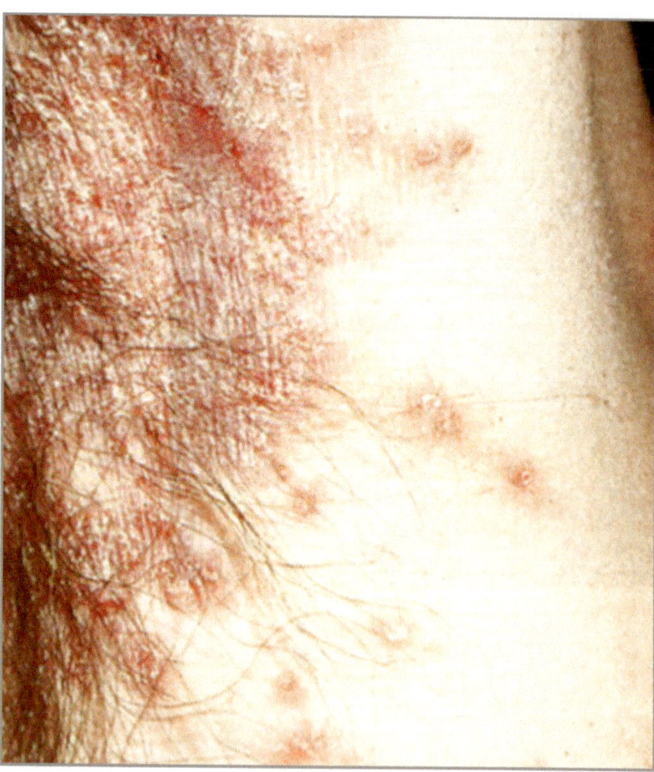

Epidermal shedding and satellite lesions are characteristic.

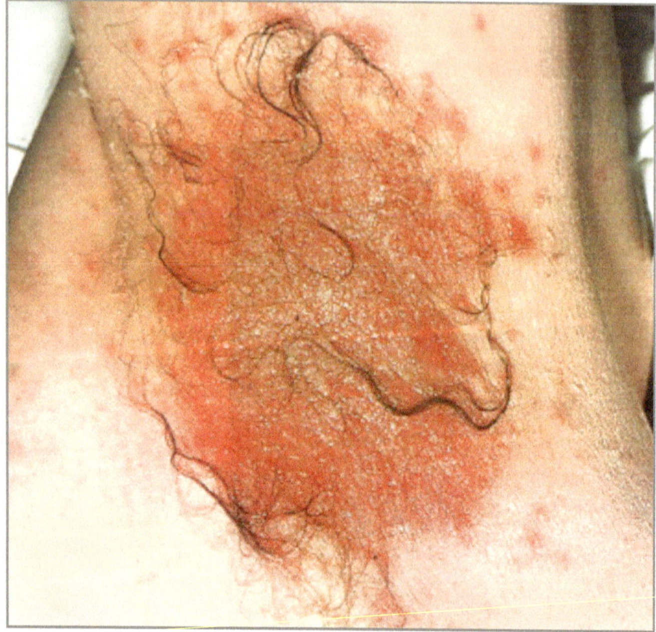

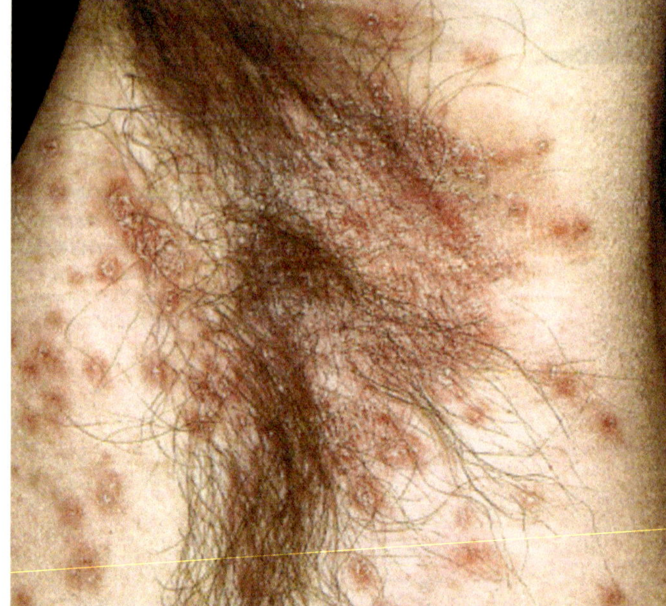

Inflammation may range from bright red and eroded to dull and scaly.

CLINICAL

- Bright pink eruption
  - Distribution:
    - Groin
    - Genitals (including penis and scrotum)

        - Intergluteal fold, buttocks
        - Axillary area
        - Submammary area
    - Surface:
        - Mace rated, desquamating (like wet tissue paper), and eroded
        - Fine, white pustules stippling central area and in satellite lesions
    - Spreading rash with irregular borders and satellite lesions
    - Severe burning and itching
- More common in:
    - Persons who perspire copiously or are incontinent
    - Obese individuals
    - Those with diabetes

TREATMENT

- General measures:
    - Wearing loose, cool clothing
    - Reduction of physical activity
    - Applying zinc oxide to reduce wetness and chafing

Do not powder with cornstarch, as it may enhance the growth of yeast.

- Drying agents
    - Effect:
        - Dry up pustules and macerated epidermis
        - Prepare skin for topical antifungal agents
        - May cure the infection by creating a dry environment hostile to the organism
    - Baths, soaks, or compresses with careful drying afterward—mainstay of therapy:
        - Tap water
        - Saline
        - Astringent (*See* page 241)

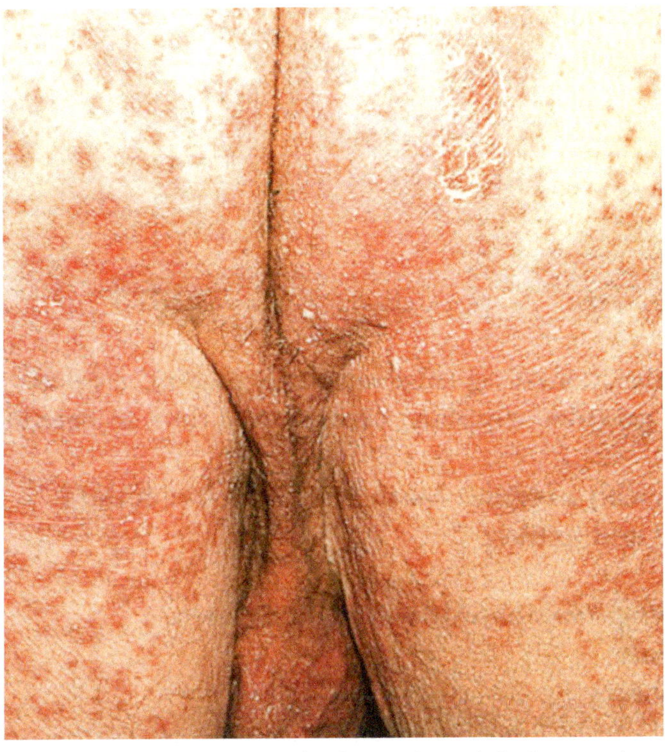

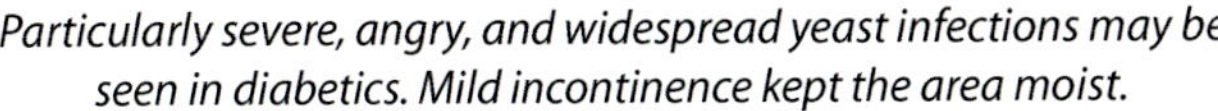

Particularly severe, angry, and widespread yeast infections may be seen in diabetics. Mild incontinence kept the area moist.

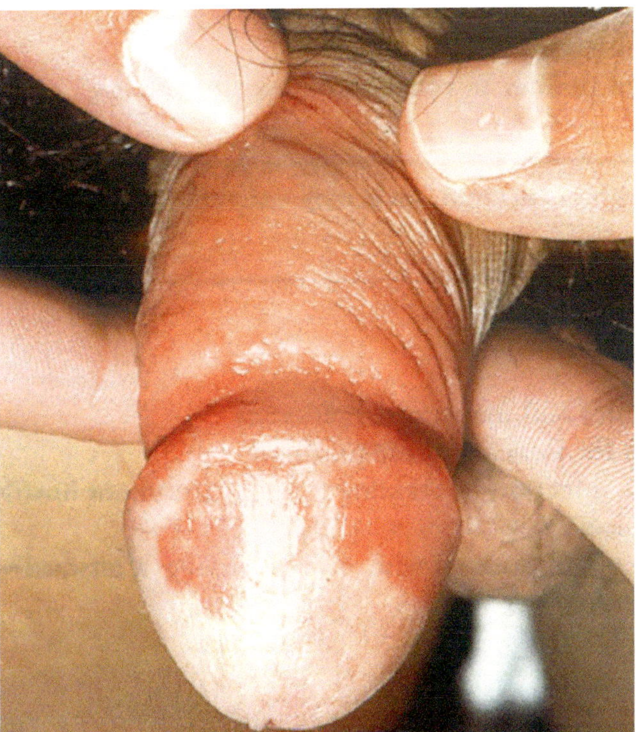

Typical bright red patch of Candida balanitis.

- Topical antiyeast medications (*See* page 236):
  - Use after lesions have been dried by baths or soaks.
  - Apply thinly twice daily for 1–3 weeks.
  - Alcohol/propylene glycol solutions are superior but may sting. They are drying agents in these moist areas and leave little residue.
  - Medicated powders are poor vehicles for the delivery of active ingredients to the skin.
- Topical corticosteroids, used *with* topical antiyeast medications:
  - This therapy relieves itching quickly.
    - Antiyeast medications used alone may take days to reduce inflammation and itching.
  - A mild preparation (hydrocortisone) is usually adequate.
    - There is good penetration in thin, moist skin.
    - Atrophy and striae may occur after just a few weeks' use of *potent* corticosteroid.
  - Lotion or solution vehicle is most pleasant to use.
  - Corticosteroid/antiyeast combination
    - Iodoquinol (Vyotone) is usually effective, but slight yellow stain noticeable on white underclothes
- For widespread or recurrent infections, use oral antiyeast medication (*See* page 236) for 1–2 weeks, until clear:
  - Fluconazole 150 mg single dose or 150 mg once weekly for 4 weeks

Griseofulvin is not effective against yeast.

Diaper Dermatitis (Diaper Rash, Nappy Rash)

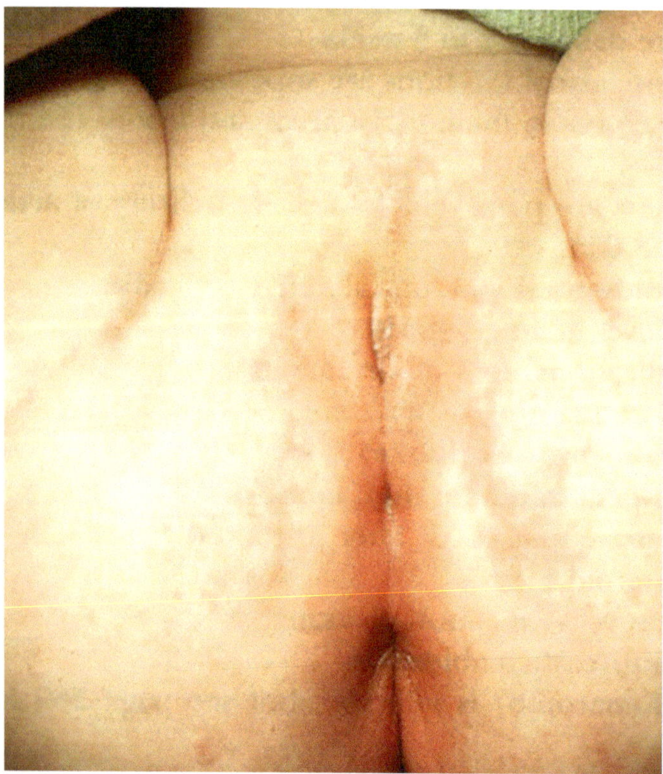

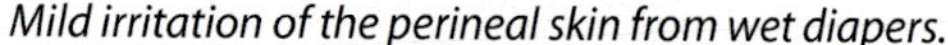

Mild irritation of the perineal skin from wet diapers.

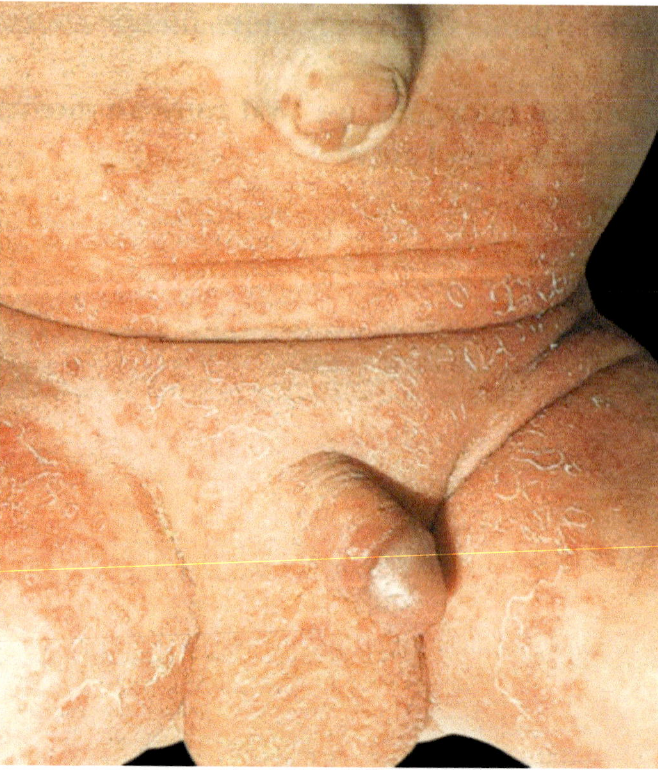

Extensive pustular and erosive yeast diaper dermatitis. Infant also had oral thrush.

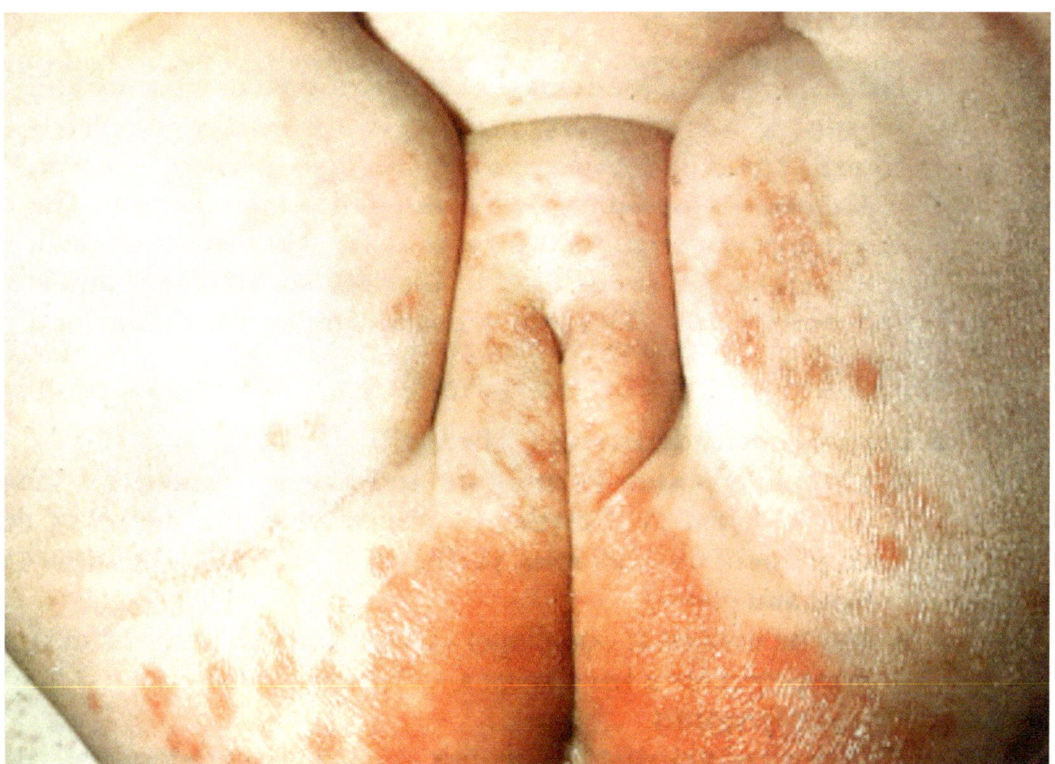

Typical yeast diaper eruption in older infant.

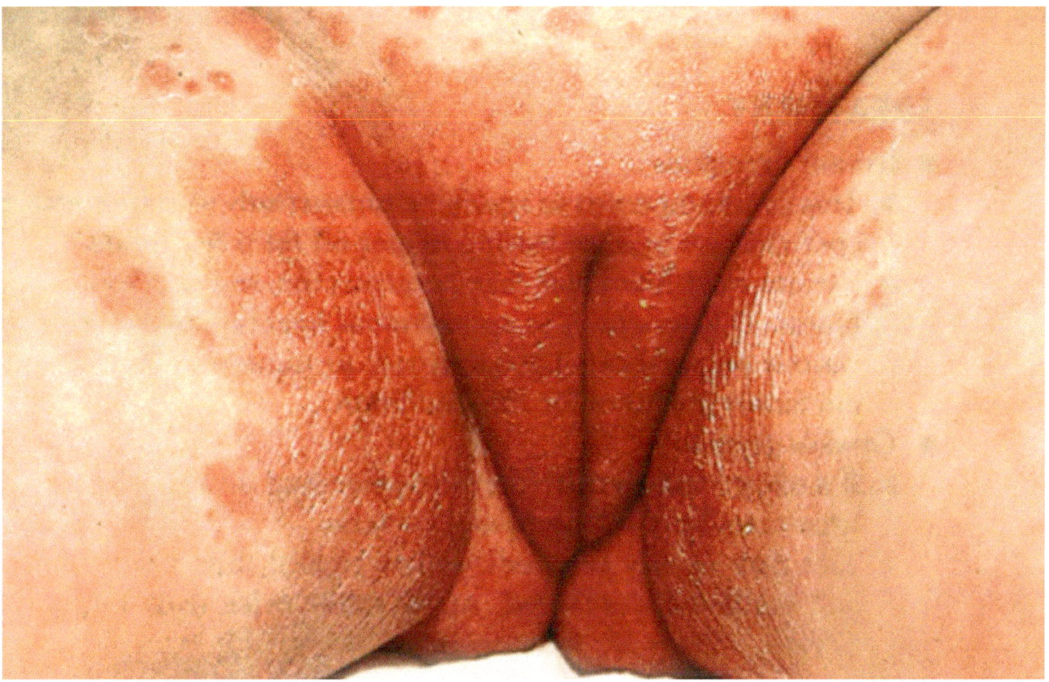

Severe, angry yeast infection and irritation. Note satellite lesions, typifying Candida involvement.

CLINICAL

The diaper area of infants is constantly exposed to moisture and irritants, so it is surprising that the skin is usually completely normal. The skin does occasionally become irritated, however, and sometimes it becomes overgrown with microorganisms. The diaper area is sometimes the site of other skin conditions, such as seborrheic dermatitis (*See* page 15), psoriasis (*See* page 117), and atopic dermatitis (*See* page 103). This section includes only the common local eruptions.

- Irritant contact dermatitis ("chafing"):
  - Chronic exposure to moisture and irritants produces a faint, poorly demarcated erythema, primarily on the domes of the skinfolds of the abdomen, perineum, and thighs. The surface is tight and glazed.
  - May be noticed at one diaper change and absent at the next or may persist for a few days at a low level of activity.
- *Candida* dermatitis:
  - In contrast to irritant dermatitis, this rash is a brighter red, consists of sharply demarcated patches with satellite lesions, and usually involves and radiates from the skinfolds. The surface is tense and shiny and may be desquamating or even pustular.
  - *Candida* dermatitis is persistent and uncomfortable.
  - This condition involves colonization by yeast from the bowel, as well as by bacteria.

TREATMENT

- Irritant dermatitis:
  - This condition tends to resolve spontaneously with frequent diaper changes or after leaving diaper off for a few hours.
  - Various mild lubricants may be protective and accelerate resolution. This tendency to spontaneous healing and response to various preparations has given rise to numerous "successful" old family remedies for this condition.
- *Candida* dermatitis:
  - If a diaper rash persists after the preceding measures, it may be supercolonized with yeast and bacteria.
  - This rash usually responds well to topical mild corticosteroid and antibiotic, combined. Apply thinly twice daily for 1–2 weeks.
    - Hydrocortisone 1% cream or lotion, followed by topical antiyeast agent (*See* page 235)
    - Hydrocortisone 1% and iodoquinol 1% cream or lotion (may leave slight yellow stain on diaper)
  - If rash persists, relapses repeatedly, or spreads, refer to a dermatologist for evaluation.

About diapers: Disposable diapers may be slightly less irritating than cloth diapers, and somewhat fewer organisms may colonize under them.

Lichen Simplex Chronicus

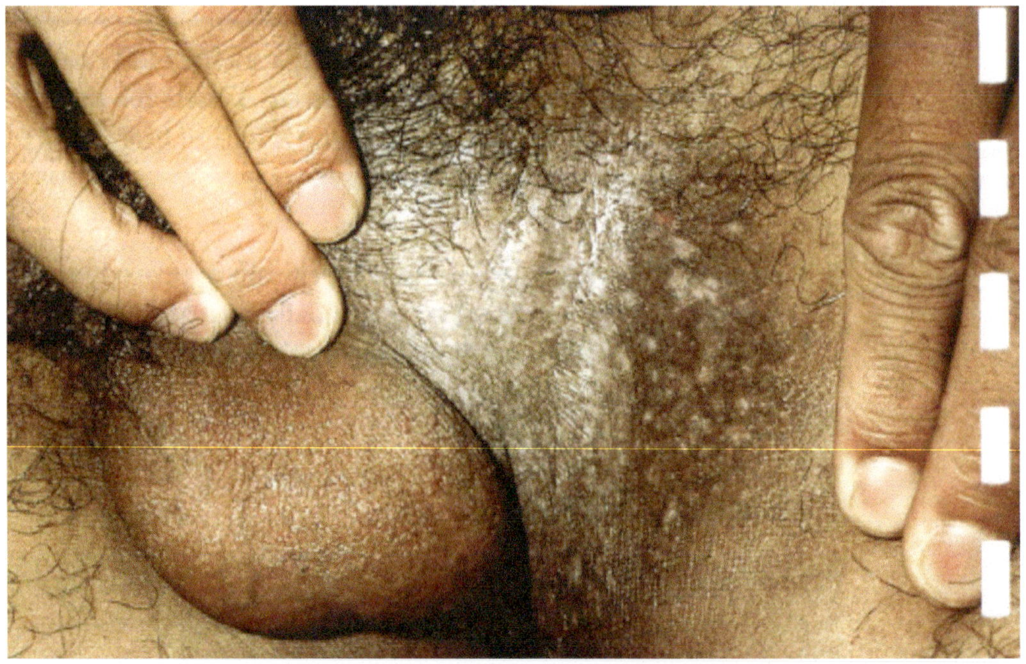

6 months of rubbing has produced this leathery, thickened skin.

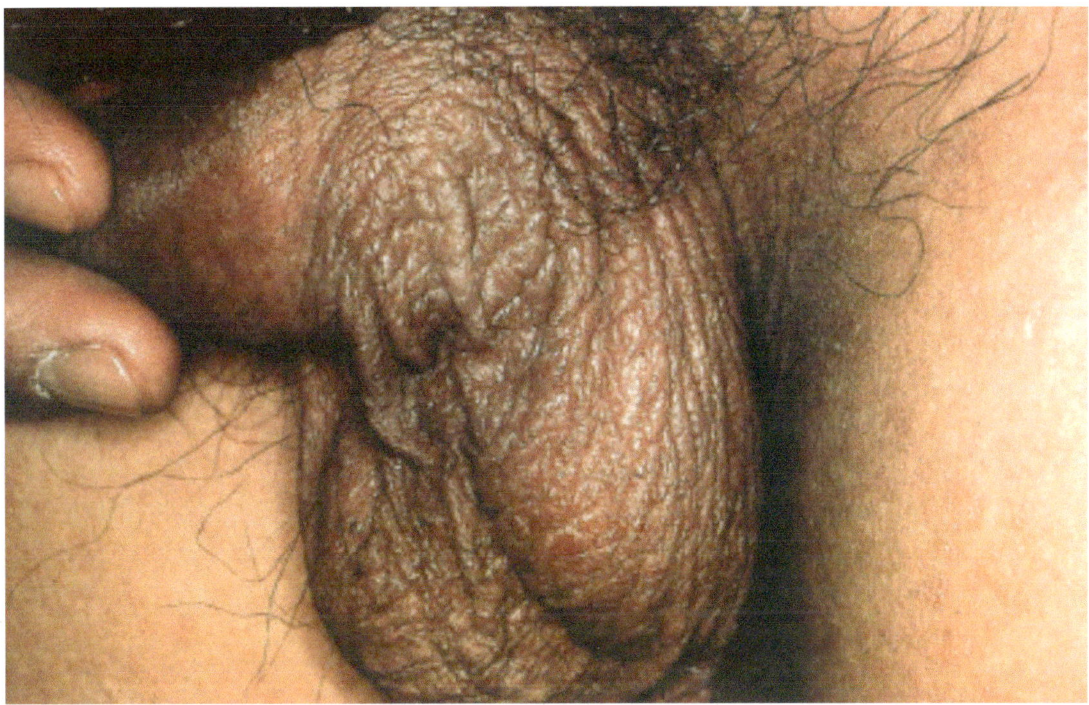

Classic lichenification is present in this patient; often unilateral.

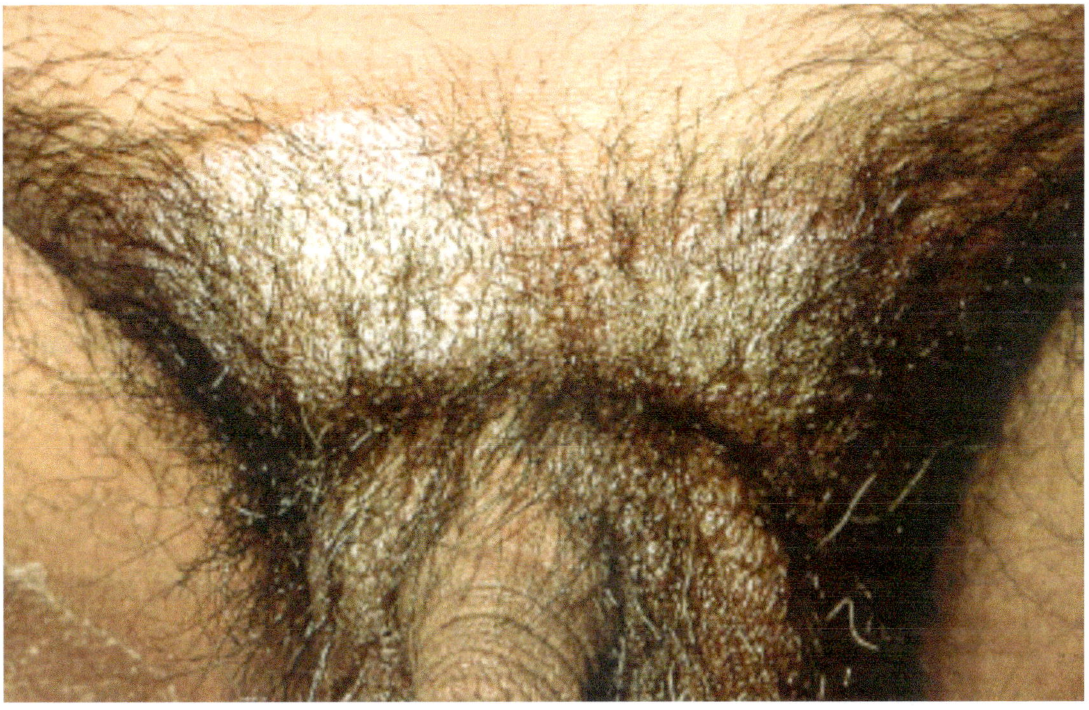

More than 3 years of rubbing, scratching, and pinching produced these lesions.

CLINICAL

- A diagnosis of exclusion: Persistent, unexplained itching and rash in absence of contactant, intertrigo, fungus, or other cause
- Lichenified plaque:
    - Elephantiasis: Thickening of entire genital skin in severe cases
- The condition may worsen in times of stress.
    - If so severe as to make skin very thick, scaly, and cracked, may represent severe psychopathology

- The condition may result from unfounded concern about genital or perianal hygiene. Some neurodermatitis is at least partially a "dishpan groin" from overzealous washing or use of antiseptics or cleansers.

TREATMENT

- General:
  - Explain role of rubbing to patients so that they may bring it to a conscious level and control it.
  - Routine hygiene during normal bathing is appropriate.
    - Keep area clean to avoid maceration and intertrigo.
    - Discourage excessive cleaning.
- Topical corticosteroids:
  - Mild- to moderate-potency creams twice daily
  - Potent creams twice daily, if the rash remains resistant, but only for a few days or weeks
    - Thin genital skin is particularly subject to atrophy from potent corticosteroids.
    - Switch to mild-potency (hydrocortisone 1%) when itching is improving or lichenification is reduced.
    - Cordran (flurandrenolide) tape protects the skin as well as delivers the corticosteroid

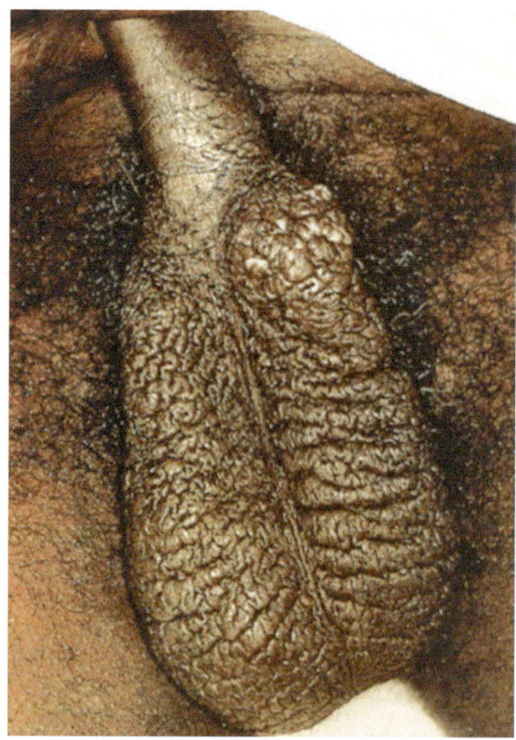

Marked lichenification is seen in this patient who constantly rubbed his genitals. A fibrotic nodule results from repeated pinching.

4 CHAPTER

Extremities

Hand Dermatitis

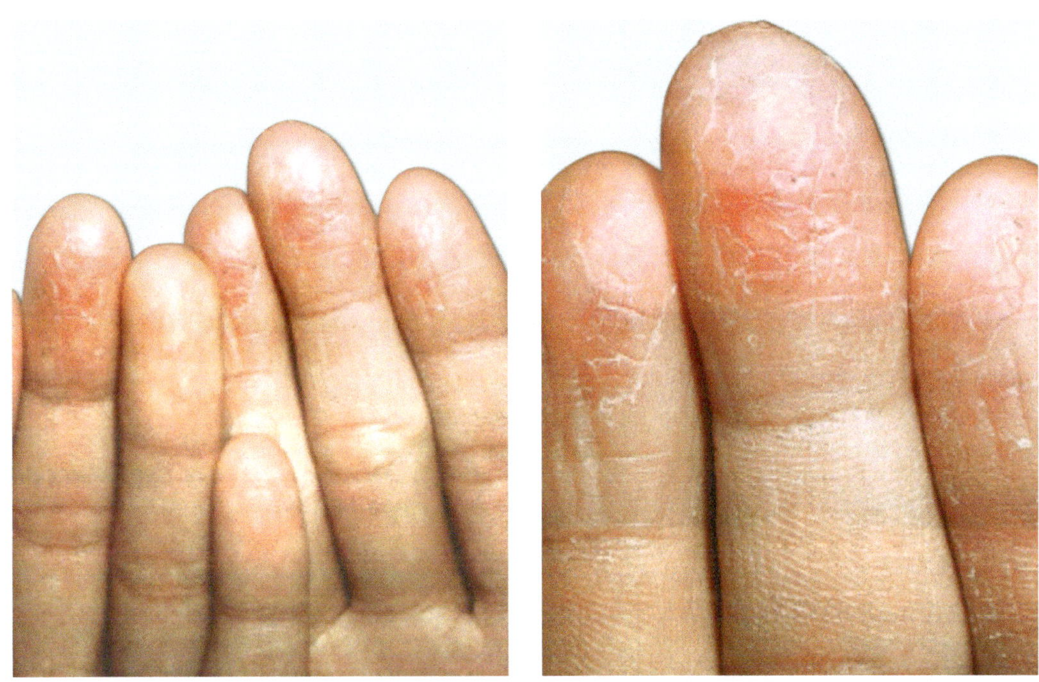

Typical "dishpan hands." Low-grade irritant dermatitis from water and cleansers. Skin is dry, tight, glazed, and cracked.

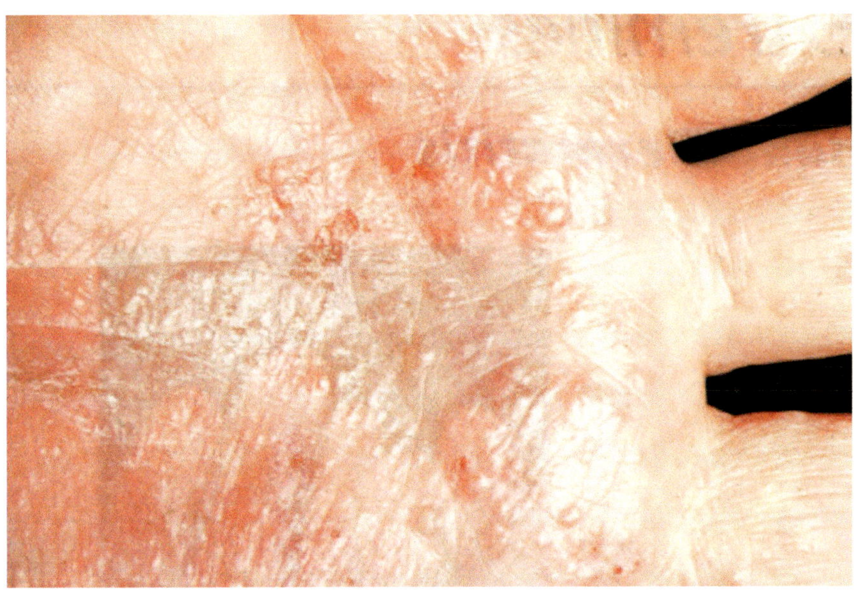

Severe dyshidrotic eczema of the fingers and palms leads to considerable fissuring and peeling.

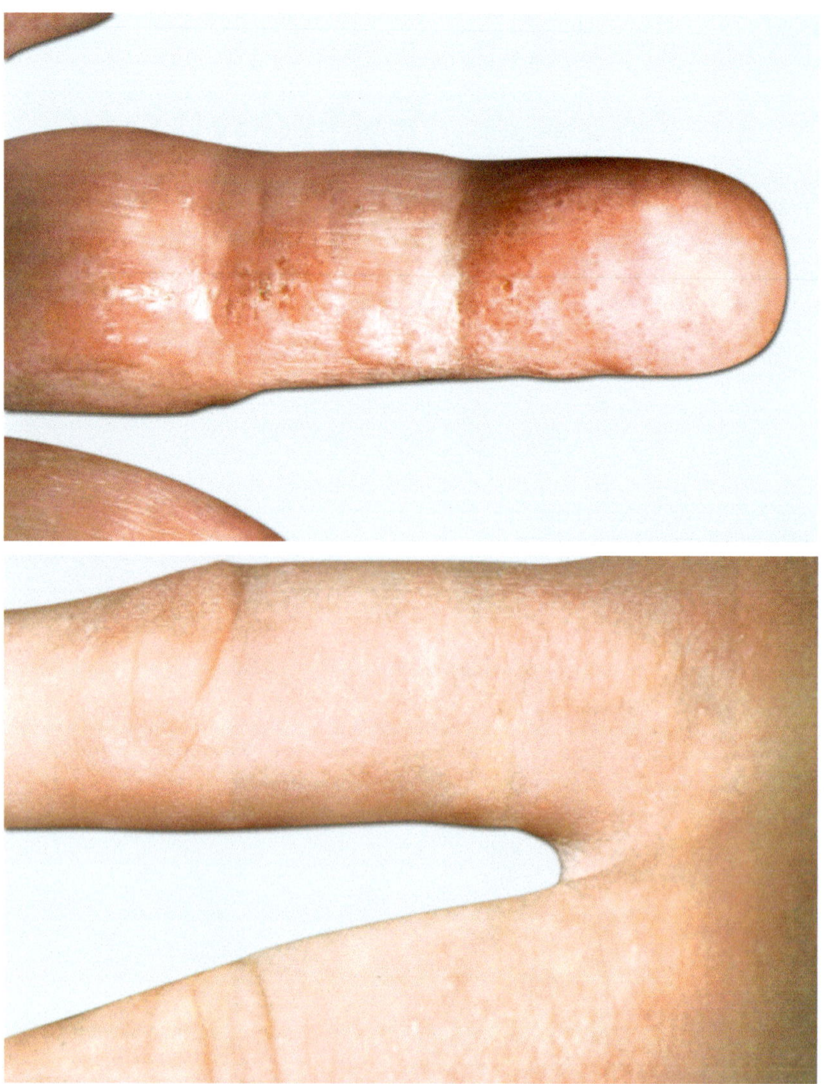

Mild dyshidrotic eczema (pompholyx) appears predominantly on the sides of the fingers.

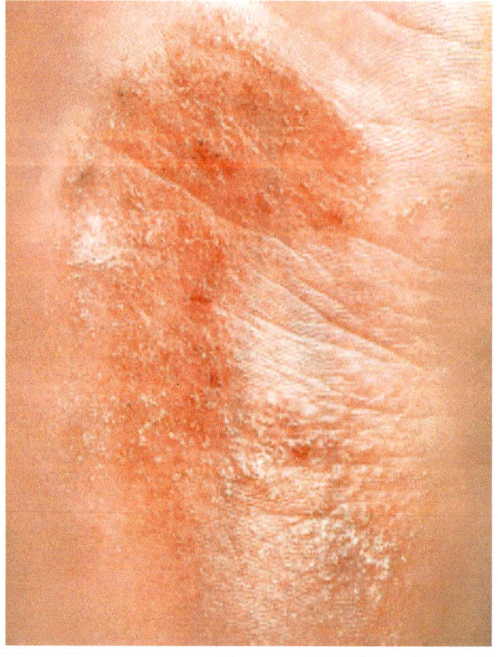

A patch of vesicles suddenly erupting on the sole in an 8-year-old with pompholyx.

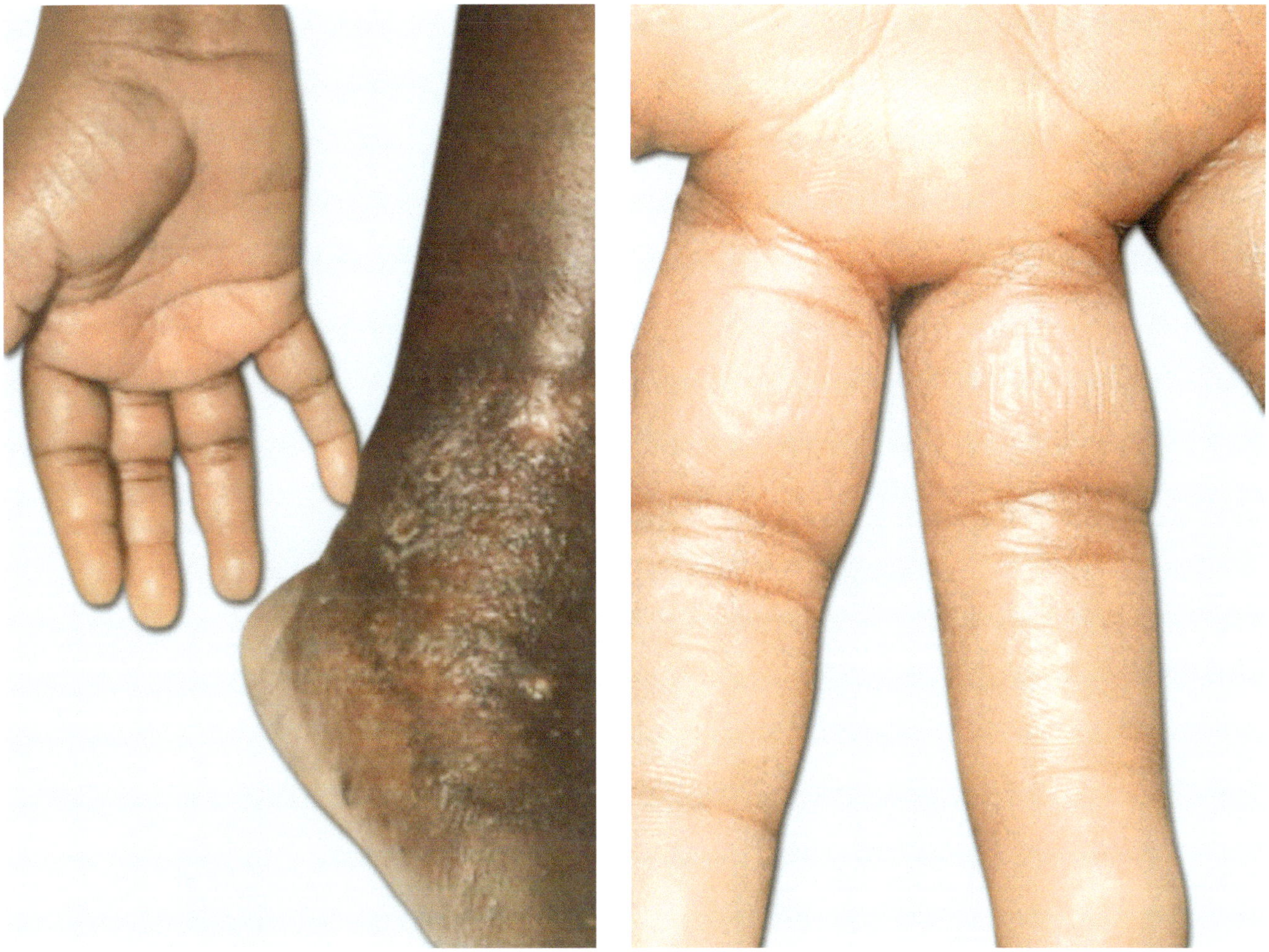

Stasis dermatitis of the ankle was followed shortly by a vesicular pompholyx-like id eruption on the palms.

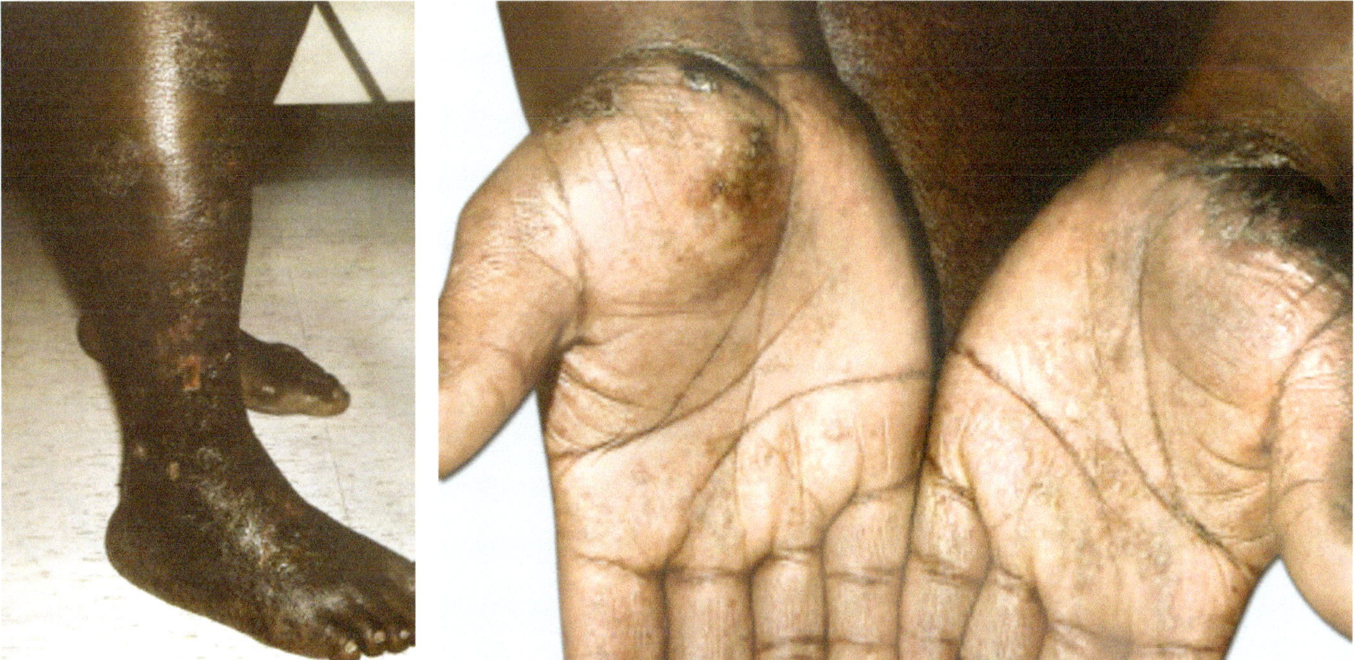

A fractured ankle led to a stasis dermatitis, then palmar id eruption.

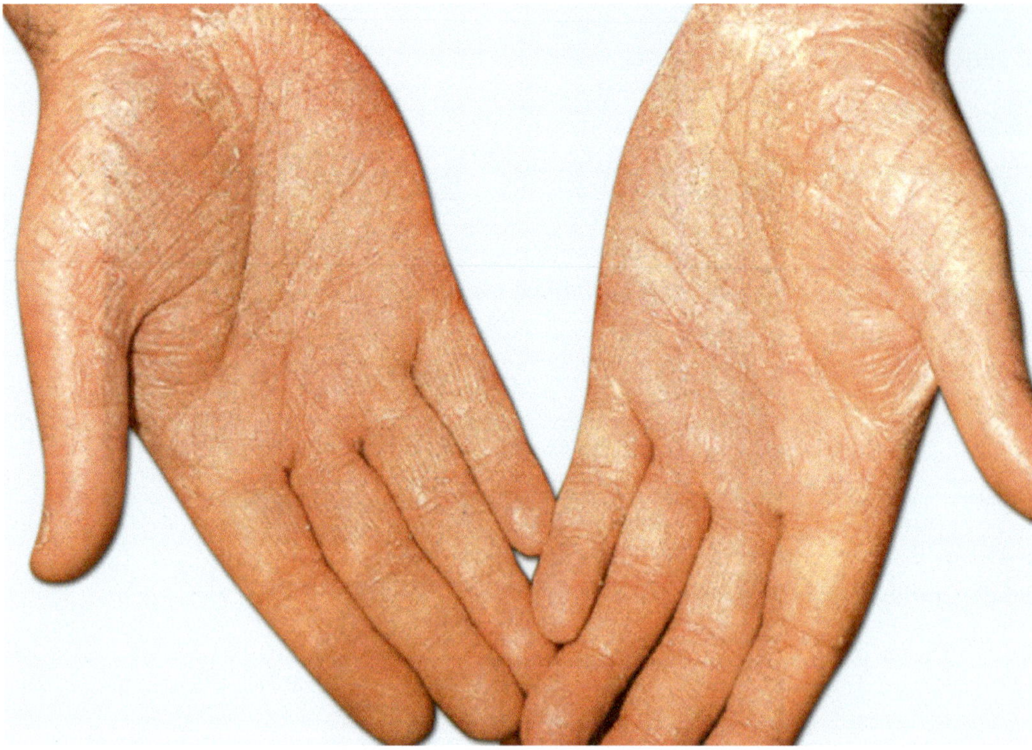

Chronic scaly psoriasis of the palms.

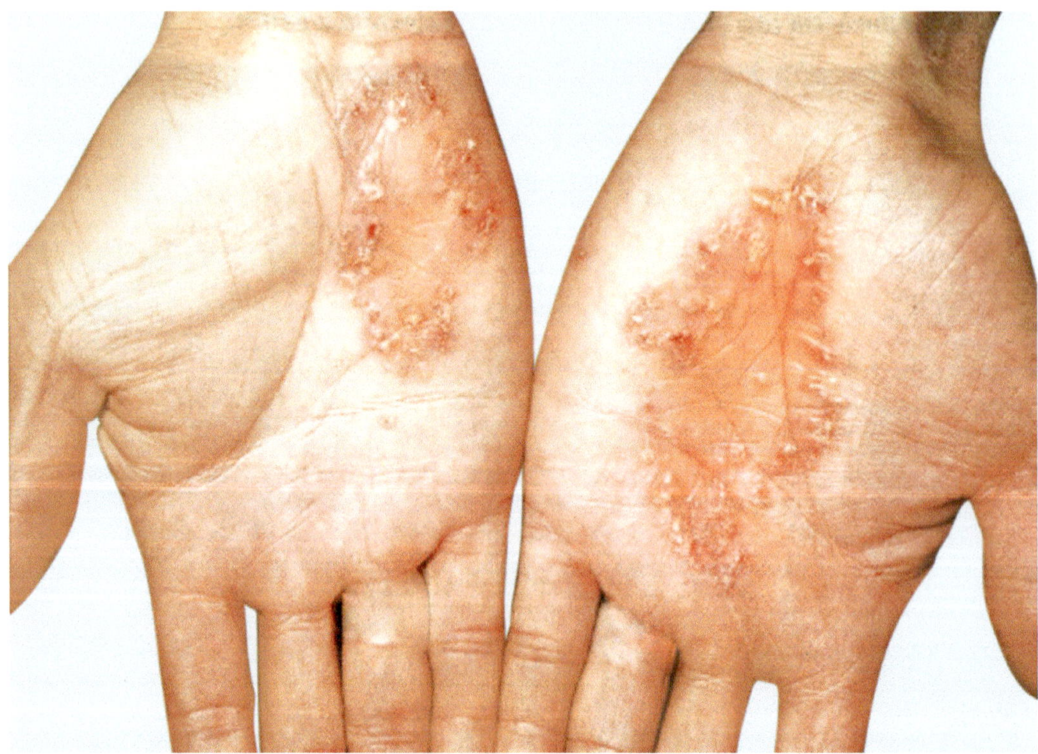

Acute pustular psoriasis of the palms. Typical psoriasis was present elsewhere. In contrast to dyshidrotic eczema, the patches are well-circumscribed and the vesicopustules are larger.

Because of the similarities in their appearance and management, these hand eruptions are discussed together:

- Irritant dermatitis
- Pompholyx (dyshidrotic eczema)
- Id eruptions
- Psoriasis

CLINICAL

- Irritant dermatitis
  - Typically, dry, glazed, cracked skin is seen on the pads, palms, webs, and dorsa of fingers.
  - Condition is induced by exposure to water, detergents, and chemicals, which alter the keratin layer, causing cracking, peeling, and inflammation.
    - Seen in "wet workers": Restaurant workers, healthcare workers, bartenders, beauticians, and the like
- Pompholyx (dyshidrotic eczema)
  - Typically, tiny vesicles erupt along the sides of the fingers and on pads and, less commonly, on palms and soles (except in children), followed by a healing, peeling phase that resembles irritant contact dermatitis.
  - This condition is idiopathic and recurrent.
    - Onset in young adults most common but may continue for decades
    - Often occurs during stress
    - Often involves history of childhood atopic dermatitis and may be a form of atopic dermatitis of the adult
- Id (autosensitization) dermatitis
  - Sudden eruption of tiny vesicles on palms, indistinguishable from pompholyx
  - A sympathetic, possibly autoimmune, reaction to a sudden inflammatory eruption of the ankle or foot:
    - Stasis dermatitis, most commonly
    - Sudden inflammatory flare of tinea pedis (*See* page 82)
- Psoriasis:
  - Psoriasis may present as a chronic hand and/or foot rash, in one of two forms:
    1. Well-circumscribed area of redness, scaling, and/or deep desquamation on palm
    2. Chronic or recurrent 1- to 3-mm vesicopustules with desquamation
- Look for typical nail changes (*See* page 120) and rash elsewhere.

When examining a patient with a hand dermatitis, always take a complete history for water exposure and past or present dermatologic disease, and perform a complete examination for evidence of atopic dermatitis, psoriasis, and rashes of the ankles and feet.

TREATMENT

- General measures:
  - Stop all lotions, moisturizers, and so on, as they often contain irritants.
  - Decrease exposure to water, cleansers, and irritants.

Protective gloves induce sweating (which macerates the skin); accumulate moisture, soap, and dirt; and may themselves be allergic sensitizers (if rubber). They should be used when handling strong irritants (e.g., oven cleaner, silver polish). Vinyl gloves are the least-irritating protection if worn over a thin cotton glove that can be changed periodically as it becomes soaked with sweat, but this is so awkward and inconvenient as to be impractical for many uses.

  - Treat inflammatory disease of the ankles, feet, and legs to control the id eruption.
- Acute vesicular eruption (pompholyx, id, pustular psoriasis)
  - Tap water or mild astringent soaks (*See* page 241) three times daily for 10–15 minutes, followed by a potent topical corticosteroid, should be administered.
  - Individual tense vesicles and bullae should be punctured, if they cause significant discomfort. A hypodermic needle or pointed scalpel blade is ideal, and patients can do it, carefully, themselves. Follow with soaking and application of topical corticosteroid.
  - Antihistamine should be given as a sedative (*See* page 243), especially at bedtime or if pompholyx attack is related to stress.
- Chronic inflammation, cracking, and desquamation
  - Topical corticosteroids are the mainstay of therapy.
    - Potent forms (*See* page 237) are needed initially and often chronically. Use less potent ones when possible.
    - Ointment form is often indicated to lubricate dry, cracked skin.
    - Apply two or three times daily, but plain lubricant may also be used several times a day.
    - Vinyl gloves (*See* page 238) can be worn over corticosteroid for a few hours a day, or overnight, in stubborn cases. Monitor closely for signs of skin atrophy, then reduce potency of corticosteroid or discontinue vinyl glove occlusion.

Tip: If only the palm is involved, cut off glove fingers for comfort.

  - Moisturization:
    - Emphasize that the patient should cease using cosmetic moisturizers, as they may contain irritants or allergens.

- If topical corticosteroids are not required (because of absence of inflammation and itching), emphasize frequent use of a thick, bland moisturizer. Lotions are too thin (mostly water) and may be drying. Use heavy creams or ointments
- Vinyl gloves worn over the emollient enhance lubrication.
  - After vinyl glove occlusion, rinse hands and immediately reapply lubricant to prevent drying.

For chronic cases, patients may need to make permanent changes in their habits and may need constantly or periodically to use lubricants or corticosteroids. Use the Patient Guides (*See* page 254) and repeatedly urge compliance.

Tinea Pedis

Tinea pedis can occur in anyone but may be more frequent or more severe in people with moist feet (excessive sweating, occlusive shoes), especially after friction and trauma (athletes). The three clinical forms are chronic plantar scaling, acute vesicular tinea pedis, and interdigital tinea pedis.

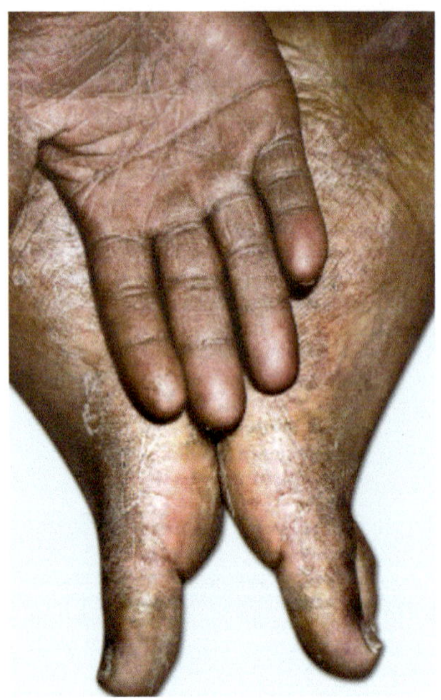

Typical "two-foot-one-hand" pattern in chronic tinea manuum. The other palm was unaffected.

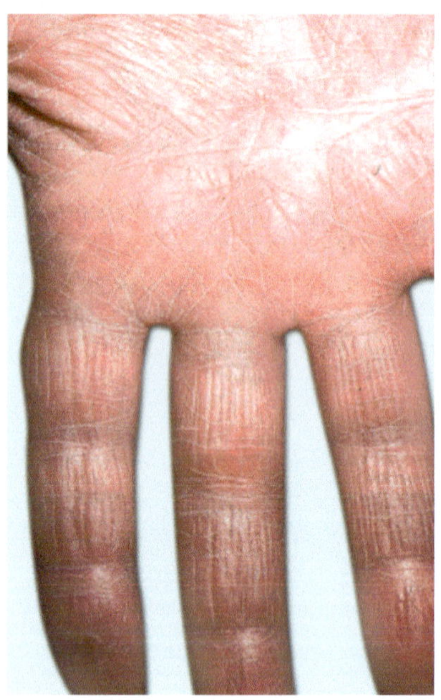

Chronic tinea of palm, sometimes described as "painter's palm," with white scale building up in skin creases, like paint after cleaning painting hand.

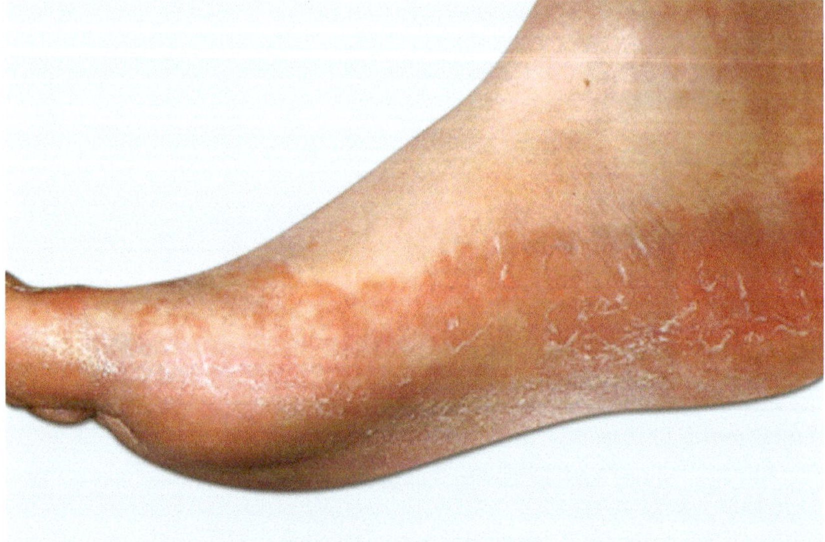

Moderately severe chronic tinea pedis with redness and scaling in "moccasin" distribution.

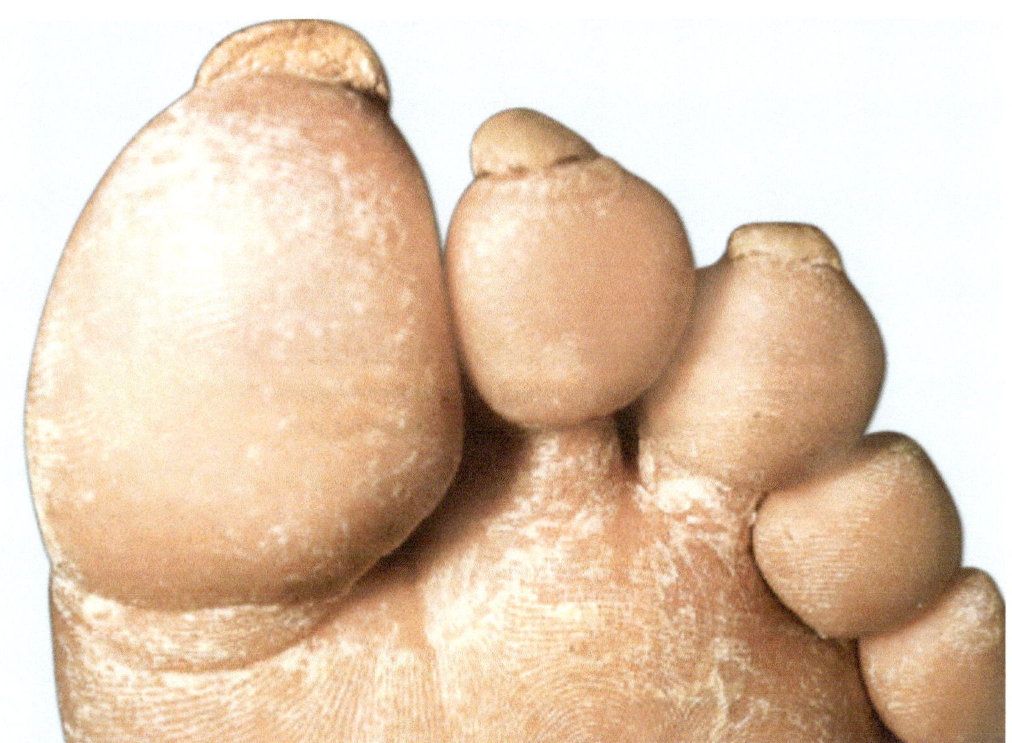

CHRONIC PLANTAR SCALING

Clinical

- "Moccasin" distribution on plantar surface and around sides of feet
  - Redness generally mild or absent
  - Scaling mild to profuse:
    - Often accentuated in normal fold lines, appearing as a white powder
    - May build up as hyperkeratosis on weight-bearing surfaces, especially around the edges of the heel
- One or more toenails often involved (*See* page 86)
- Itching usually absent
- Difficult to find organism on potassium hydroxide (KOH) examination (*See* page 226)

Treatment

In 10–20% of individuals, there is a constitutional incapability of mounting an immune response to the organism *Trichophyton rubrum,* so it exists peaceably on the foot and usually recurs (from environmental contamination or persistent skin spores) even after adequate treatment. Emphasize to the patient that no cure is expected only suppression of symptoms. Treatment is for amelioration of symptoms or to improve appearance and is not a medical necessity.

- Keratolytics (*See* page 244):
  - Chronic application minimizes or abolishes scale, thus reducing organism population.
  - These agents are a useful adjunct to topical antifungal agents.
  - Keratolytics are rarely curative.
  - Apply ointment or gel thinly once or twice daily or as necessary.
    - Salicylic acid 6% in propylene glycol gel
  - These products may be irritating, especially on nonplantar skin.
- Topical antifungal agents (*See* page 235):
  - Chronic applications minimize or suppress eruption.
  - These agents are sometimes curative.
  - Apply cream or solution twice daily; powder form is not very active.
  - There is occasional development of resistance to these agents.

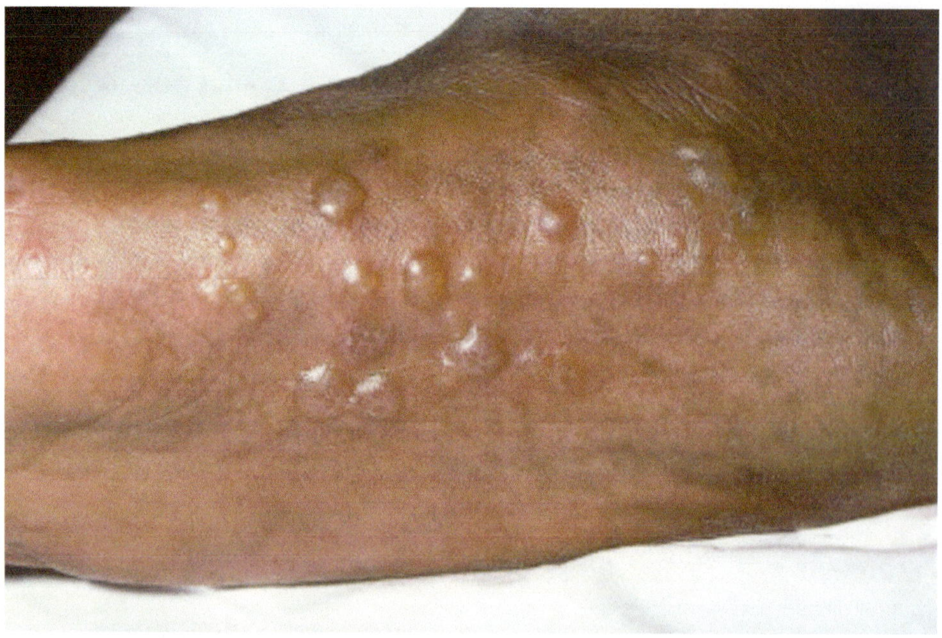

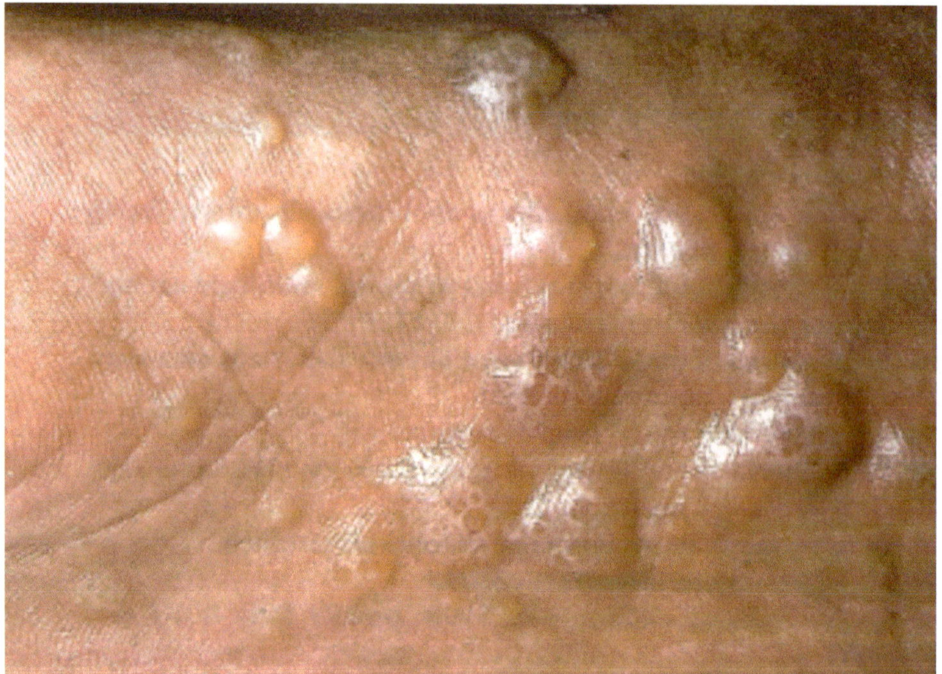

Acute vesicular tinea pedis. Close inspection of vesicles shows that they are multilocular, unlike unilocular friction blisters.

- Systemic antifungal agents are suppressive but rarely curative. Possible side effects make use rarely justified.
  - Fluconazole 150 mg daily for 2–6 weeks
  - Itraconazole 200 mg twice daily for 1 week
  - Griseofulvin microsize 1 g daily or ultramicrosize 750 mg daily for 4–8 weeks:
    - Griseofulvin may be less effective than other oral antifungals

ACUTE VESICULAR TINEA PEDIS

Clinical

- Sudden eruption of pruritic or painful blisters:
  - Often occurs abruptly in teenagers, which may induce immunity from further infections
  - Sometimes occurs on background of chronic scaling tinea

  - Small individual vesicles or, characteristically, multilocular bullae
  - Often follows, by 1–2 days, sweating and friction to soles (athletes)
- Positive KOH examination result is difficult to obtain (*See* page 226) because inflammation kills organisms.
  - Roof of blister is removed, soaked in KOH several minutes, and examined.
  - Blister fluid is serum, which does not contain organisms.

Treatment

Acute tissue reaction (blisters) kills fungi, so treatment is aimed at treating the inflammatory reaction itself.

- Decrease sweating by minimizing occlusive footwear and friction
- Soaks or baths should be used two or three times a day for a few days to dry up blisters.
  - Tap water
  - Astringents (*See* page 241)
  - Dry thoroughly after soaks
- If tense blisters are painful, carefully puncture and drain blisters with a clean needle.
  - Blister top settles onto eroded base and serves as dressing. **Do not remove blister tops,** as they promote healing.
  - Continue soaks until blisters are dry to reduce chance of secondary infection.
- A potent topical corticosteroid helps to relieve itching.
- Specific antifungal therapy is usually not necessary because inflammation kills organisms. If chronic scaling remains, treat as described in the preceding section.

INTERDIGITAL TINEA PEDIS

Clinical

- Erosion, scaling, and fissuring in toe webs:
  - Fourth web is most common
- Usually itchy, burning, or painful
- More common in people with sweaty feet or occlusive footwear
- Marked malodor often noticeable
- Represents maceration with colonization by fungi and gram-negative bacteria
  - Often occurs in absence of tinea of sole

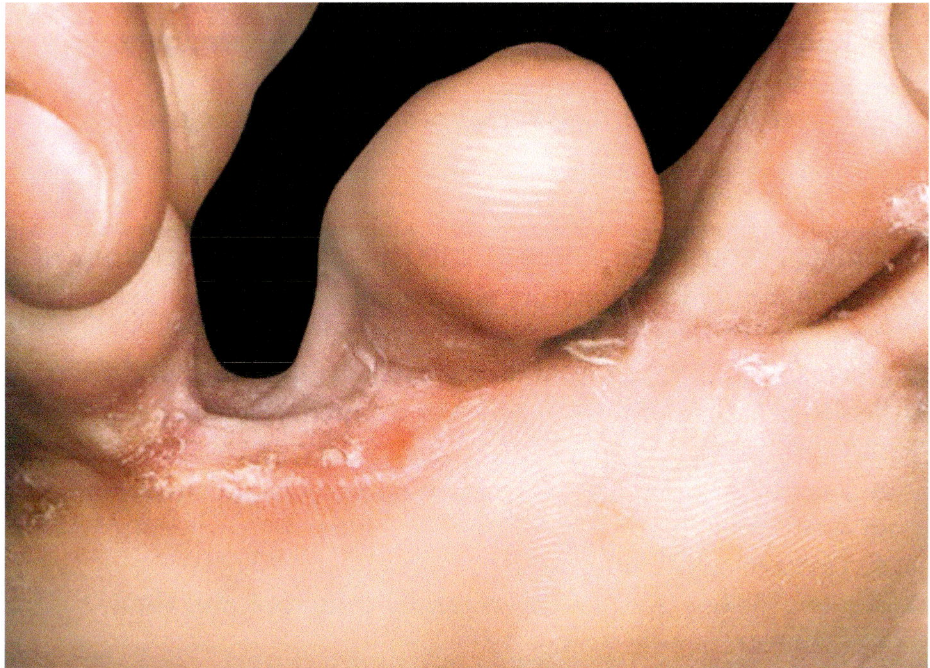

Itchy, eroded, and malodorous interdigital tinea.

  - KOH examination result (*See* page 226) often negative on first attempt but usually positive after repeated attempts
  - Gram-negative bacteria may cause burning and offensive odor

Treatment

Because the primary contributing problem is superhydration and maceration, the cure can be effected by drying, without specific therapy aimed at the fungi or bacteria.

- General measures:
  - Light, loose, and nonocclusive footwear:
    - Sandals
    - Absorbent cotton socks (any color)
  - Thorough drying after bathing
  - Reduction of sweating with topical sweat inhibitors:
    - Aluminum chloride solution 20%
    - Tannic acid powder
- Drying agents:
  - Soak feet twice daily for 10 minutes, then dry well
    - Water
    - Astringent solution (*See* page 241)
  - Drying paints may be applied twice daily with cotton-tipped applicator
    - Aluminum chloride 6–20%
- Antimicrobial agents
  - Antifungal solution (*See* page 235) (drying vehicle) applied twice daily
  - Econazole cream—an antifungal agent with some antibacterial properties, which may be more effective than other topical antifungals
  - Combined antifungal and antibacterial therapy:
    - Antifungal agent and mupirocin
  - Oral antifungals—often not beneficial

Onychomycosis

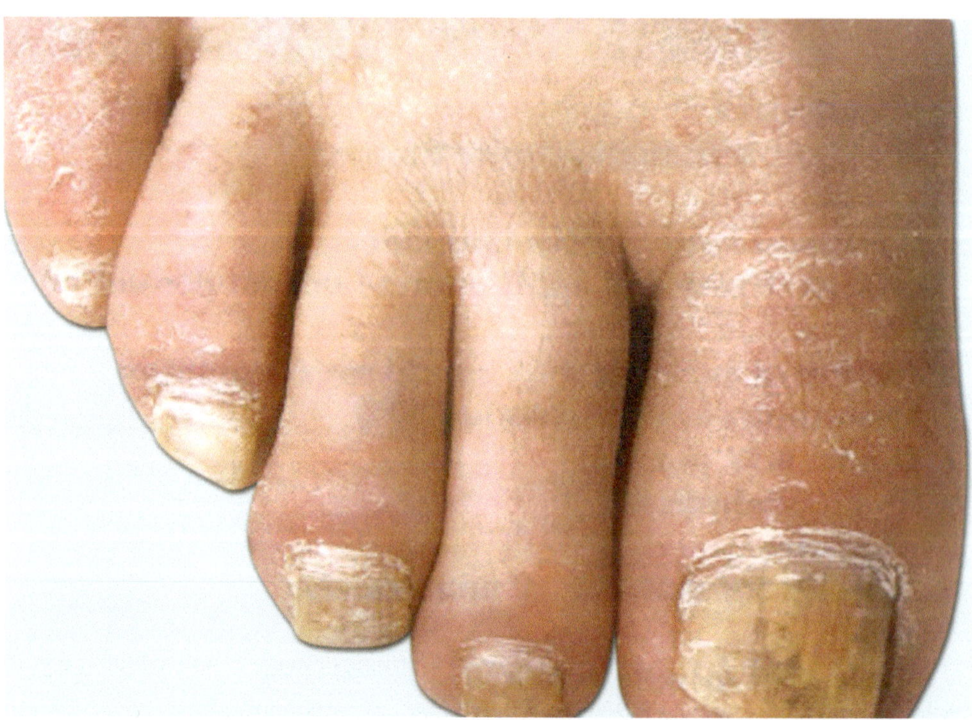

Nails of patient shown on page 83 are thickened and have accumulated crumbly subungual debris.

CLINICAL

- Infection of the nail and/or the nail bed with dermatophyte (ringworm) fungi:
  - Many species can cause infection.
  - Secondary colonization with nonpathogenic fungi is common.
  - KOH examination and fungal culture results are often negative, even with excellent technique.
  - Histology and Periodic acid-Schiff (PAS) staining are predominantly used for diagnosis
- Clinical characteristics:
  - Distal nail edge onycholysis (separation of nail plate from nail bed) with yellowish thickening of nail plate and accumulation of tan crumbly debris beneath separated portion of nail
    - Distal edge of nail may split and crumble and eventually shorten considerably through "erosion."
    - Nail may thicken, become elevated and grossly distorted, and be painful from pressure of shoes.

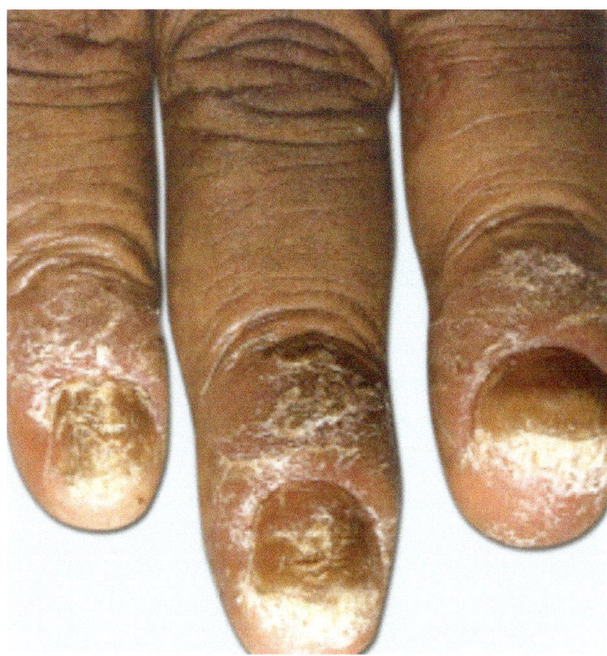

This diabetic patient had particularly marked nail and skin involvement with dermatophytes.

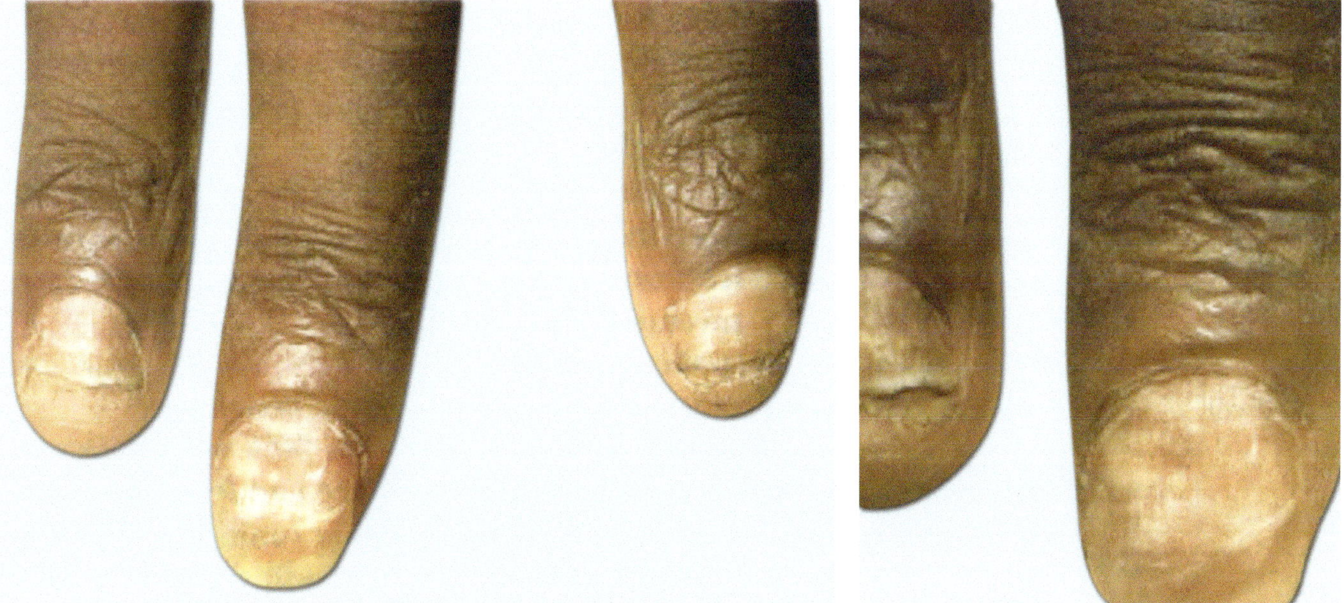

Chronic indolent onychomycosis caused only slight thickening and longitudinal striation of these fingernails.

    - Black or greenish subungual color may occur from secondary colonization by nonpathogenic fungi (e.g., *Aspergillus*).
  - Condition is often seen in association with tinea pedis or tinea manuum.
  - Toenail involvement is much more common than fingernail involvement.
    - May occur in single nail (often great toenail) or in multiple nails
    - If isolated and skin is unaffected, may be secondary to traumatic damage to nail, which is a portal for infection
  - Usually lasts a lifetime; rarely heals spontaneously:
    - More nails may become involved with passage of time, especially if skin of soles and palms is affected.

TREATMENT

- General:
  - Continuous treatment of chronic palm or sole tinea (*See* page 82) possibly decreases the likelihood of nail infection.
  - Well-established onychomycosis, especially of the toenails, is difficult to cure, and it is best to warn the patient of the poor prognosis and the possibility of relapse.
  - After discussion, the patient might decide to forgo treatment.
    - Keep the nail neatly clipped and buffed flat (with file or pumice stone) for cosmetic appearance and to prevent painful pressure by shoes.
- Topical therapy:
  - Most topical agents are of little benefit.
    - Efinaconazole 10% solution (Jublia) once daily for 48 weeks
    - Gently spread the solution completely around the toenail (toenail bed, folds, hyponychium, and undersurface of the toenail plate) with the attached applicator brush and let dry thoroughly.
- Systemic antifungal agents (*See* page 235):
  - These agents are associated with a high likelihood of response (85%), but some nails may not respond.
  - Relapse rate for toenails is very high (80%) within a few years after therapy is stopped.
    - Relapse rate lower (50%) for fingernails
  - Course of therapy is prolonged with the use of some agents (until nails clear).
    - About 12 months for toenails
    - About 6 months for fingernails
  - Side effects are possible (*See* page 236).
  - All agents are expensive.
  - Because of long duration of therapy, possible side effects, and high relapse rate, oral agents are used with reluctance for onychomycosis of the toenails (which is essentially a cosmetic problem) but are worth a try for onychomycosis of the fingernails (where not only is cosmesis more important, but intact nails are necessary for picking up small objects).
    - Itraconazole: In the United States, the approved course is 200 mg daily for 6 weeks for fingernails, 12 weeks for toenails. More commonly suggested is 200 mg twice daily for 1 week; repeat every 4 weeks for 2 months (fingernail) or 3 months (toenail).
    - Fluconazole: The course for this drug is 150 mg weekly until clear (an unapproved use in the United States). Its success and cost are comparable to those of itraconazole.
- Nail avulsion: Removal of a single involved nail sometimes allows a normal nail to grow again in its place.
  - The relapse rate is high, especially if more than one nail is involved or if the sole is involved and not treated.
  - Treat with topical antifungal solution or oral antifungal agent during regrowth.
  - Surgical avulsion is standard but should be performed only by a trained practitioner.
    - To do this, use ring block anesthesia (without epinephrine), apply a tourniquet, use a periosteal elevator to separate the entire nail plate from the nail bed and cuticle, pull the nail out of the matrix with hemostat or pliers, then gently curette the bed to remove infected debris. Lightly cauterize bleeding points, but do not curette or cauterize matrix, as that may permanently prevent nail growth. Remove tourniquet and have the patient soak the digit two or three times daily in warm water or astringent for 2–4 days (until oozing stops).

Note: See page 89 for *Candida* paronychia, which may be confused with onychomycosis.

Paronychia

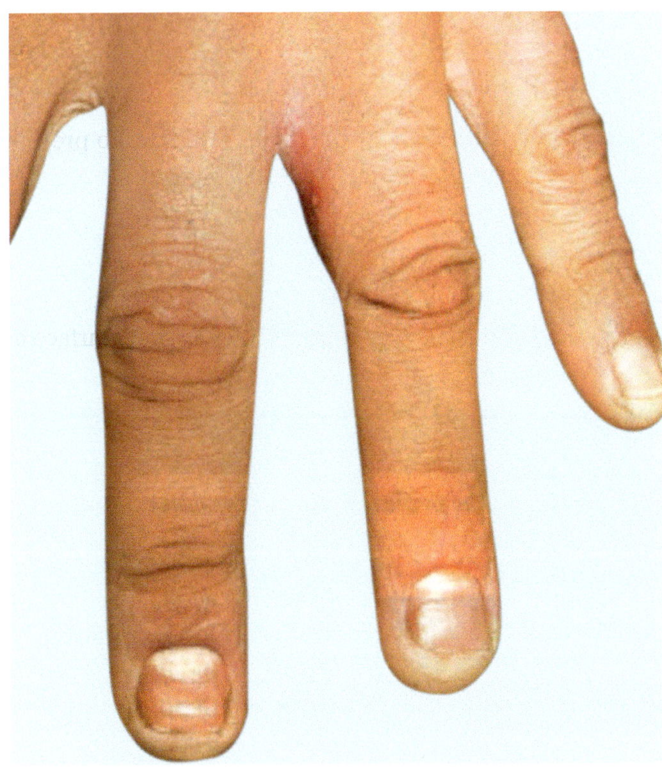

Mild puffiness of paronychial tissues. Note that nail dystrophy occurs only distal to the point of cuticle absence.

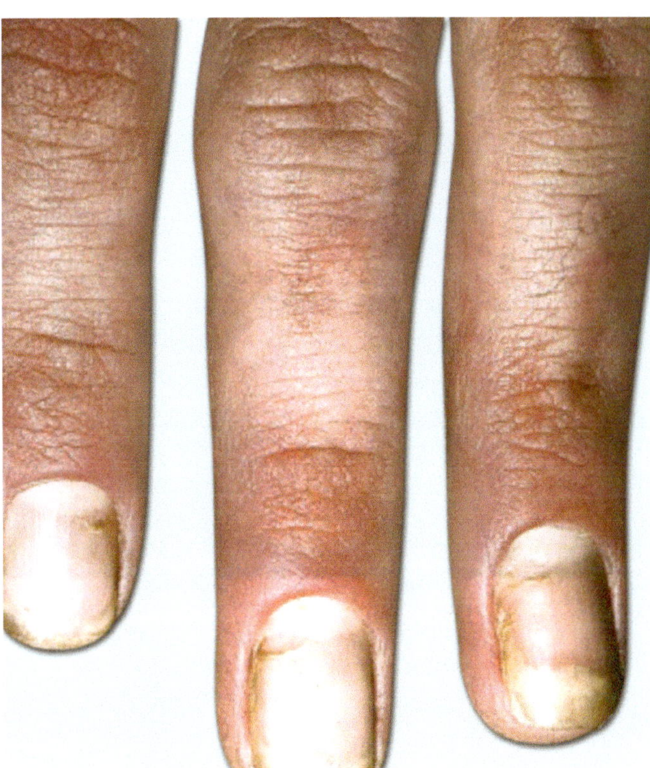

Slightly more inflamed periungual folds in a bartender, who also has onycholysis (separation of distal part of nail plate from nail bed).

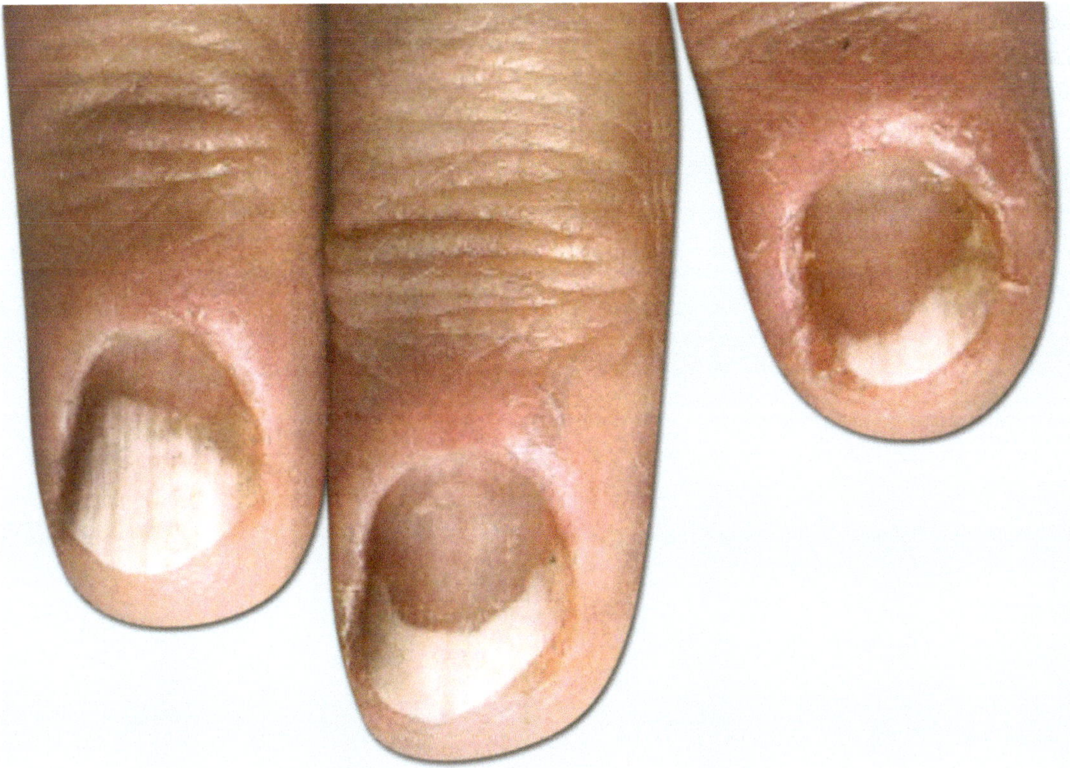

Marked paronychia and onycholysis in a professional hairdresser.

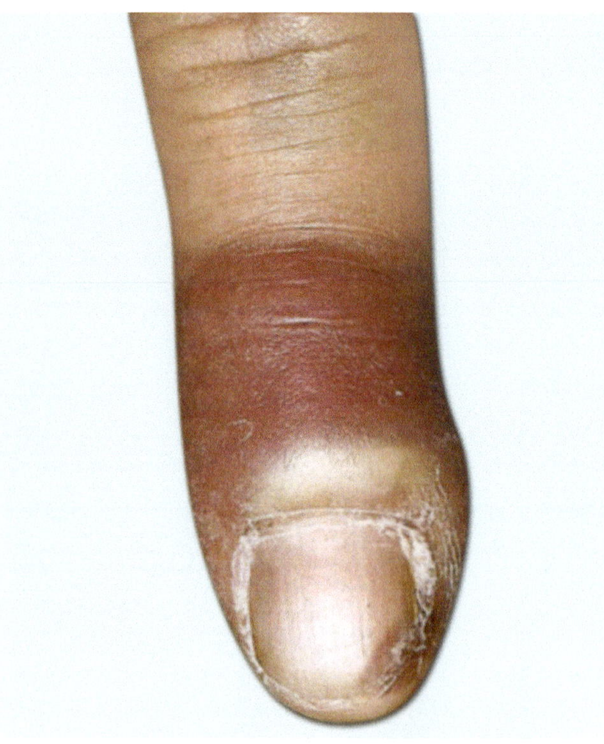

Acute, painful bacterial paronychia. Should be incised and drained where pus is visible.

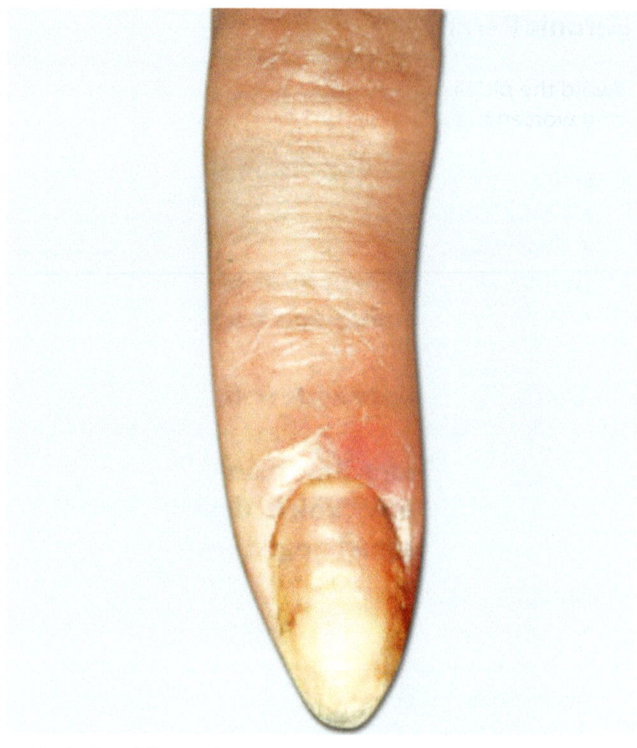

Marked nail dystrophy in this chronic Candida paronychia, which also has an area of acute bacterial paronychia.

CLINICAL

- Acute bacterial paronychia:
  - This condition is characterized by sudden development of redness, pain, and swelling, usually at side and posterior corner of nailfold. Central pustule may develop.
  - Lymphangitic streaking, chills, and fever may develop.
  - *Streptococcus* is the usual causative organism.
- Chronic paronychia
  - Mild to moderate redness and edema of posterior and lateral fingernail folds (rare on toes)
  - Absence of cuticle with retraction of nail folds away from nail plate
  - Mild to severe nail plate dystrophy, with horizontal ridging and discoloration

A related condition is distal onycholysis (separation of nail plates from nail bed). This may appear as opaque whiteness or as a yellowish or green stain (from secondary fungal or *Pseudomonas* colonization).

  - Caused by the following sequence of events:
    - Excessive water exposure (as with a bartender or beautician) softens the cuticle and it pulls away from the nail.

Vigorous manicuring of cuticles greatly contributes to this process.

    - Continued water exposure prevents reformation of cuticles and encourages the colonization of *Candida* and bacteria under the posterior or lateral nail fold.
    - The presence of *Candida* and bacteria prevents reformation of cuticle.
  - The condition is usually only mildly tender, but painful acute bacterial paronychia occasionally develops, which drains pus and resolves, leaving the chronic process unchanged.

TREATMENT

Acute Paronychia

- Incise and drain, if possible. Often just carefully detaching and lifting the cuticle at the involved site with a thin blade allows drainage.
- Follow incision and drainage with soaks (*See* page 241), three times daily for 1–2 days to enhance drainage.
- Use oral antibiotics that suppress streptococci (e.g., penicillins and cephalosporins).

Chronic Paronychia

Avoid the pitfall of assuming the presence of a chronic bacterial infection and prescribing soaks. Such treatment can prolong and worsen the condition.

- General measures:
  - Minimize water exposure—a change of jobs or furlough from job may be indicated
  - Wearing rubber or vinyl gloves over thin cotton gloves and changing them when wet is helpful but inconvenient
- Drying agents are the treatment of choice.
  - These products dry out the "cave" under the posterior nail fold, and the colonizing organisms cannot survive in the absence of moisture.
  - A thin liquid should be applied with an eyedropper or from a nozzle squeeze bottle twice daily, especially after finishing wet chores.
  - Popular agents are:
    - Thymol 2–4% in 70–90% alcohol (must be compounded by a pharmacist)
    - Aluminum chloride 6–20% in alcohol
    - If these are irritating, the patient may need to use a mild corticosteroid lotion or cream when appropriate.
- Antifungal agents:
  - Antiyeast materials in solution (alcohol-based, drying) should be applied twice daily
    - Clotrimazole
    - Miconazole
    - Ciclopirox
    - Ketoconazole
  - Antiyeast materials in creams may be successful but often fail because they are occlusive and cause maceration.

Even with successful treatment, it will take 2–3 months for the cuticle to reform, signaling a cure. An additional 6 months may pass before the dystrophic nail grows in normally. Emphasize to the patient the importance of continuing to avoid water and persisting with treatment.

Periungual Warts

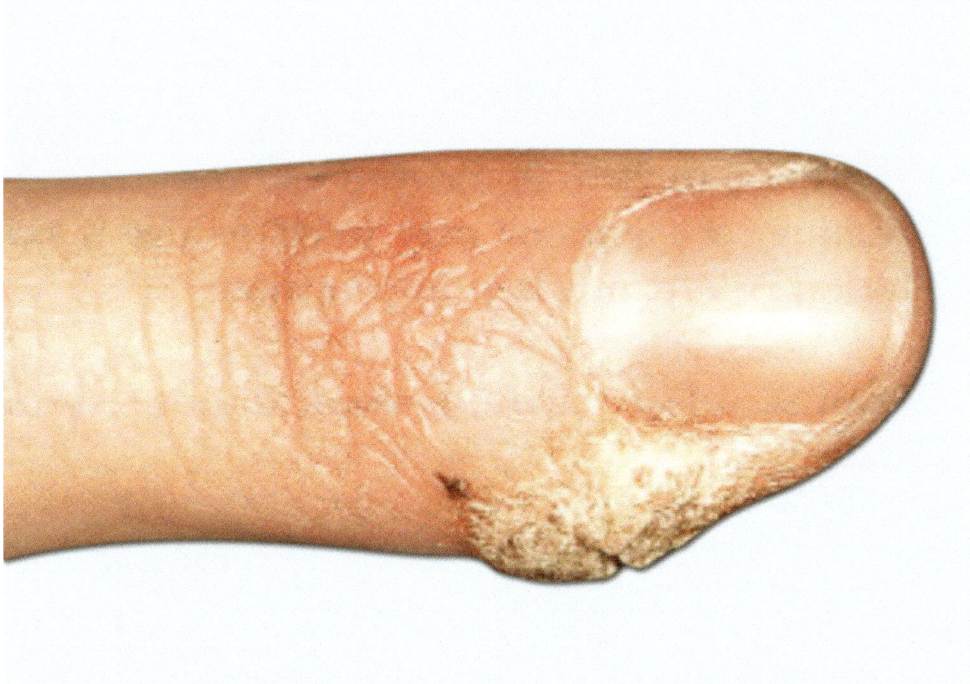

Large wart on lateral nail fold has not clinically extended under the nail plate.

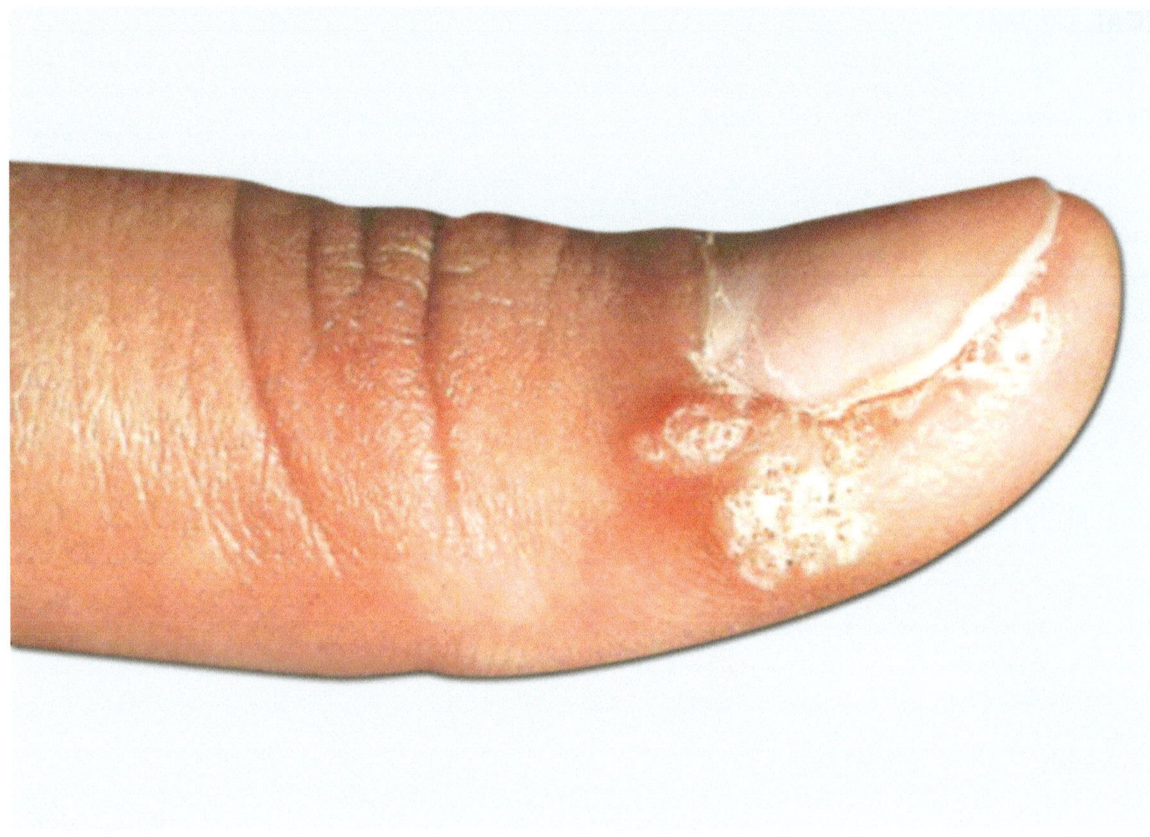

Wart tissue is present under the edge of this nail.

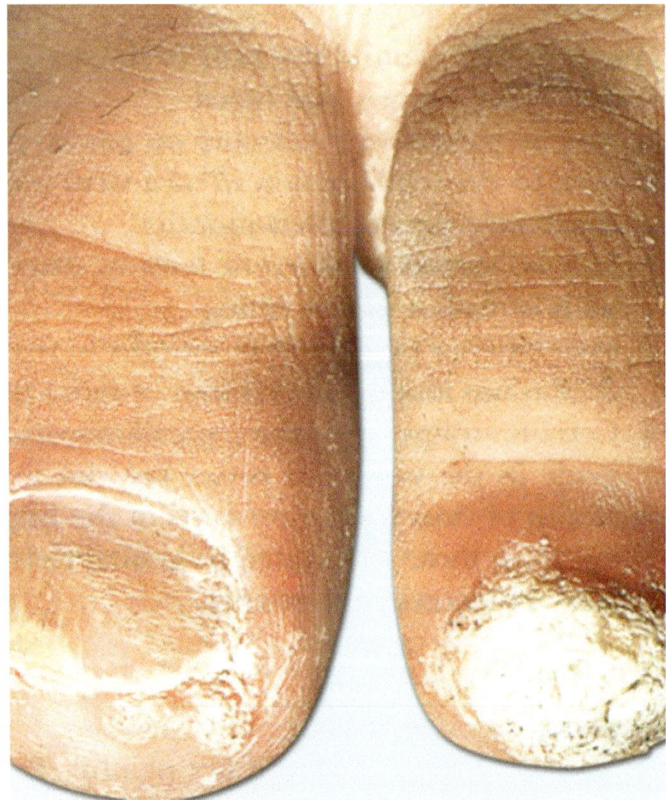

Wart is growing under the distal edges of these toenails and has almost replaced one nail bed.

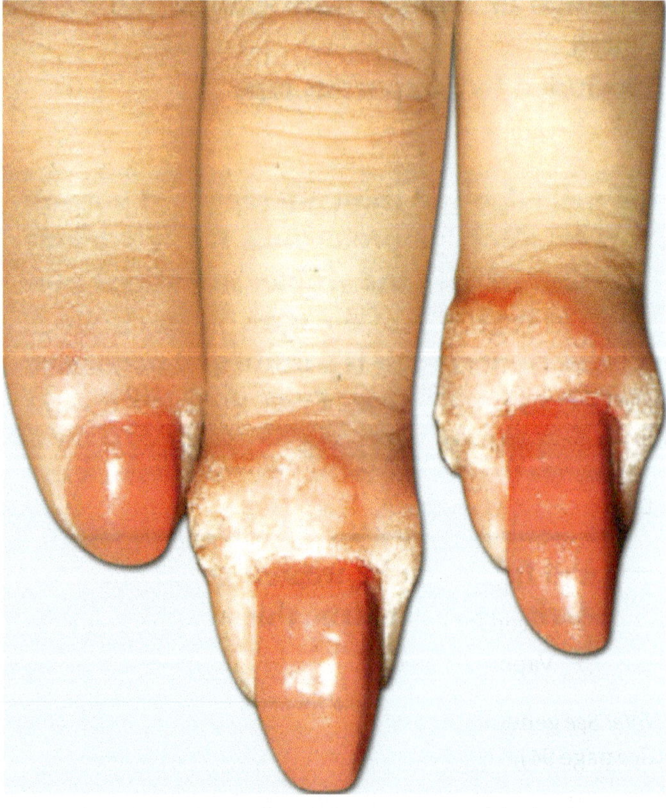

Extensive periungual warts in a teenager with leukemia.

CLINICAL

- Warty growths around the nails of fingers and, rarely, on the toes:
    - May crack, fissure, and bleed
    - May be painful with pressure on paronychial tissue or nail bed
- Caused by the implantation of wart virus into skin
    - Incubation period is a few months.
    - May be spread to adjacent nails by direct contact or to other nails by nail or cuticle biting
    - Spontaneous involution in months to years:
        - May last months in children or more than a decade in adults

TREATMENT

- General:
    - No treatment necessary if not painful (Patient Guides, *See* page 255).
    - Stop nail and cuticle biting.
- Palliative:
    - Keratolytic agents should be applied twice daily to reduce bulk and keep the wart soft.
    - More effective if occluded by nonporous tape.
- Destructive

> Warts under the distal nail edge and those on the distal portion of the lateral nail folds usually have projections that go deeply under the nail. Destruction of only the visible, superficial portion almost always results in regrowth of the wart. To be curative, destructive therapies must be deep; this is painful and may cause slight deformity of the periungual tissue. Even then, cure rates are <50% after one treatment.

> Warts on the proximal nail fold must be treated gently to avoid permanent injury to underlying nail matrix; this would result in permanent nail deformity.

- Cryotherapy (liquid nitrogen by cotton-tipped applicator):
    - For warts on posterior nail fold, treat lightly at 2- to 3-week intervals to avoid permanent matrix injury (may get temporary nail deformity). Two or three treatments are usually sufficient.
    - Warts under the distal areas must be frozen deeply for >30 seconds, which is a very painful process; this is about 30% curative after several biweekly treatments.
- Surgical curettage is curative in >50% of cases if it is thorough. The procedure: administer ring block anesthesia, tourniquet, cut nail back several millimeters behind visible wart tissue, curette deeply (often near bone), and electrodesiccate thoroughly. The area is surprisingly nontender after anesthesia dissipates, though healing may take place with loss of periungual tissue bulk.

> Do not perform this on *posterior* nail fold (it is likely to permanently damage matrix).

- Laser destruction is tidier and perhaps more effective than surgical curettage, but it is much more expensive. It is reserved for warts that are particularly refractory to treatment.
    - Vapor plume may contain intact wart virus, which is of uncertain danger to the operator and staff.

Note: See general discussion of warts (*See* page 199), facial warts (*See* page 47), genital warts (*See* page 57), and plantar warts (*See* page 94).

Plantar Warts

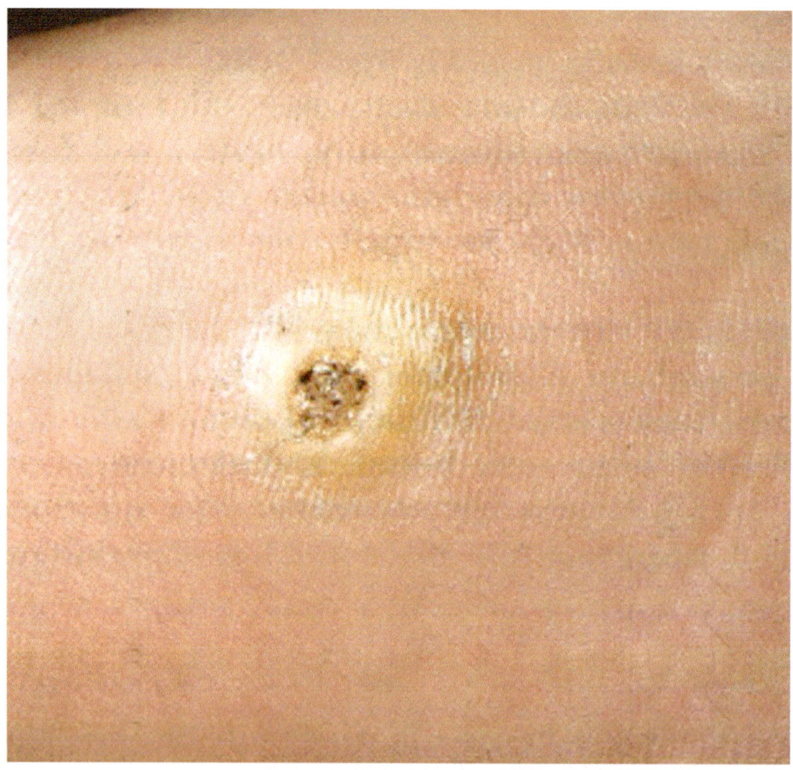

Typical isolated plantar wart surrounded by callus.

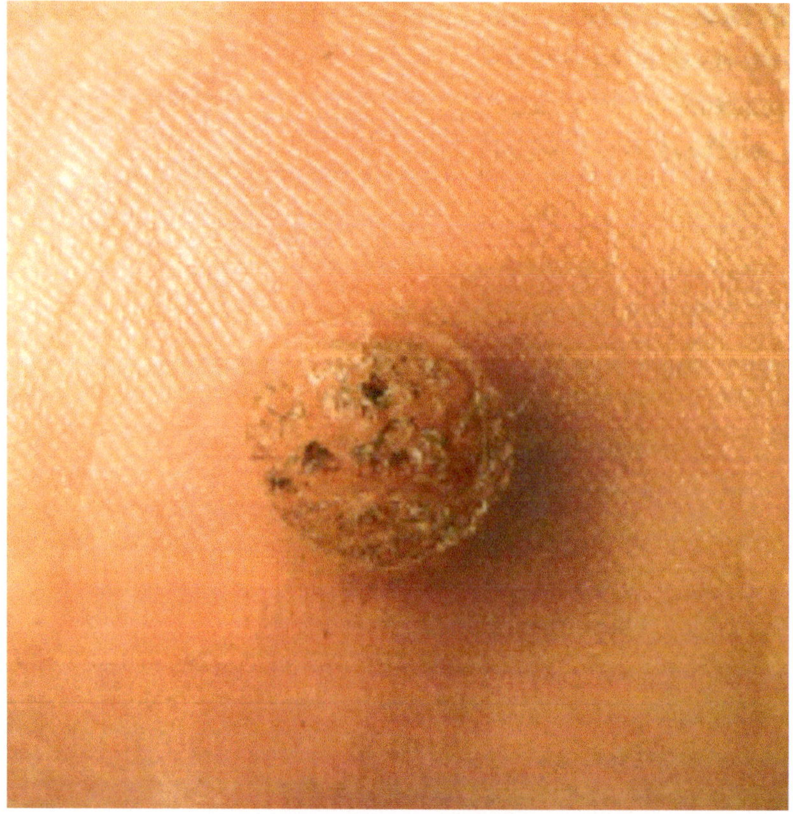

This protuberant plantar wart was painful during walking. Pressure caused irritation of surrounding skin.

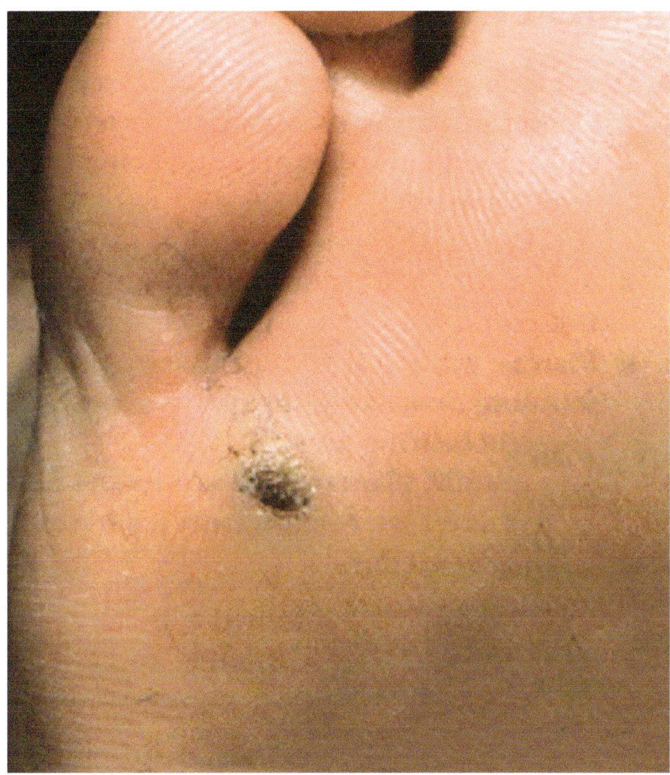

Sometimes capillaries in the wart clot, often heralding spontaneous resolution.

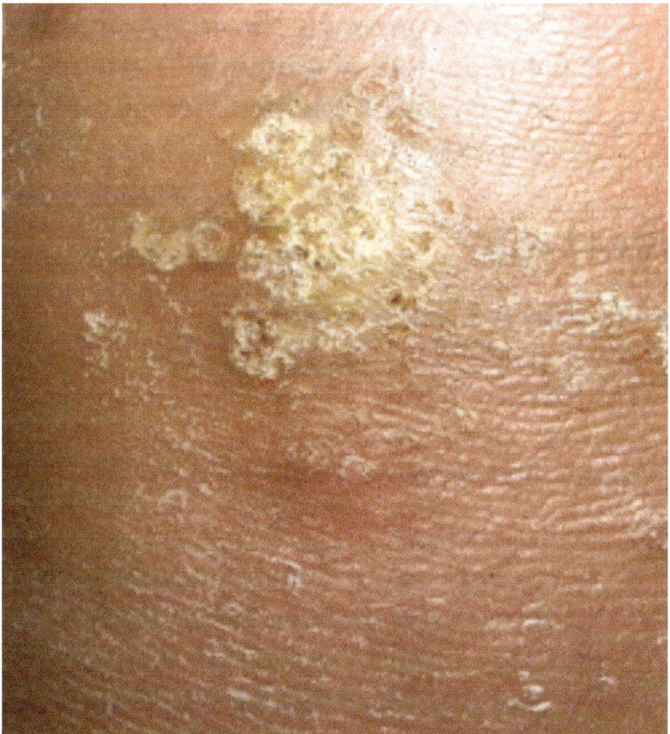

Mosaic plantar wart is a cluster of perhaps a dozen single verrucae.

CLINICAL

- Discrete or grouped firm, keratotic masses on the sole
  - Center of wart mass has granular, crumbly, pitted surface.
    - Tiny, dark dots, representing clotted capillaries, are occasionally present.
  - A callus of surrounding normal skin is usually present.

- A "mosaic" wart is one covering a large area with multiple central cores.
- Plantar warts may be asymptomatic or may be painful when standing or walking (as space-occupying mass), especially if on a weight-bearing area.
  - Typically, plantar warts are tender upon lateral pinching (as well as direct, firm pressure), and corns are tender only upon direct pressure.

▪ A viral infection of epidermal cells:
- Incubation period is thought to be a few months but may be much longer.
- New warts can seed from the initial one, either early in the course of the first wart or after months of its existence.
- Spontaneous involution occurs when immunity to wart virus develops.
  - Occurs after months or years.
  - Duration generally shorter in children than in adults.
  - Development of immunity is variable: Some individuals have only one wart briefly; others are plagued with various warts for years.

TREATMENT

▪ No effective specific antiwart virus medications exist. Therapy, therefore, is either palliative or destructive. Destructive therapy may yield a cure of one or two isolated warts. Mosaic warts nearly always recur after such treatments, so only palliative therapy is recommended for this type of wart.

▪ Palliative therapy:
- Keeps warts asymptomatic until spontaneous resolution occurs. (There is a risk that new warts may seed from the original during this time.)
- No treatment is necessary, if wart is asymptomatic.
- Apply a keratolytic (keratin-softening) agent (*See* page 244) overnight every few days, so that the keratin becomes soft and can be easily scraped off.
  - Salicylic acid 40% plaster
  - Salicylic acid 16% and lactic acid 16% in flexible collodion
- The patient can pare the wart with a knife or scalpel or grind it down with a nail file or pumice stone.
- Many physicians favor alternating this keratolytic therapy with drying by formalin soak or compress on subsequent nights, claiming that this speeds removal of keratin and even shortens the duration of the wart.

▪ Destruction of wart tissue

If only wart or epidermis is damaged, then healing will occur without a scar. **If the dermis is damaged, a scar will result. A scar on the sole, especially on the weight-bearing area, can be painful permanently. This rare outcome is particularly tragic, as the wart will heal eventually without treatment.**

- Cryotherapy is rarely successful with just one treatment because of the depth of the wart, although repeated treatment, or treatment after keratolytic treatments (see previous therapy method) may be successful.
  - Considerable pain is a major drawback for several days, especially when walking.
  - Scarring is rare unless treatment is too deep.
- Repeated parings (every 1–2 weeks in the office) or several weeks of keratolytic treatment may thin the wart to the point at which acid (trichloroacetic acid 60%) repeatedly applied by pointed wooden applicator may eradicate it.
  - Recurrences are common.
  - Skill is required to avoid dermal injury.
- Curettage and chemical cautery (trichloroacetic acid 60% or phenol 88%) or *light* electrocautery after local anesthesia is successful about 80% of the time for isolated (single) warts.
  - Local anesthesia of sole is painful.
  - Postoperative tenderness may be considerable for a few days, and healing may take 2–3 weeks.

Excessive curettage or cautery could result in painful scar.

- Laser destruction is tidier and perhaps more effective than surgical curettage, but it is much more expensive. It is reserved for warts that are particularly refractory to treatment.
  - Vapor plume may contain intact wart virus, which is of uncertain danger to the operator and staff.

▪ For Patient Guides on warts, *See* page 255.

Stasis Dermatitis

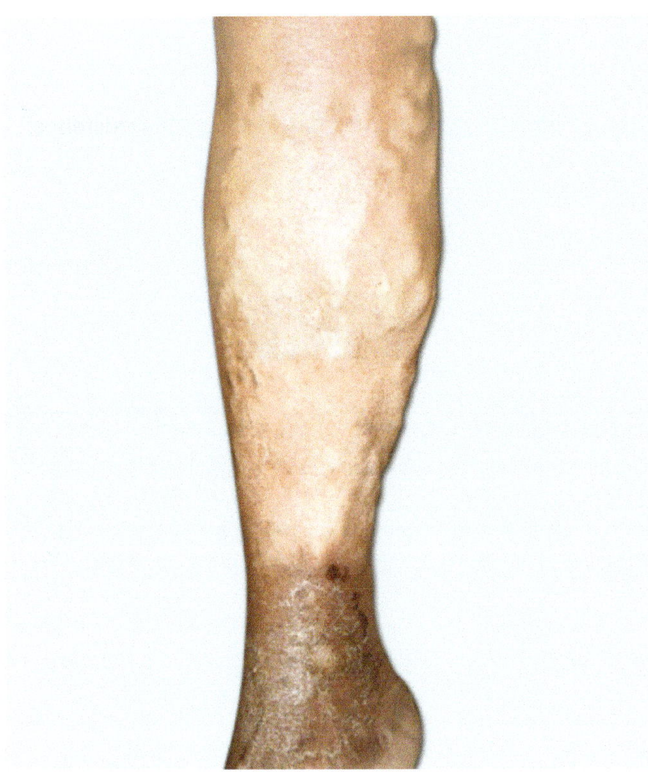

Obvious varicose veins and chronic stasis dermatitis of ankle.

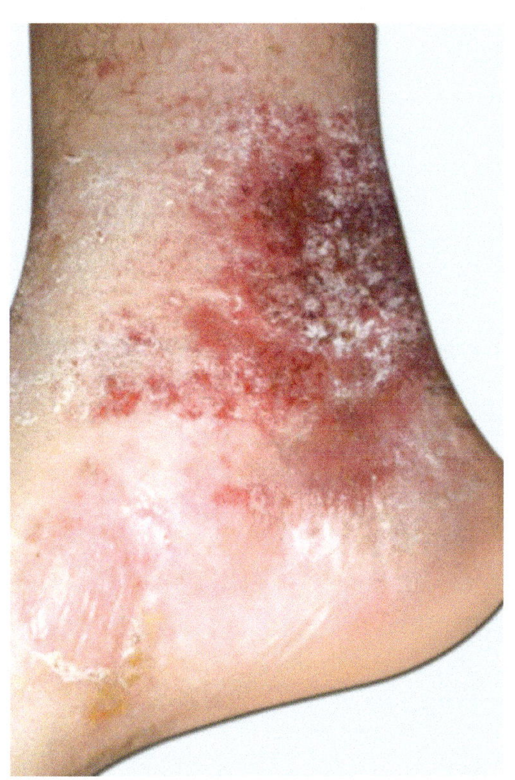

Early (5 days) acute stasis dermatitis over the most distal perforator vein connecting the deep and superficial systems.

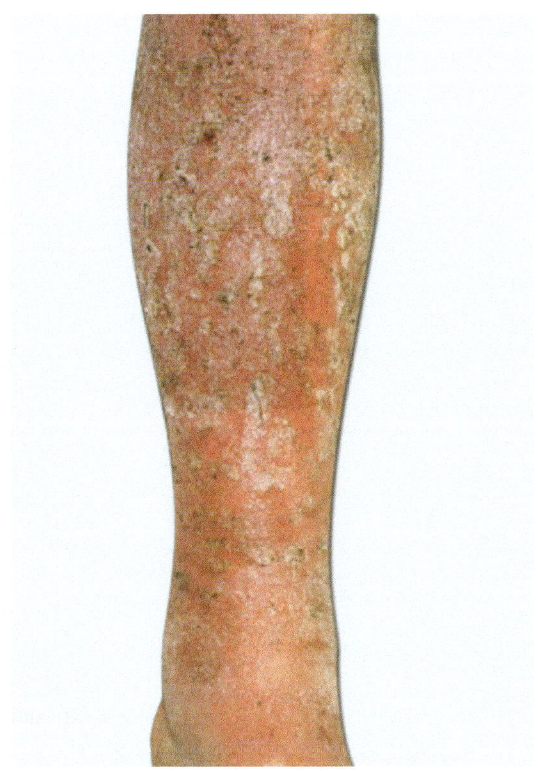

Very widespread acute stasis dermatitis rapidly enlarging from original site on ankle.

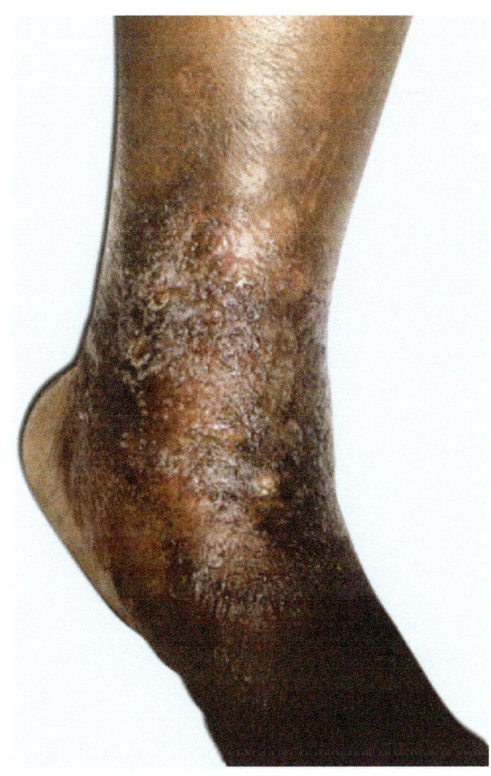

Widespread stasis eczema on a quite swollen ankle.

CLINICAL

- Caused by increased hydrostatic venous pressure:
  - More common in people who stand for prolonged periods
  - Usually a rash and/or ulcer on medial side of ankle where the most inferior perforator connects deep and superficial venous systems and hydrostatic pressure is greatest
  - Veins and valves may have been damaged by clots, infection, or injury.
- Eruption:
  - Eruptions may range from mild pink or pigmented to raging, angry red; oozing necrosis and ulceration may occur.
  - There may be a local spread on the leg or distant id (autosensitization) dermatitis, especially on the hands (*See* page 81).
  - Lichenification and neurodermatitis may supervene after stasis element has remitted.
  - Secondary infection (usually staphylococcal) may occur.
    - Increased oozing and crusting
    - Pain

TREATMENT

General: Reduction of venous pressure is paramount. Educate the patient to avoid stress on malfunctioning veins.
- The patient should minimize standing still (walking is not harmful because muscle action pumps blood through veins).
- Recommend that the patient use an ottoman or pillows to elevate feet when sitting. This lowers gradient back to the heart and unkinks veins compressed when the knee is bent.
- If standing is necessary, wear support hose, surgical support stockings, or custom-measured elasticized stocking to minimize dilatation of veins.

- To treat dermatitis
  - Ascertain the diagnosis:
    - If oozing: Soaks, baths, or compresses (*See* page 241) three times daily for 15 minutes
      - Discontinue when dry
  - Topical corticosteroids
    - These may be mild to potent, depending on degree of inflammation.
    - Do not use potent preparations longer than necessary, to avoid atrophy.
    - Ointment form is more lubricating and contains fewer sensitizers.
  - Zinc oxide (Unna's) boot
    - Do not use if oozing is copious.
    - This treatment may be mildly soothing.
    - Application of Unna's boot may be cumbersome; makes wearing of shoes and bathing difficult.
    - This may be applied over topical corticosteroids.
    - Change every 2–7 days.
- To treat ulcers:

This is one of the most diverse areas of treatment in medicine. Treatments include oral zinc, topical zinc oxide, gold leaf, benzoyl peroxide, hyperbaric oxygen, and many others. Mild ulcers respond to elevation, soaks, and time. Severe chronic ulcers may respond to repeated application of an Unna's boot.

  - Modalities shown to hasten healing of ulcers:
    - Grafting:
      - "Pinch" or "postage stamp" grafts to base of ulcer
      - Excision and split-thickness graft
    - Repeated application of especially prepared, banked porcine skin grafts

Specific instructions for the use of these modalities are beyond the scope of this book and should be sought elsewhere.

- Treatment of secondary bacterial infection:
  - Prevention and cure of superficial infections may be achieved by:
    - Soaks and baths (*See* page 241)
    - Benzoyl peroxide (*See* page 234)
    - Topical antibiotics (*See* page 235)

Caution: Topical antibiotics containing neomycin are frequent sensitizers in this setting.

  - Deeper or stubborn infections require systemic antibiotics.

Lichen Simplex Chronicus

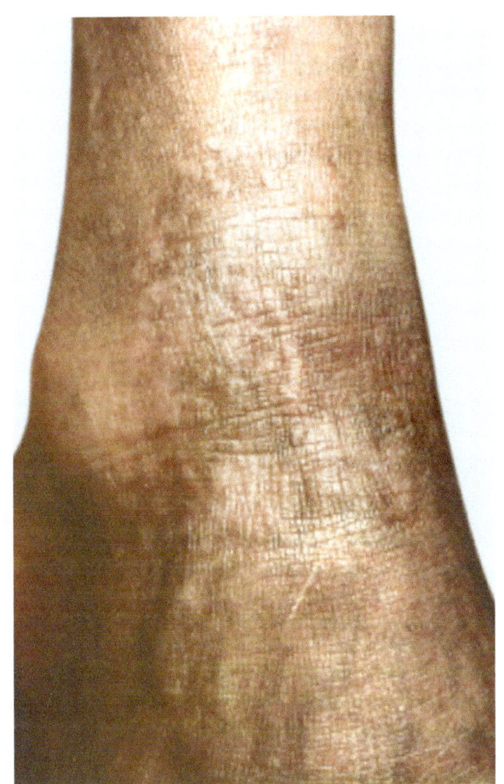

Lichen simplex chronicus of ankle that patient has been rubbing for 10 years , especially when tense.

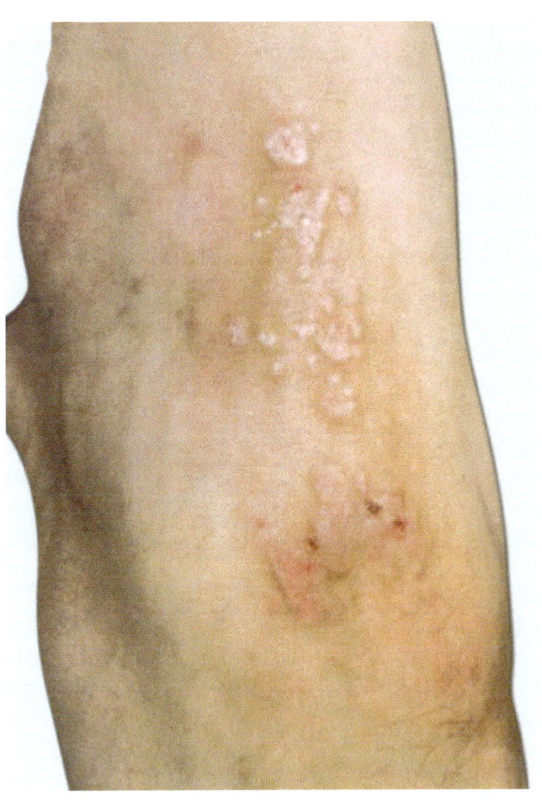

The anterior surface of the ankle has been rubbed for months, producing this hobnail type of lichenification.

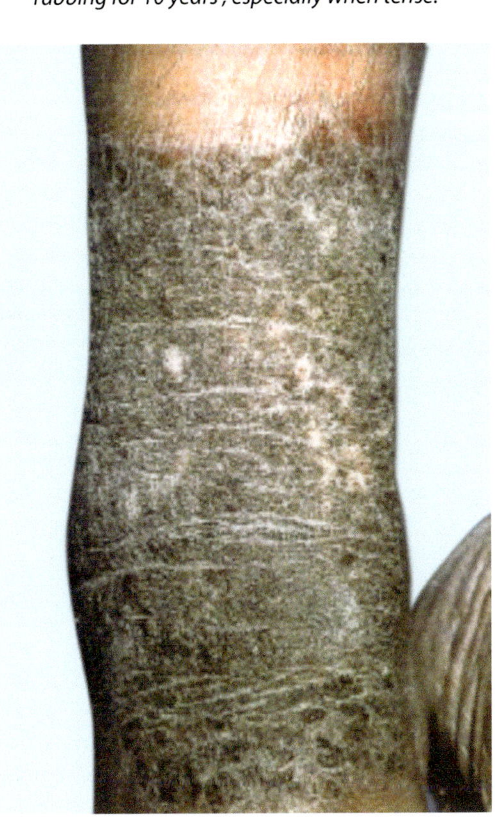

Years of vigorous rubbing and scratching produced a leathery, scarred dermatitis.

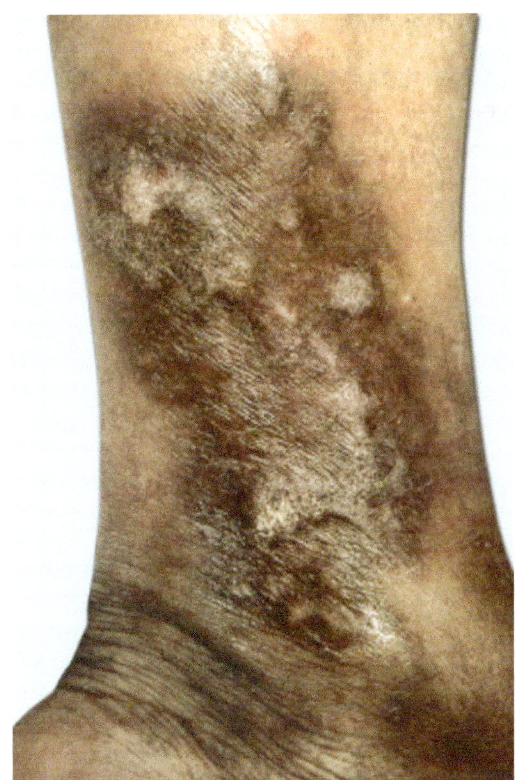

Massive lichenification verging on self-mutilation.

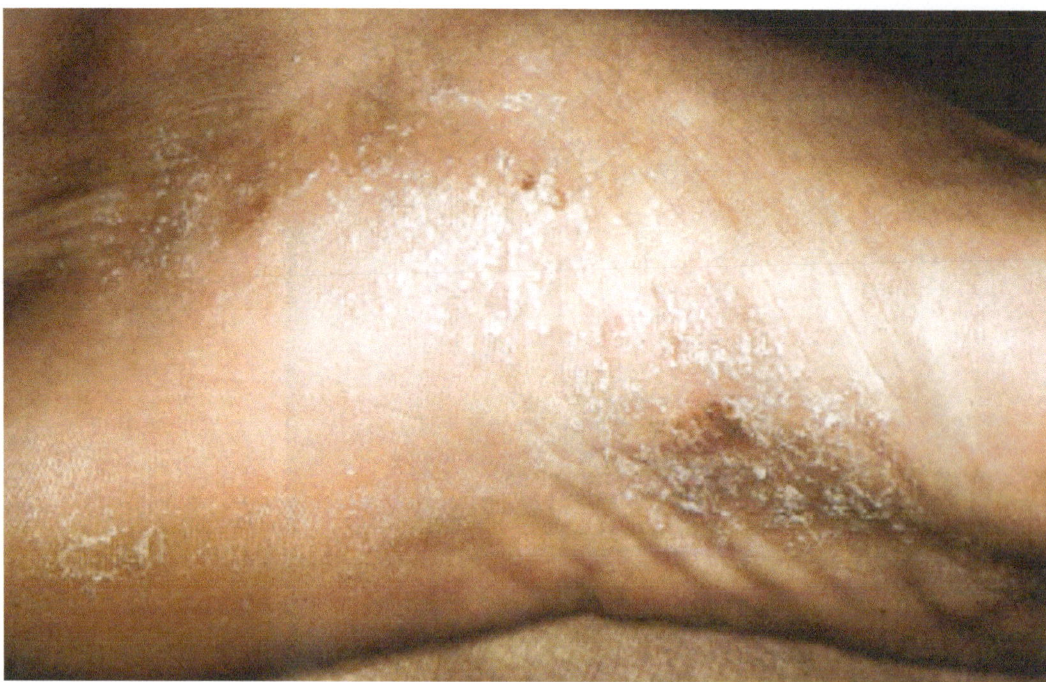

For 2 years, this man rubbed this linear area in his instep by slipping a finger along the side of his foot under the side of his shoe.

CLINICAL

- Thick, lined, well-circumscribed lichenified patch:
  - Often hyperpigmented
  - Usually solitary
  - Location
    - Lateral and medial sides of ankle
    - Lower shin
    - Occasionally, on the dorsum or instep of the foot
- Seen more commonly in:
  - Older men
  - Women, usually on neck or arms
  - Adults who had atopic diseases as children
  - South-East Asians
- Rarely in children
- Results from an unexplained itch-scratch cycle:
  - It often worsens in times of stress.
  - Often the rubbing and scratching are unconscious.
- One plaque of psoriasis may mimic lichen simplex chronicus.
  - Look in other body locations for signs of psoriasis.

TREATMENT

- General:
  - Even though the disease may be associated with stress, it is impractical to treat only by reducing stress because once the disease is established, the lichenified skin itself itches.
  - Making the patient aware that rubbing or scratching maintains the disease may bring the rubbing to a conscious level.
- External corticosteroids:
  - Reduce itching and reverse inflammation and lichenification
  - Creams and ointments:
    - Potent ones are usually necessary.
    - In the beginning, the patient should apply agent every time there is itching, so that the rubbing habit may be converted to a medication habit.

- Usually apply twice daily.
- Slow improvement is noticed over several weeks.
- Using a milder preparation as lesion thins to normal thickness will prevent atrophy.
- Occlusion over topical steroid:
  - Greatly enhances effectiveness of drug
  - Prevents rubbing
  - Corticoid-impregnated tape (Cordran) a convenient system for small lesions
- Intralesional injection of corticosteroid (*See* page 240)
  - Usually effective in resistant cases
  - May need to be repeated at monthly intervals
- Tars (*See* page 244):
  - May be applied alone or with corticosteroid
  - Mild anti-inflammatory effect
- Systemic agents:
  - Corticosteroids *not* indicated
  - Antihistamines or tranquilizers:
    - Drowsiness often makes these agents impractical for daytime use.
    - These products are useful at bedtime, if patients scratch in their sleep.

Nummular Eczema

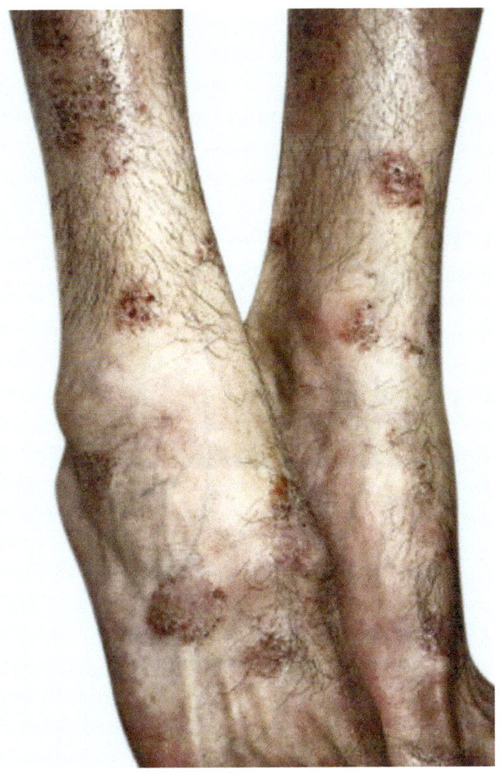

Typical scattered coin-like lesions of indolent dermatitis in nummular eczema.

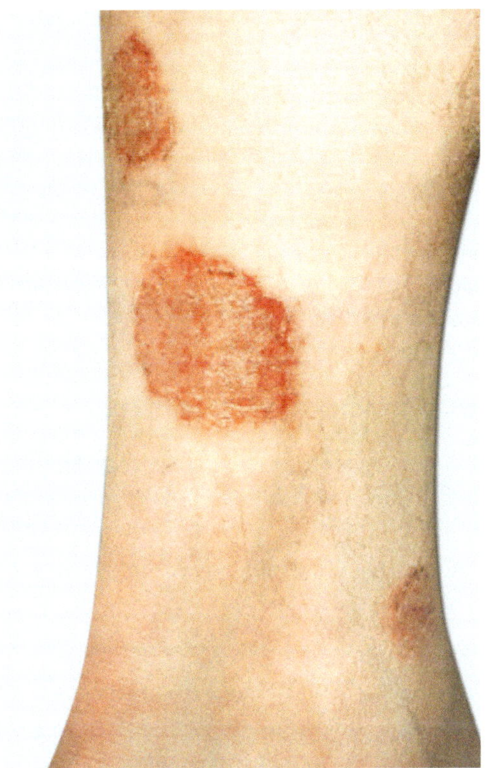

Inflammation and dryness may lead to fissuring of lesions.

CLINICAL

- Coin-shaped ("nummular"), moderately well-demarcated patches of subacute dermatitis:
  - Predominantly on legs but may occur on arms and trunk
  - Patches are occasionally enlarging and becoming confluent.

- Usually very itchy
- Typically in middle-aged men
- Often associated with dry skin:
  - Increases in dry weather
  - Worsens with excessive bathing
- Idiopathic

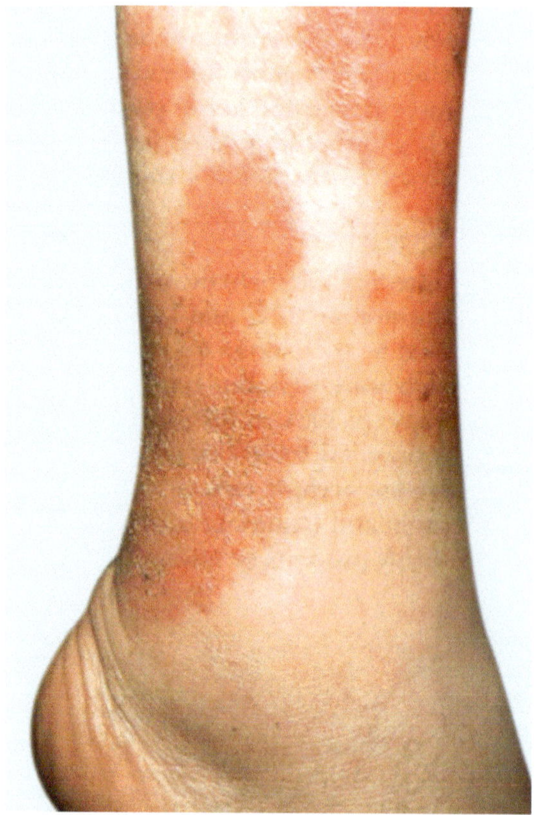

Round patches made up of inflamed puncta are not unusual.

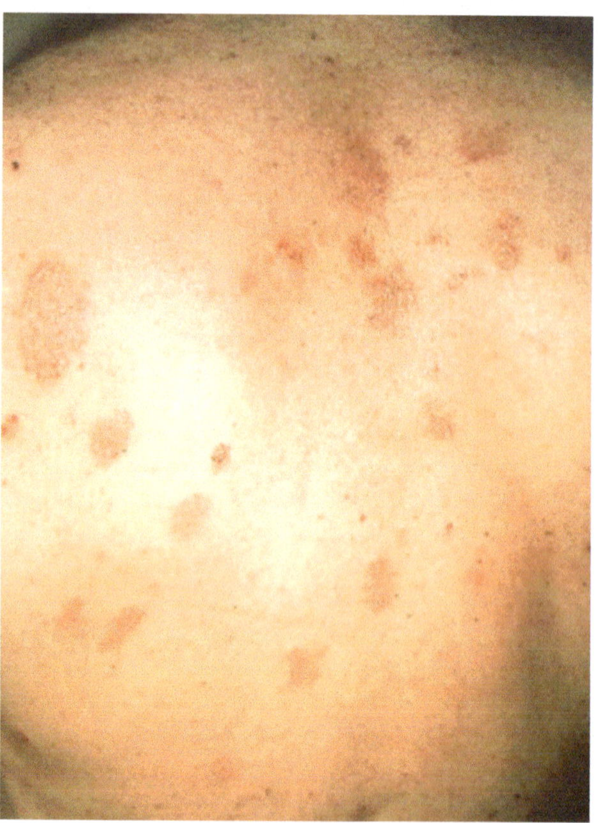

Patients with nummular eczema of the trunk usually have similar lesions that appeared earlier on the legs or arms.

TREATMENT

- In nummular eczema, there is often a paradox of clinical appearance and response to therapy: The mild-appearing dermatitis requires potent treatment.
- Corticosteroids:
  - Potent topical corticosteroids are often necessary.
    - Use milder agents for maintenance.
  - Ointments provide better potency and lubrication.
  - Occlusion (Cordran tape**)**
  - Systemic corticosteroids should be used briefly for stubborn cases.
- Prevention and treatment of dry skin (*See* page 111):
  - Probably prevents or minimizes nummular eczema

5 CHAPTER

Trunk and Generalized

Atopic Dermatitis

Note: Many patients and physicians use the word "eczema" for atopic dermatitis, but eczema is merely a synonym for "dermatitis" and should have a qualifier preceding it (e.g., stasis or contact).

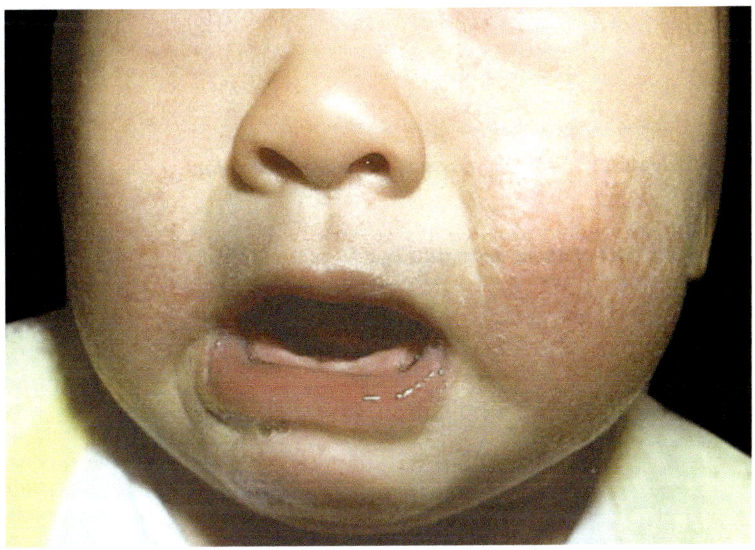

Early acute atopic dermatitis as typical "chapped cheeks" in an infant.

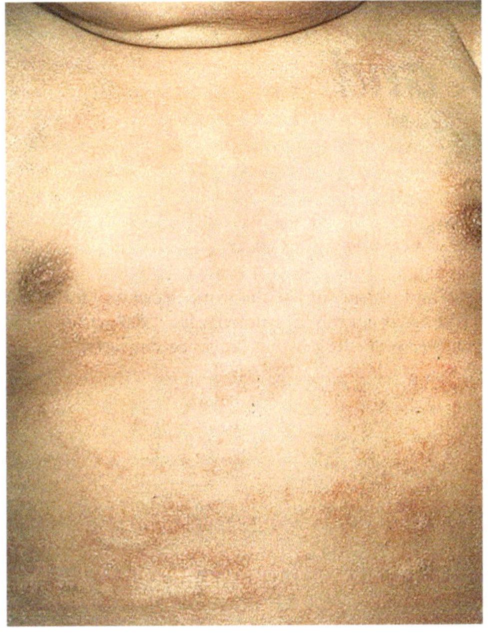

Early scattered atopic eczema of the trunk of an infant.

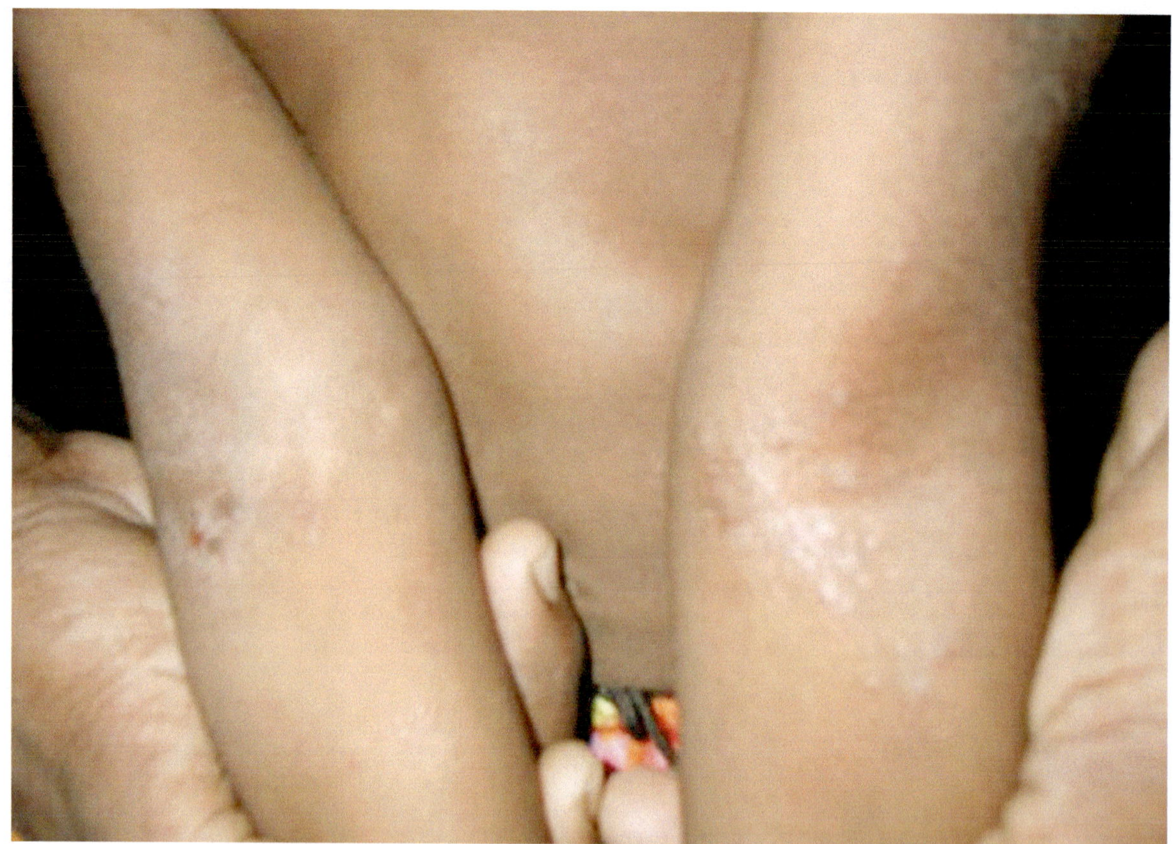

Atopic dermatitis in flexors.

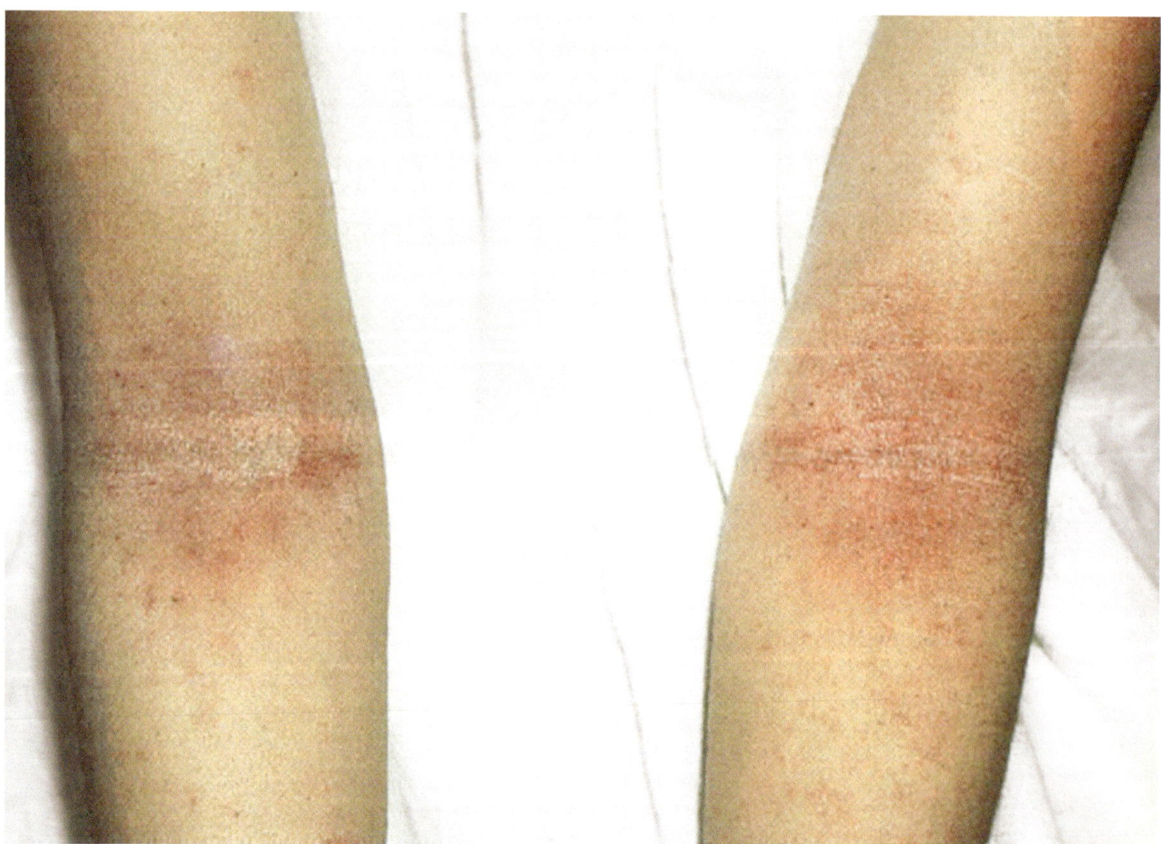

Acute flare of atopic dermatitis in a 10-year-old child.

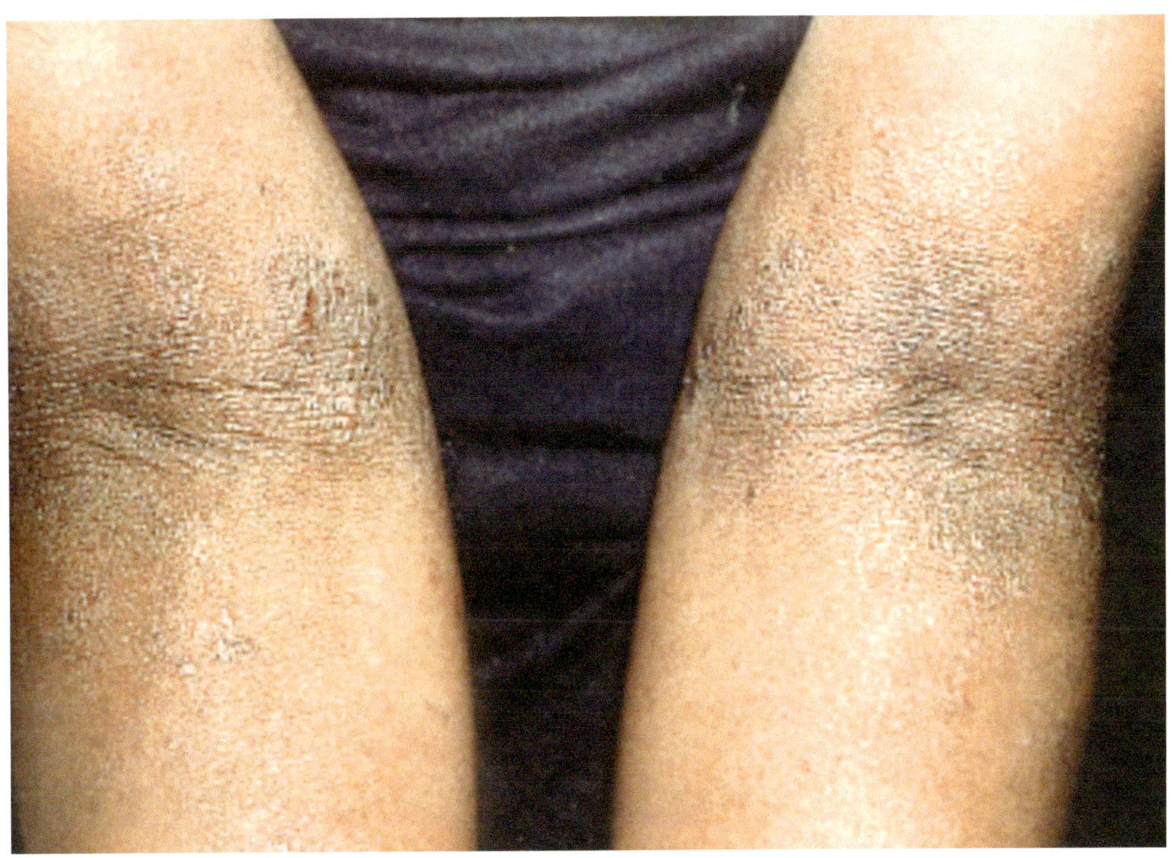

Chronic lichenified atopic dermatitis in a 10-year-old child.

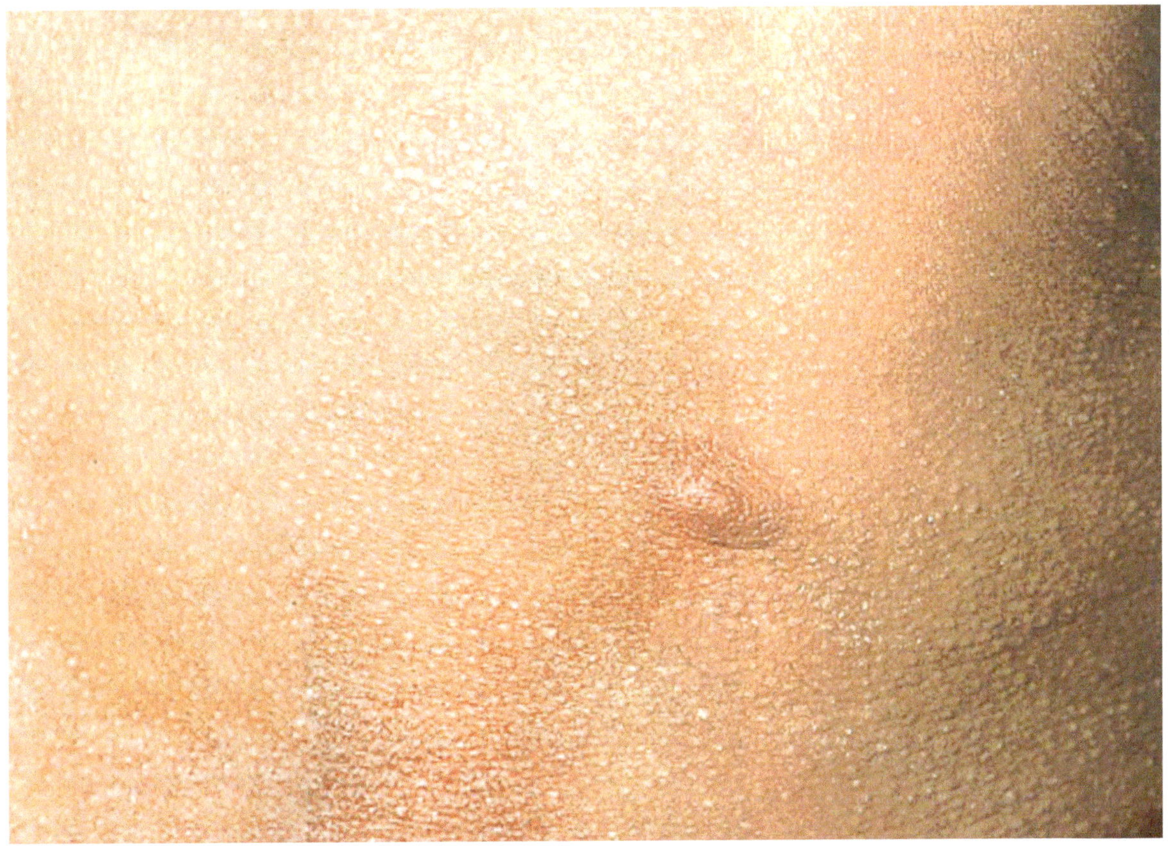

Mild papular eczema in a child.

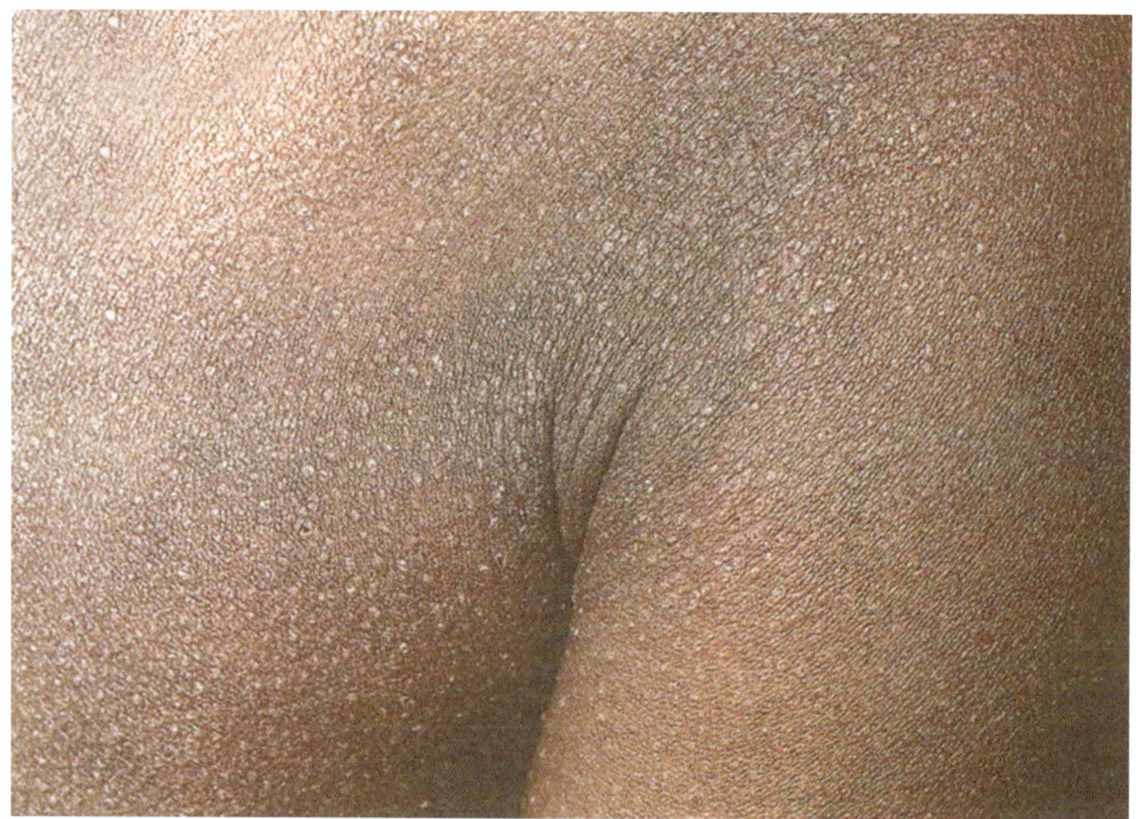

Severe papular eczema in a child.

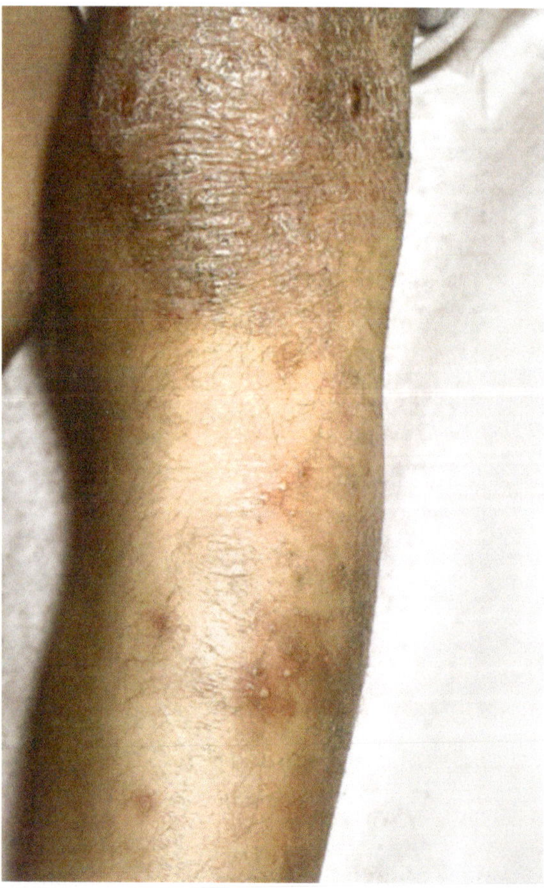

Infected eczema of knee with staphylococcal pustules on skin.

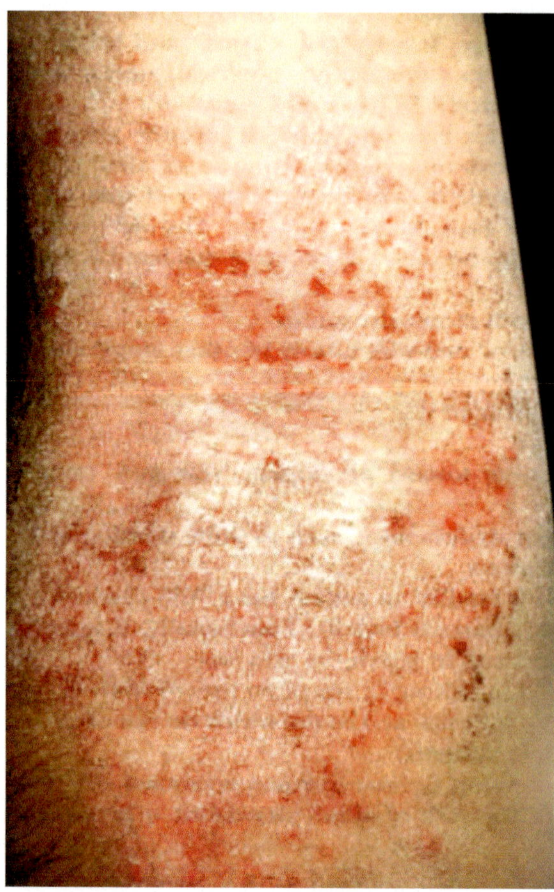

Severely infected flexural atopic dermatitis.

CLINICAL

- Atopic dermatitis is a complex inherited condition, the appearance of which varies greatly and which can change with age and environment. The rash can be bright red, edematous, and oozing; it can be chronic, lichenified, and hyperpigmented; or it can be a mixture of both. Typical clinical patterns are:
  - *Infantile* atopic dermatitis is subacute (red and oozing) and appears on the scalp, face, trunk, and extensor sides of the extremities, with onset between 2 and 6 months of age. Itching may make the infant irritable and hyperkinetic.
  - *Juvenile* atopic dermatitis follows the infantile stage or occurs de novo after 1 year of age. It is typically chronic and lichenified, occurs in flexural sites (antecubital, popliteal, neck), is very itchy, and is characterized by flares and remissions.
  - *Adult* atopic dermatitis may be persisting juvenile atopic dermatitis or a chronic dermatitis appearing years after juvenile dermatitis has cleared. It may be flexural or it may appear particularly on the face, hands, or both. The dermatitis in many adults with or occupational hand eczema is atopic.
- Stigmata associated with atopic dermatitis:
  - Family history and/or personal history of other atopic diseases (rhinitis and asthma)
  - Dry, flaky, and easily irritated skin
  - Hyperlinear palms
  - Increased propensity toward developing heat rash (miliaria, *See* page 140)
  - Peripheral vascular dysfunctions, such as white dermographia
- Etiology and mechanisms
  - Atopic dermatitis is familial (a patient has a 70% chance of developing it if both parents had it). Functionally, it is best to regard it as a condition in which the skin has:
    - A low threshold to itching (a symptom provoked by dryness, rough clothing, solvents, and so on, which do not cause itching in nonatopic patients)
    - An ability to develop dermatitis when scratched or rubbed (most or all of the rash of atopic dermatitis is produced *by* scratching)

Itching and scratching can occur during sleep, aggravating the dermatitis and causing restless sleep.

  - The relationship of atopic dermatitis to allergy is complex.
    - Favoring immunologic mechanisms are the following: occurrence in persons with true allergic disease (asthma, hay fever), usually increased serum levels of immunoglobulin E (IgE), decreased sensitization to *Rhus* antigen, and frequent positive results for intradermal skin tests. There is some evidence that breastfed infants have less severe atopic dermatitis than do bottle-fed babies, but data are conflicting.
    - Against an allergic mechanism are the following: occurrence in persons with normal or absent serum levels of IgE, no correlation of skin test results with provoking agents, no benefit from withdrawal of suspected allergens in the vast majority of patients, and no response to hyposensitization therapy. Diet manipulation may be of partial benefit in a small percentage of infants and young children, but the benefit is usually modest, the diet may be very hard to follow, and, as the child grows older, he or she often can eventually tolerate the food that in infancy caused a problem.
  - Anxiety and tension often contribute to increased itching and scratching, aggravating the dermatitis.
- Skin infections by bacteria and viruses are more common or widespread in individuals with atopic dermatitis. This susceptibility is probably due to the multitudes of breaks in the physical barrier of the skin, but atopic patients also suffer transient dysfunctions of neutrophils and lymphocytes (while the dermatitis is flared), which may contribute to susceptibility.
  - Secondary bacterial pyodermas (*See* page 159) are common in atopic dermatitis, with 95% of eczema patients carrying *Staphylococcus aureus* on their skin. True infection may be manifested as:
    - Increased itching and resistance of the dermatitis to previously effective therapy
    - Scattered, tiny erosions in the dermatitis sites; itching is more intense with mild tenderness present
    - Obvious pyoderma with redness, pain, oozing, and yellow crust formation
  - Viral infections of the skin can become widespread and even systemic and life-threatening.
    - Herpes simplex can quickly spread from its small, localized site to involve wide areas of skin, usually resolving in 1–2 weeks, but viremia, pneumonia, and meningitis can occur.
    - Molluscum contagiosum may multiply to hundreds of lesions but resolves in 6–12 months.

TREATMENT

- Educate the patient and the family about the constitutional nature of the condition (*See* Patient Guides, page 250) and of the fact that the skin will itch when subject to various physical stimuli and that scratching will provoke the rash. Point out that you will instruct and treat to prevent itching so that the patient will be comfortable and have little or no rash. Telling patients that "allergens" do not influence the rash will relieve feelings of guilt and prevent repeated and frustrating attempts to find its "cause". Guilt is also relieved by mentioning to patients that, although the rash may flare with anxiety and tension, that is also true for most diseases, and "nerves" do not "cause" atopic dermatitis.

- Prevent irritation of the skin:
  - Dry skin itching is common in atopic patients, especially in dry climates or in cold climates in heated buildings (in which relative humidity is very low). Prevention and care of dry skin is important. It is discussed fully on page 111 and consists of:
    - Adequate but not excessive bathing is advised; baths and showers should be short and not extremely hot. Mild superfatted soaps should be used sparingly (e.g., just in axillae and groin) instead of detergent and deodorant soaps. Light lotions may be used as a soap substitute. Application and removal of a light lotion as a bathing substitute is messy and unnecessary.
    - After bathing, replacing skin oil with an oil, cream, or ointment is advised; lotions (*See* page 111) are pleasant to use but often contain too little lipid to be adequately moisturizing.
    - Moisturize dry skin with an oil, cream, or ointment (*See* page 111) once or twice daily, as needed. For very dry skin, a thick ointment is necessary.
  - Avoid unlined wool and polyester clothing, as they are physically rough and irritating and may cause itching. *(Note:* This is not a wool allergy.) Cotton and cotton blends are the least irritating types of clothing materials.
  - Minimize or avoid jobs, chores, or hobbies requiring excessive skin contact with grease, dirt, and solvents, or excessive water exposure (photographic developing, ceramics, automobile repairing, hairdressing, dishwashing, and so on). Protective vinyl gloves, worn on top of cotton gloves, should be worn with any wet work.
  - Avoid hot, humid jobs or climates if heat rash occurs readily, as it does in 10–20% of atopic patients. Thick ointments may provoke heat rash in these individuals.
- Topical treatment of dermatitis
  - Soaks are rarely needed.
    - The dermatitis is rarely acute and vesicular.
    - Anything drying the skin, such as soaks, may provoke dermatitis.

Topical corticosteroids (*See* page 239) are the mainstay of therapy.

-
  -
    - Do not hesitate to use potent topical corticosteroids for acute, severe, or thickly lichenified dermatitis, as they can stop itching after 30 minutes of use and their short-term use is safe.
    - Mild-potency corticosteroids (e.g., hydrocortisone 1%) are adequate for mild disease or for maintenance after use of a potent corticosteroid.
    - A corticosteroid of moderate potency may be necessary for maintenance in severe cases.
    - Use an adequate lubricating vehicle (ointment or thick cream) in dry dermatitis, in which a thin vehicle (lotion or solution) may worsen drying.
    - Use occlusion with caution, as it may provoke heat rash and enhance bacterial growth.
  - Topical calcineurin inhibitors (tacrolimus and pimecrolimus) and the boron-based phosphodiesterase 4 (PDE-4) inhibitor crisaborole are of some value
- Systemic treatment
  - Oral antibiotics are indicated when clinical signs of infection (see earlier) occur. Taking a skin culture is of little use because more than 90% of atopic patients carry *S. aureus* on their skin, especially in the rash, and its presence does not indicate active infection.
  - Oral or intramuscular corticosteroids.
    - These agents are associated with an excellent response, but, as this seems such an easy "fix," many patients will "shop around" to continue treatment.
    - If the patient's condition does not respond to topical treatment, referral to a dermatologist is the next step.
  - Although antihistamines are not directly antipruritic (*See* page 243), they will deaden perception of itching and promote comfortable sleep.
    - Especially useful in agitated children for the first few days of treatment with topical corticosteroids
    - Useful at bedtime if the patient is sleeping poorly because of itching and scratching
    - Nonsedating antihistamines (e.g., fexofenadine) of no benefit

Dry Skin (Xerosis, Asteatosis, and Winter Itch)

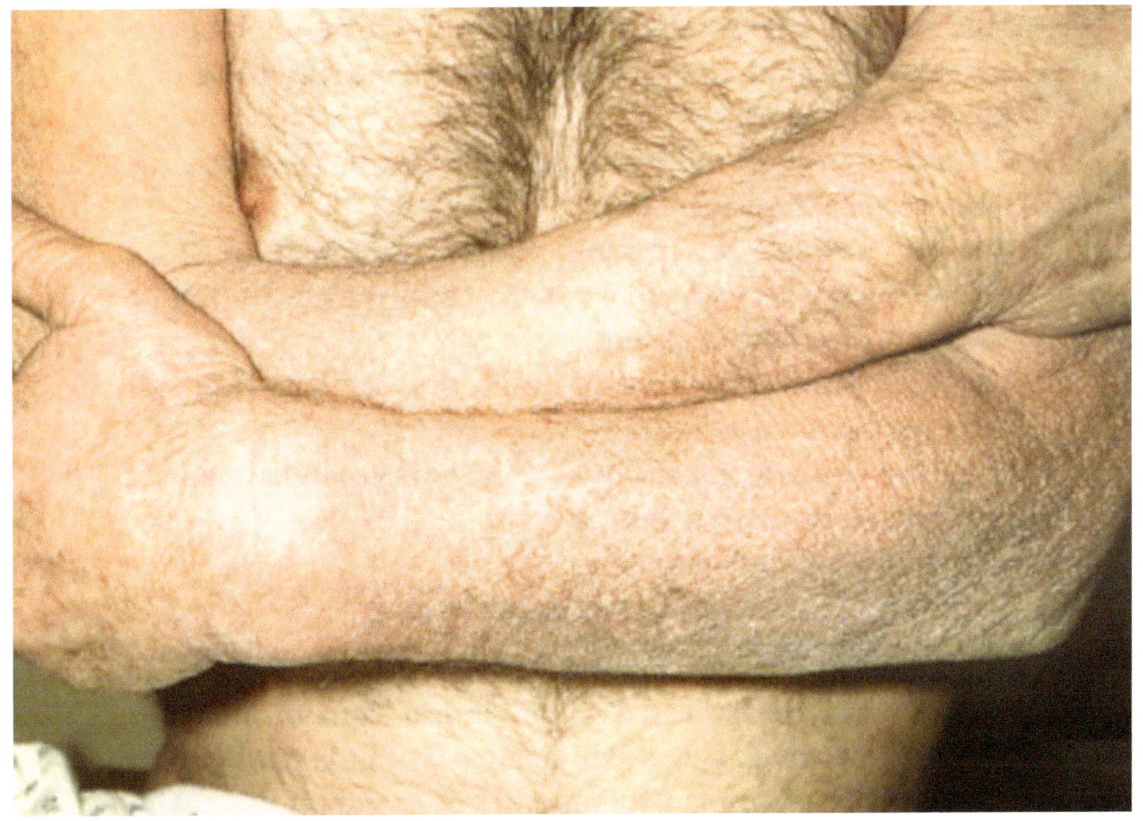

Marked dry skin of arms and trunk.

Xerosis with "eczema craquelé," or cracks in keratin layer.

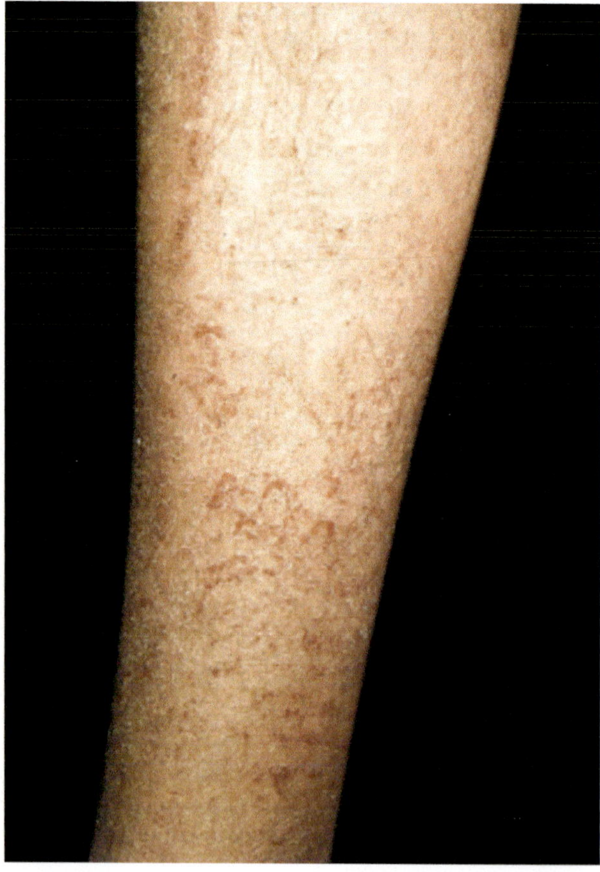

Xerosis with hemorrhage in keratin cracks; sometimes mistaken for petechiae.

CLINICAL

- Typically, this condition consists of moderate to severe itching of legs, predominantly with the appearance of dry, scaly skin.
  - May have marked itching with normal-appearing skin

By far the most common cause of pruritus without rash.

  - Other common sites are arms and trunk, but face and moist, flexural areas are spared
- A tendency to dry skin is inborn but is often not expressed until middle age or later.
  - More common in atopic patients (*See* page 103)
  - Unmasked and exacerbated by dry weather, typically in winter when central heating causes extremely low interior humidity
  - Exacerbated by bathing, as water and soap leach oil from the skin and cause "dishpan body"
- Helpful diagnostic clues are:
  - Patient describes itching as intense
  - Itching often flares a few minutes after patient goes to bed. Itching is "all over" but usually absent on face, scalp, and in flexural areas.
  - Itching ceases when patient is in the bath or shower for several minutes; the skin becomes hydrated.
    - Often leads patient to bathe more, causing more drying
  - Itching "explodes" 15–30 minutes after bathing as skin dries out.
  - Resolution occurs during humid weather or when the patient visits a warm, humid climate.
- Xerotic eczema is a condition in which dry skin may be so severe as to crack and fissure, becoming red and inflamed in the fissures (eczema craquelé), or to develop scattered, round areas of subacute eczema (nummular eczema, *See* page 101).

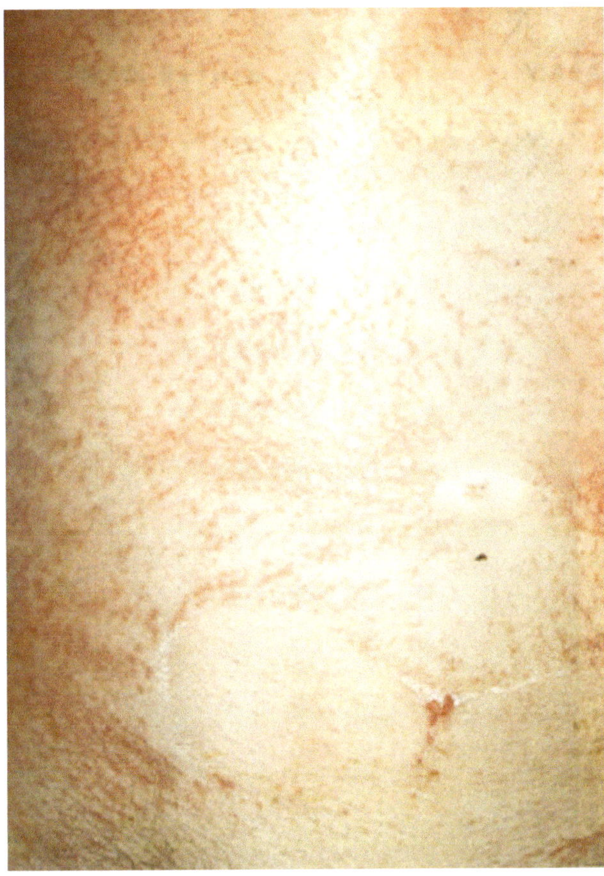

Severe xerosis with cracking and hemorrhage in a patient repeatedly washed in the hospital. Note sparing where dressing occluded the skin.

TREATMENT

- Patient Guides, *See* page 251.
- Environmental manipulations are impractical. Interior humidity can be raised only by the addition of gallons of water to the air in each room each day. A large humidifying unit on a central hot-air heating system may be sufficient in a well-insulated house. Placing pans of water on radiators is of negligible benefit.
- Practical treatment consists of decreasing washing and of applying moisturizers.
- Washing, without subsequent moisturization, causes the skin to become drier and drier. Water alone can cause significant drying (persons who swim regularly may become very dry; they often erroneously attribute the dryness to chlorine in the water).
    - Frequency of bathing should be less than daily, especially in the elderly (sweating, oil output, and body odor decline with age, fortunately).
    - In showers, baths, and other forms of bathing, water temperature should be moderate—not extremely hot—and duration should be short.
    - Mild oilated or superfatted soaps are less drying than regular and deodorant bath soaps. Pure soaps efficiently remove oil and are drying. Amount and duration of sudsing should be minimal and concentrated mostly in fold areas (e.g., legs and arms need little soaping).
- Moisturizers should be applied immediately after bathing, and once or twice daily to dry-skin areas. It is recommended to apply moisturizers to wet skin, followed by gentle towel drying. Thin applications are sufficient and are more pleasant for the patient, which encourages compliance. Moisturizer selection is important. The ideal moisturizer is a thick, *pure grease* (e.g., petrolatum), because of its occlusive properties. However, this is sticky and objectionable to many patients. Also effective and usually acceptable are *water-in-oil thick creams,* such as hydrated petrolatum and aqua-aquaphor (Eucerin). Plain, stiff, canned vegetable shortening (e.g., Crisco) is similar in texture and just as effective; however, it is unattractive to most patients! Thinner oil-in water *vanishing creams* are pleasant to use but leave enough lubricant only for mildly dry skin. Even less satisfactory are lotions, which contain mostly water and are sometimes drying to the skin.

- Occlusion
  - Severe dry skin may be stubborn and not show improvement with moisturizers. To obtain fast results, apply moisturizer, then occlude with plastic wrap overnight, if possible. A vinyl exercise suit may be used for arms and legs. In the morning, bathe lightly and reapply moisturizer.

This is useful as a diagnostic test and to convince the patient that itching is from dry skin. Cessation of itching when the skin is hydrated rules out metabolic causes (uremia, diabetes, internal malignancy) and scabies.

- Topical corticosteroids, in an ointment base, are used if there is xerotic or nummular eczema (*See* page 101).

Contact Dermatitis

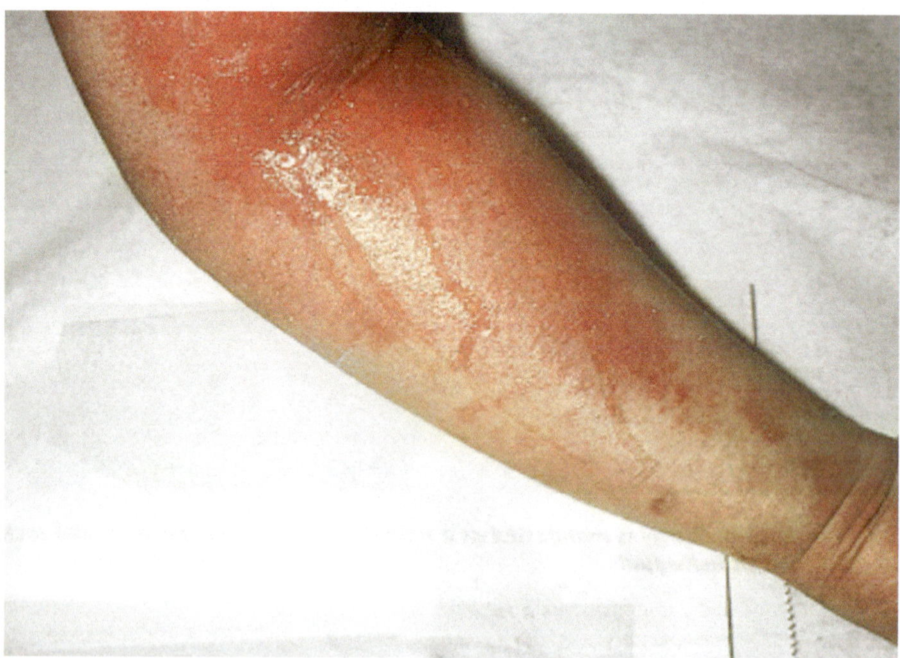

Acute weeping allergic contact dermatitis to topical anesthetic "anti-itch cream."

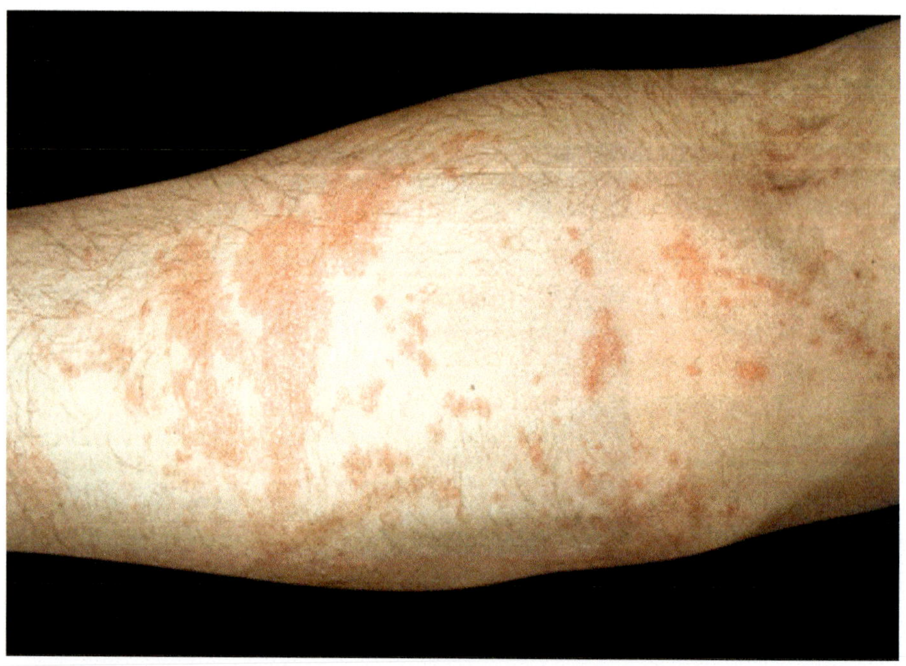

Typical linear allergic dermatitis from Rhus plant contact. Lines result from brushing of branches as a person walks through underbrush.

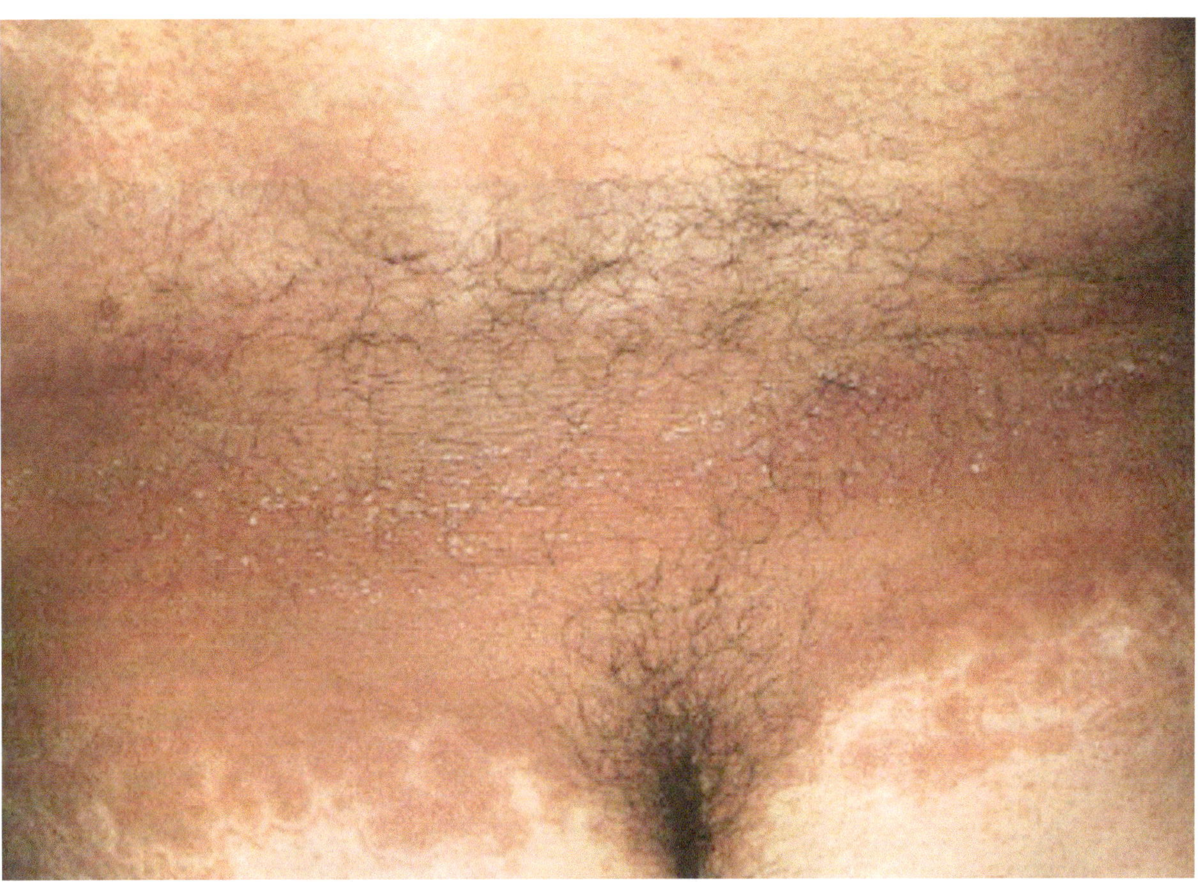

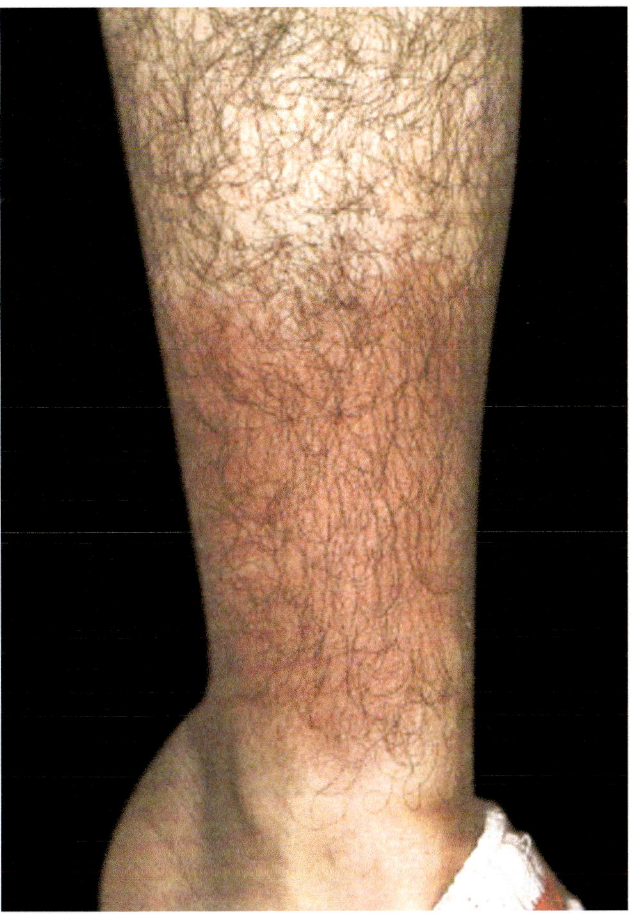

Rubber allergy is manifested as a reaction to elastic in underwear and socks in this individual.

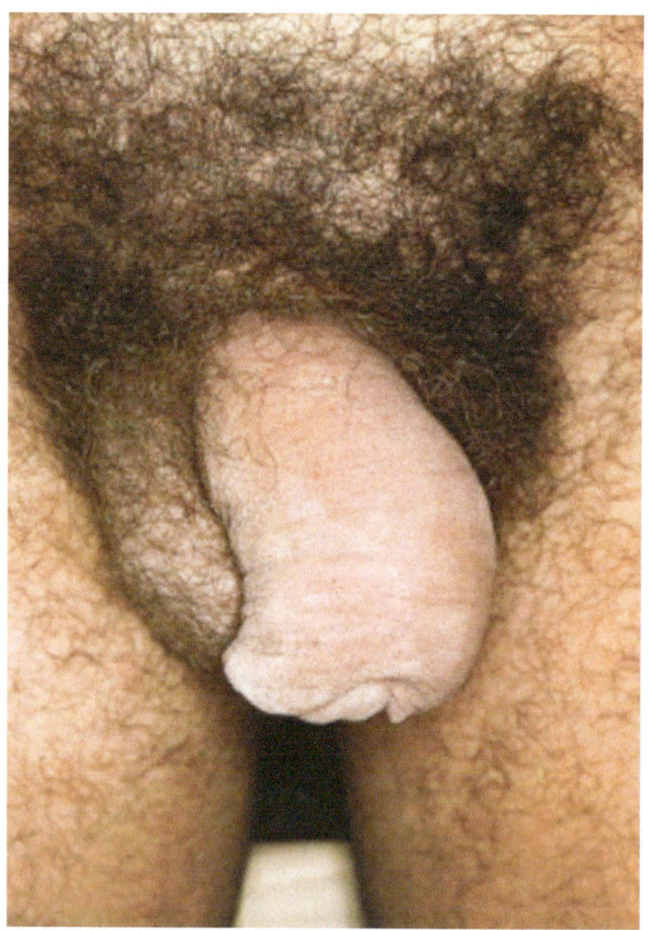

Rhus allergy. Antigen is carried on hands to seemingly protected sites.

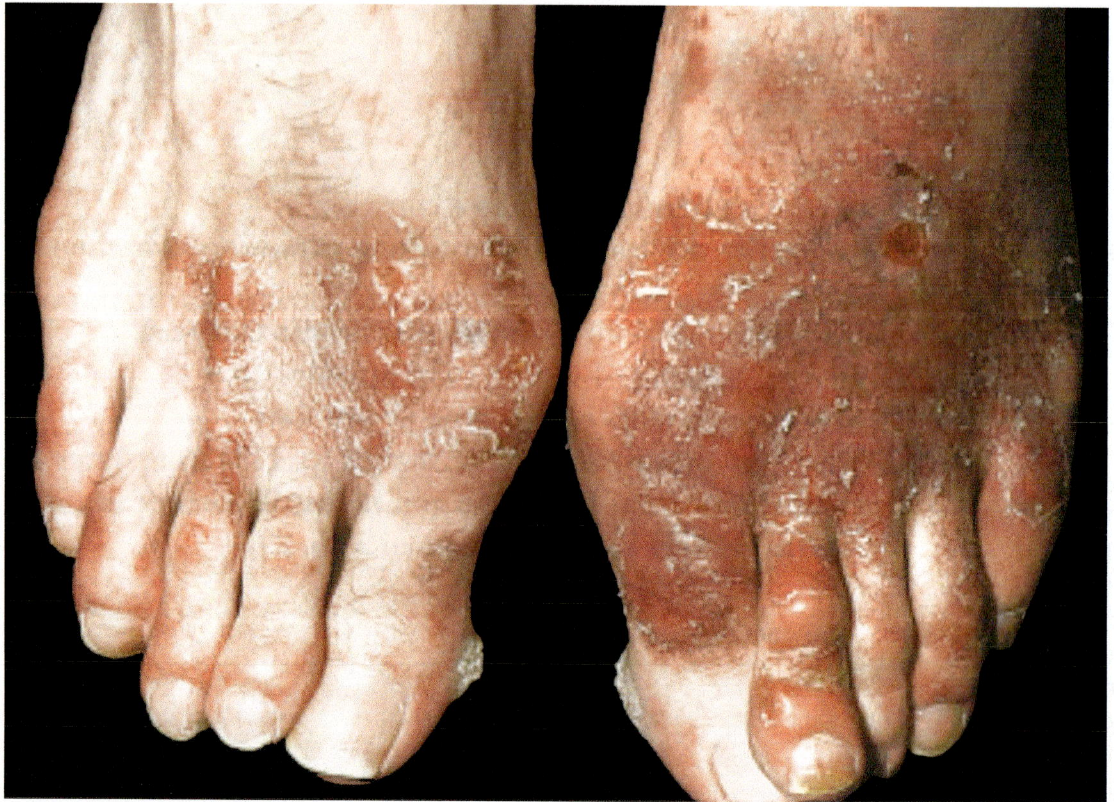

This patient is allergic to the leather in his shoes. He earlier had reacted under a leather watchband.

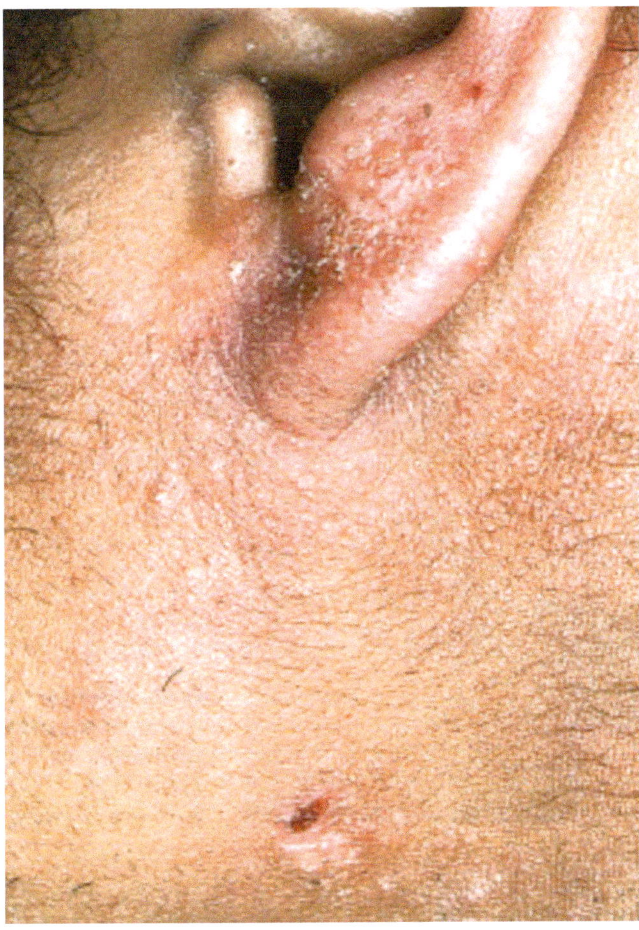

Contact dermatitis in a person allergic to nickel in jewelry (earring).

CLINICAL

- There are two forms:
  - i. Irritant
  - ii. Allergic
- Irritant contact dermatitis is more common.
  - Occasionally occurs acutely, with one exposure, as a chemical burn
  - More commonly occurs slowly with chronic exposure
    - Dryness, scaling, fissuring, and mild inflammation
    - May require years of exposure or just days
    - Most common type: Hand dermatitis (*See* page 77) from water and cleansers or from moisturizers and industrial chemicals
    - Also occurs on face from cosmetics (*See* page 19)
- Allergic contact dermatitis varies with cultures and environments.
  - Because sensitization is required, allergic contact dermatitis infrequently occurs on first exposure to allergen.
    - With some potent allergens, if exposure is constant, patients can develop sensitization and react in as few as 10 days.
    - Patients may become sensitized on first exposure, after many exposures, or never, depending on unknown host factors and the potency of the antigen (*Rhus* plants sensitize 60–80%, rubber sensitizes 0.01%).
  - For *Rhus* plant antigens (poison oak, poison ivy, mango rind), topical medications, and liquid antigens, reaction is often an acute vesicular dermatitis.
  - For leather, rubber, and nickel, reaction is often a low-grade chronic dermatitis.
  - The *first time* an individual reacts acutely, the rash usually starts 1–4 days after contact, new lesions may occur for 10 days, and the eruption commonly lasts 2–3 weeks.
  - With *subsequent exposures* and reactions, the rash often starts earlier, new spots appear for only a few days, and resolution occurs in 7–10 days. However, the course may be prolonged, similar to that of the primary reaction.

The daily development of new lesions, especially in primary attacks, has given rise to the myth that scratching or blister fluid "spreads" the reaction. In reality, the antigen becomes fixed to skin proteins in about 15 minutes. Before that time, it can be washed off to prevent or diminish a reaction. After that time, the fixed antigen cannot be removed. Excess antigen can be washed off with water and soap (no special soap is necessary unless the antigen is a chemical or medication in an unusual base). Excess antigen can be spread by rubbing, until it becomes fixed. The new lesions developing days after the rash began represent areas that were exposed to less antigen initially or a variable immunologic response.

- Diagnosis of allergic contact dermatitis is by history and by the presence of an eruption in patterns suggestive of the causative agent. Local factors determine the most common culprits. In the United States,
  - *Rhus* plant allergy is by far the most common and often occurs in linear patterns from the brushing of stems against the skin during gardening or walking in underbrush or on the face or genitals, where hands deposit allergen.
  - Rubber sensitization occurs from shoes and under elastic (underwear).
  - Nickel dermatitis occurs from jewelry.
  - Topical medicament dermatitis occurs from antibiotics, benzocaine, antihistamines, and preservatives.

Allergic contact dermatitis rarely occurs before 10 years of age. In children, contact dermatitis is usually irritant: wool and soap "allergy" in children is always mildly irritant, usually in atopic children with low itch threshold (*See* page 103). Allergic reactivity diminishes in the elderly.

- Patch testing is performed in persistent, puzzling cases. Refer the patient to a dermatologist experienced in this procedure.

TREATMENT

- General:
  - Determine cause and suggest avoidance.
  - For chronic irritant hand dermatitis, refer to page 81 for complete discussion.
  - If substitution (e.g., leather and rubber) is difficult, refer the patient to an experienced dermatologist, who usually knows of sources of substitutes.
  - In jewelry dermatitis, many patients can tolerate high-grade gold and silver, which are low in nickel. If they cannot, they may coat jewelry with urethane varnish for "special occasions." Clear nail polish is sometimes suggested but wears off more easily.
- Mild-to-moderate dermatitis is treated with topical corticosteroids (*See* page 237).
  - Vehicle:
    - Ointments for dry, scaly, and fissured dermatitis
    - Solutions for scalp or moist fold areas
    - Creams may be used but are less potent.
  - Potency:
    - Potent corticosteroid for inflamed, itchy, and/or thickened dermatitis
    - Mild-to-moderate potency for mild dermatitis or after the condition has improved through treatment with a potent preparation.
- Acute, vesicular, and/or widespread dermatitis (prototype is *Rhus* plant allergic dermatitis)
  - A small area can be treated with soaks, baths, or compresses three times daily for 10–20 minutes.
    - Use tap water or astringent solutions (*See* page 241).
    - Follow soaks with potent topical corticosteroid.
  - Widespread or severe dermatitis (edema of face or hands, difficulty in sleeping) usually responds only to *systemic corticosteroids.*
  - Be sure to establish any history of glaucoma, hypertension, diabetes, and so on, and monitor if appropriate. Warn the patient of possible gastric irritation and psychological side effects (depression, euphoria, and depersonalization) during short-term use.
    - The oral route is as fast as the intramuscular; the benefit starts in 12–16 hours.
    - For adults, dosing usually starts at 40–60 mg of prednisone or equivalent taken in the morning. This may be taken with food to minimize gastrointestinal upset.
    - If there is no benefit in 36–48 hours, increase the dosage to 100 mg daily for several days.

- Corticosteroids help edema, redness, and itching but often do not completely clear the rash. *Note:* New, but mild spots of rash may appear during treatment, especially in the primary attack. Warn patient of this possibility to minimize disappointment.
- If *primary attack,* administer the initial dose for about 5 days, then slowly taper off over 2–3 weeks. If the medication is discontinued too soon, the rash will flare (as immune reaction is not complete).
- If *repeated attack* (patient has had recent eruptions), it may be possible to taper off the treatment over 10–12 days.

If it has been some years (>10) since the last attack, a new attack is more likely to behave as a primary attack and last 3 weeks.

- Widespread lesions may also be treated with baths and soaks (*See* page 241), especially if vesicular.
- Oral antihistamines or sedatives may be used at bedtime to aid sleep.

- Desensitization is not effective or practical.
  - In the United States, over-the-counter oral *Rhus* preparations exist for supposed desensitization. They do not work and often cause gastrointestinal upset and perianal dermatitis.
  - Experimental desensitization has been achieved but is difficult and must be continued as long as there is risk of allergen exposure.

Psoriasis

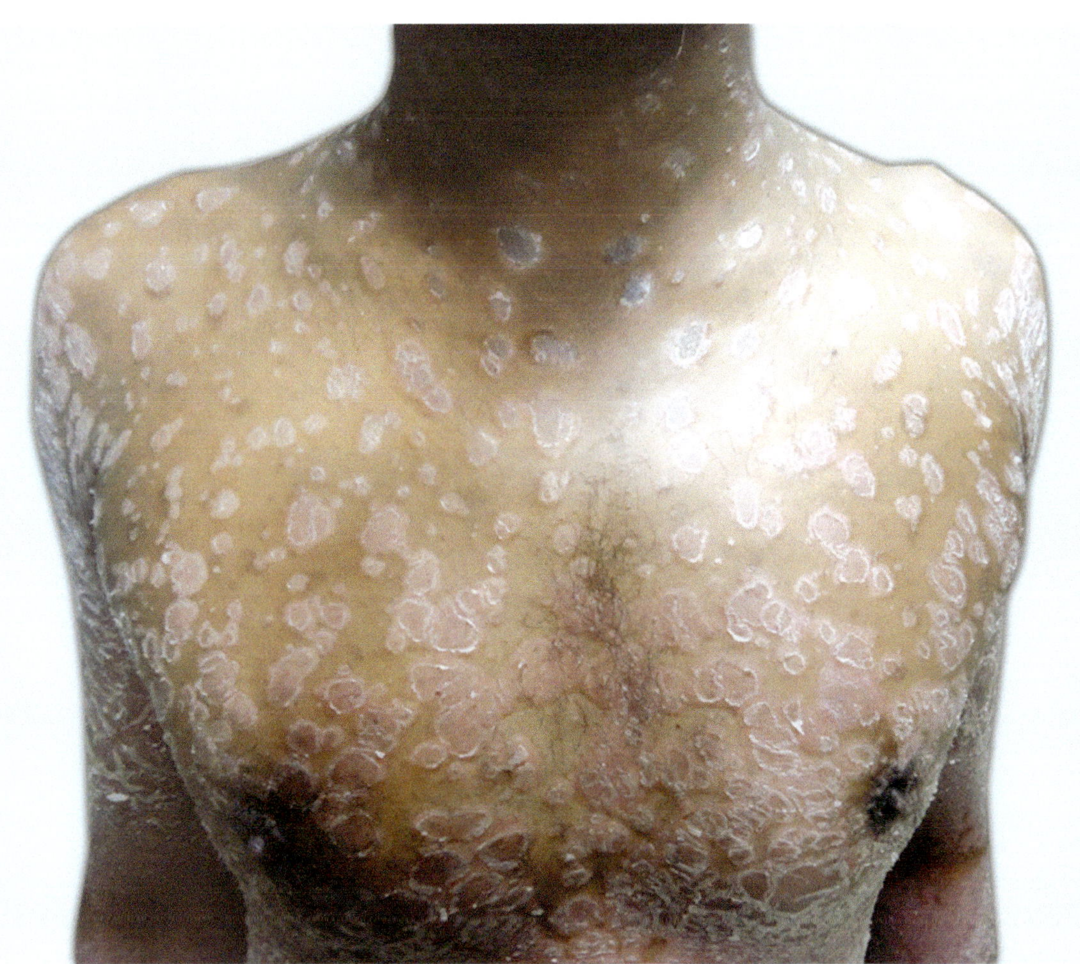

Psoriasis triggered by beta-blocker in an adult. Note the varying stages, guttate papules, plaques, and lichenoid hue.

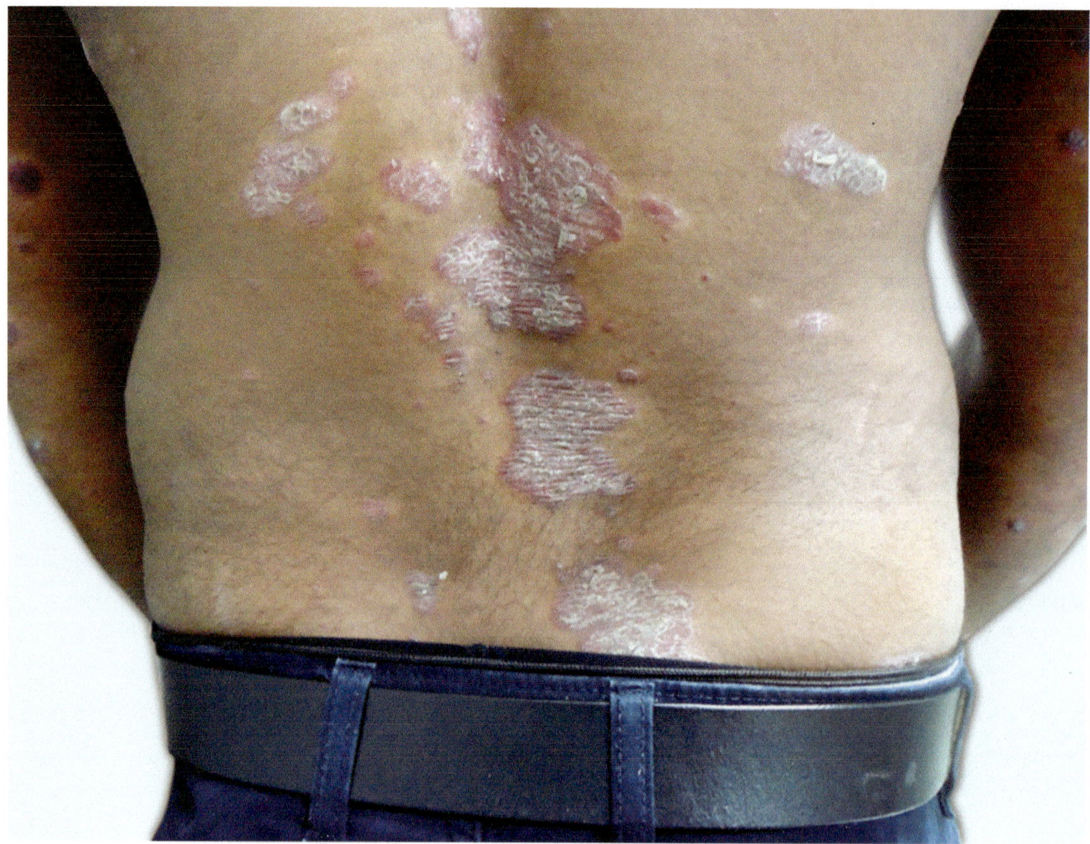

Salmon pink plaques with silvery scales of psoriasis, showing uniform appearance.

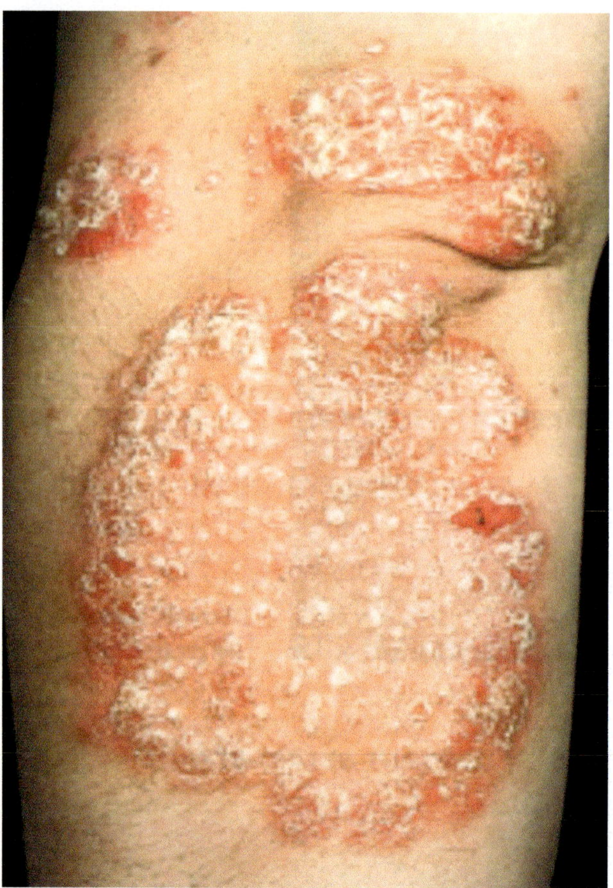

Typical bright red scaly plaque of psoriasis with silvery scale over a joint.

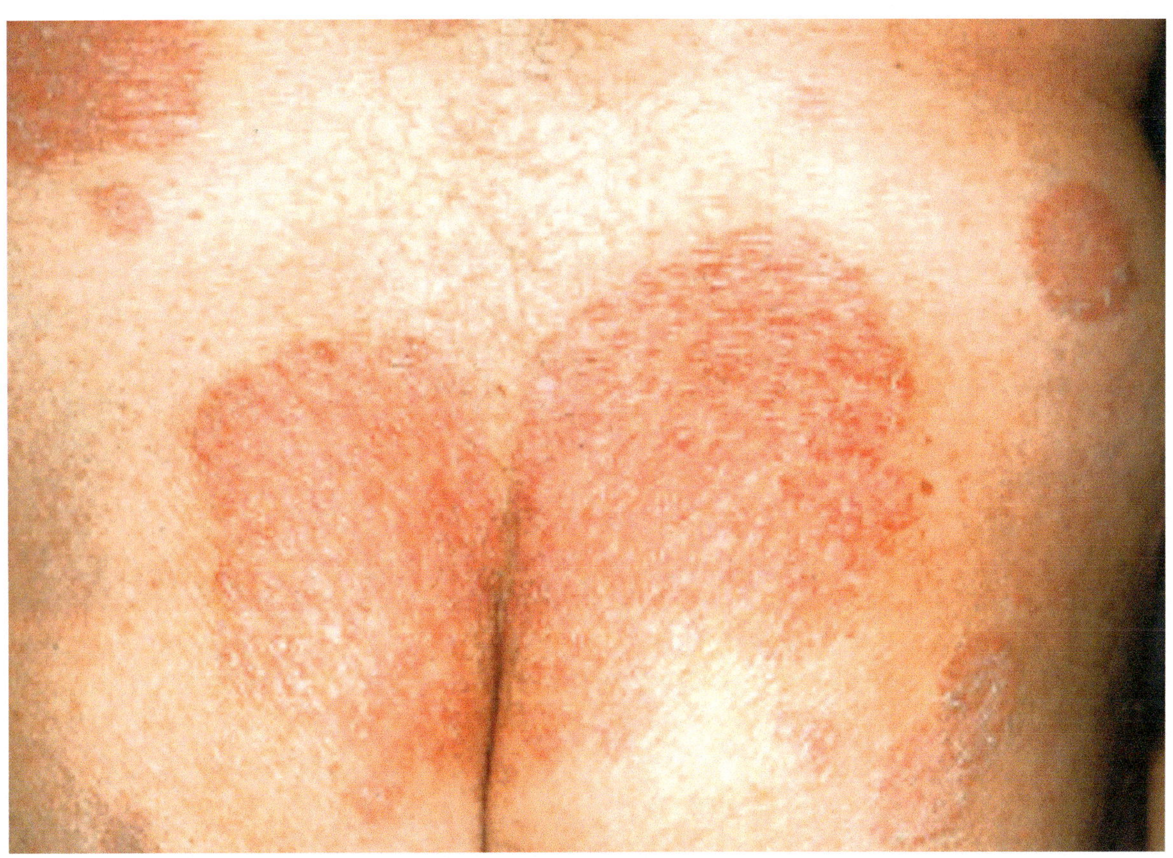

Mild, widespread plaque psoriasis, may show little scaling.

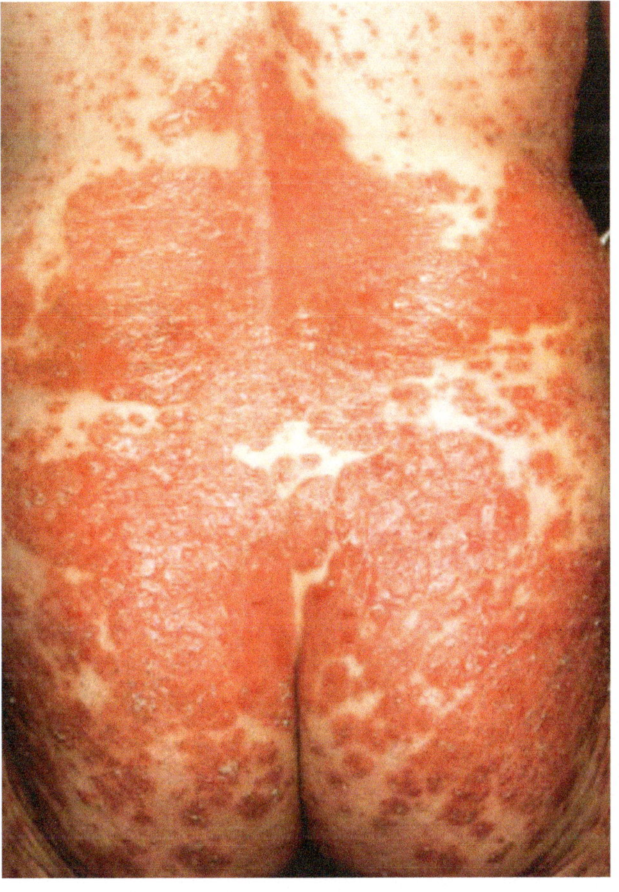

Acute, angry flare of psoriasis.

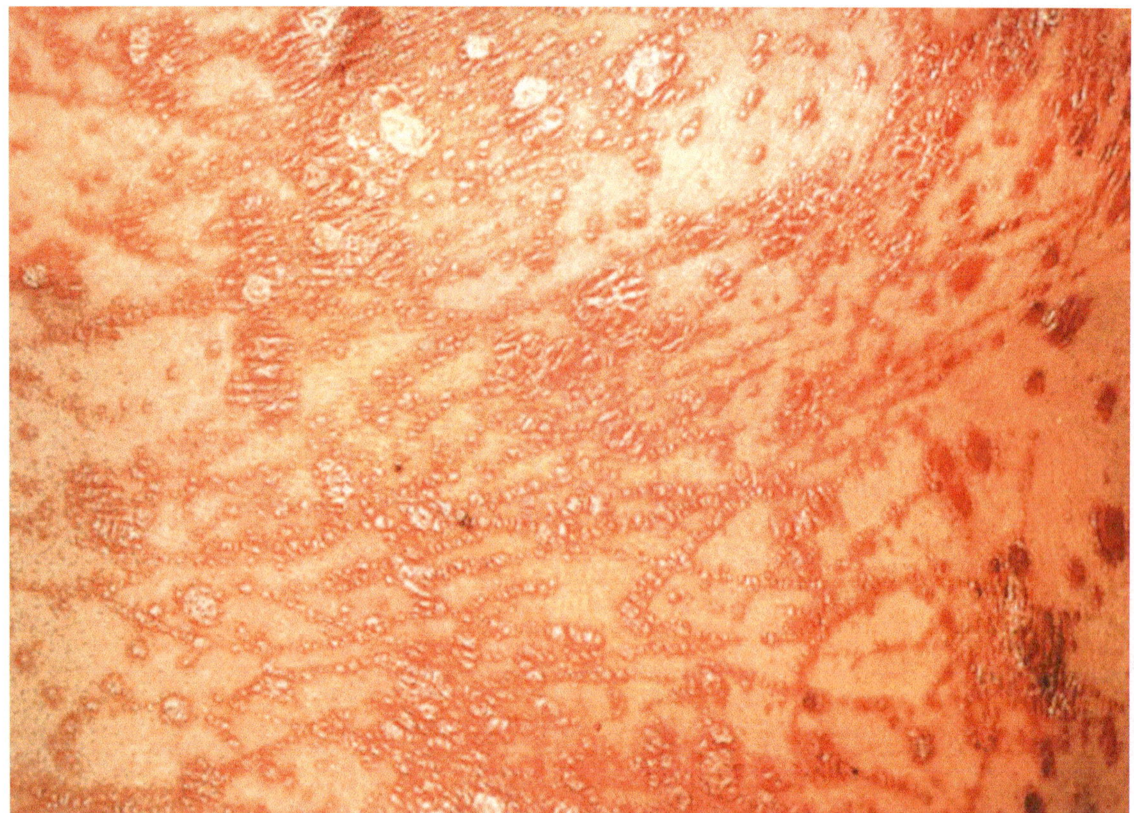

Koebner phenomenon, or development of psoriasis at sites of trauma, in this case, scratching.

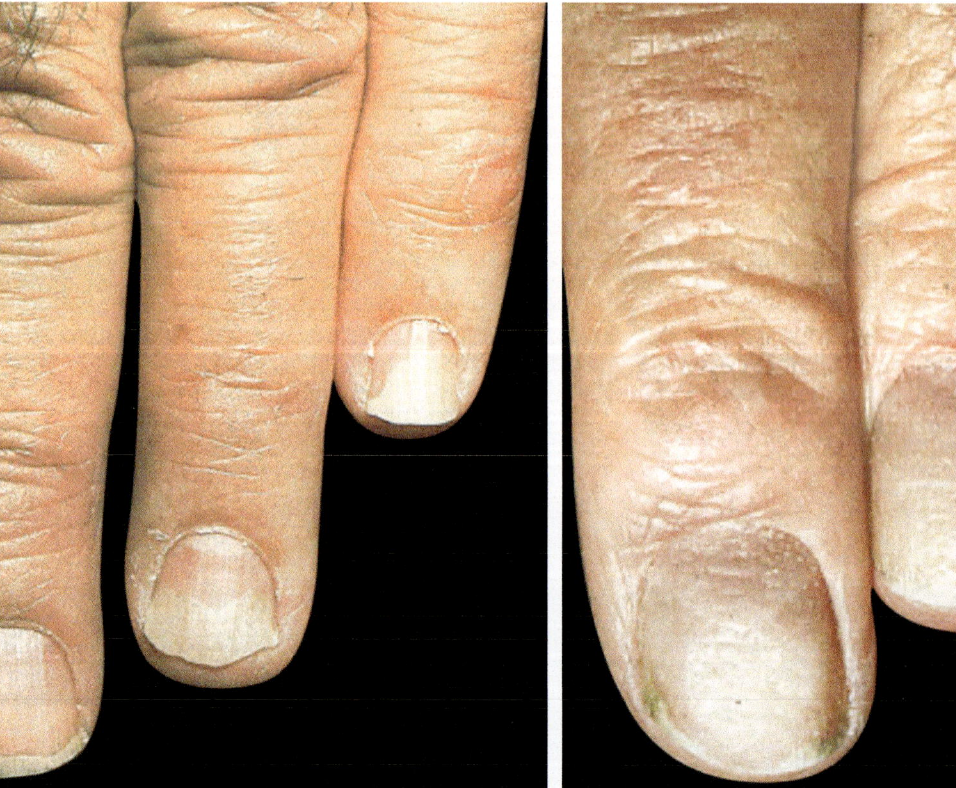

Nail changes in psoriasis may include onycholysis (lifting of distal edge of nail plate from the nail bed), accumulation of subungual debris, and pitting of the nail surface.

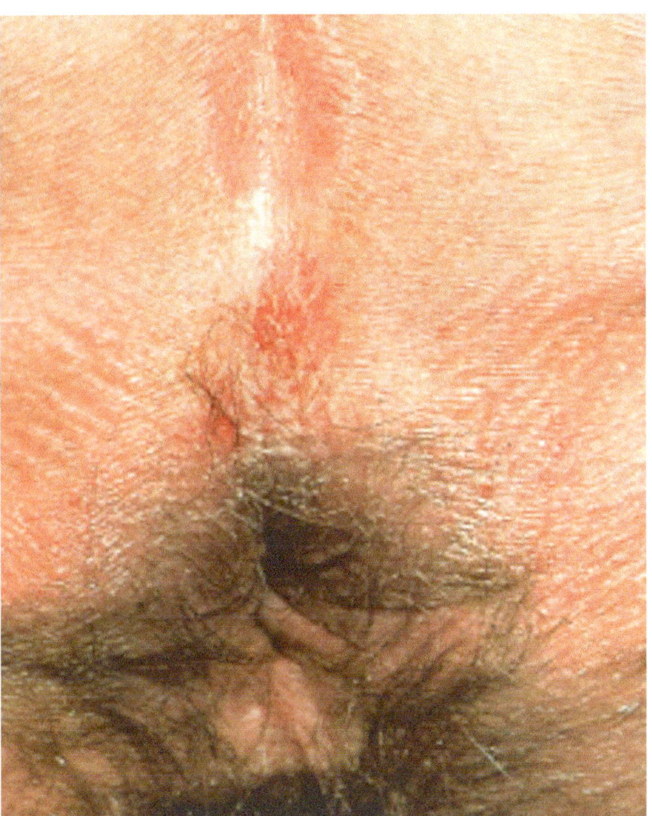

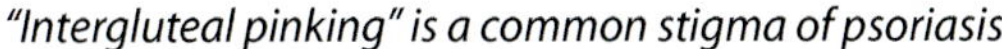

"Intergluteal pinking" is a common stigma of psoriasis.

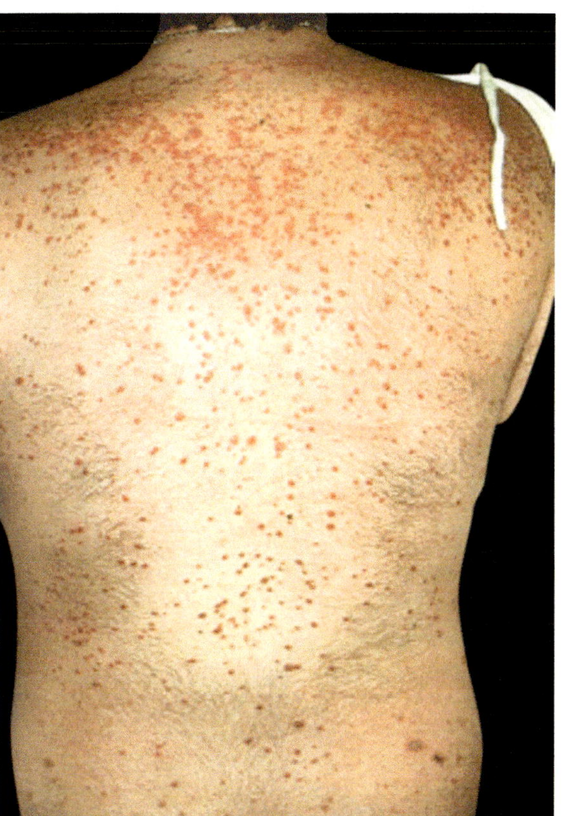

Guttate or droplike psoriasis on trunk. Eruption often follows a streptococcal pharyngitis.

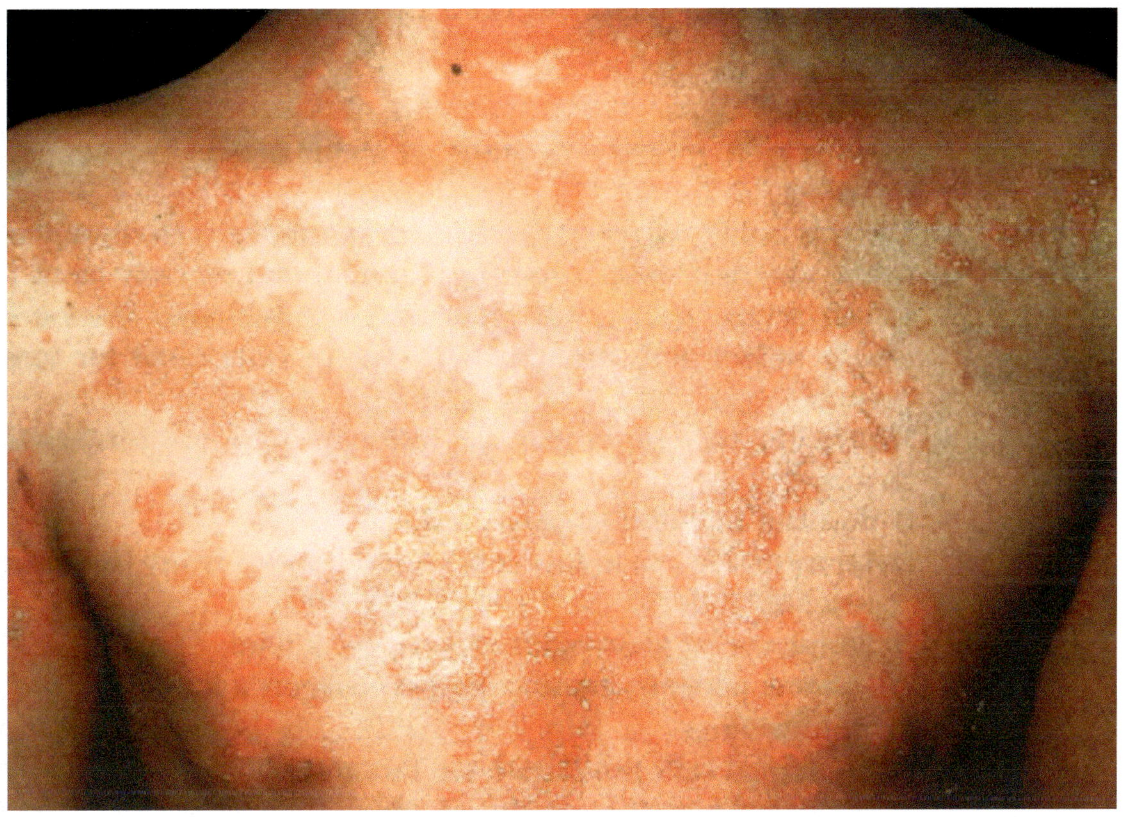

Acute, widespread pustular psoriasis. Often the eruption is bright red with bizarre patterns and pustules predominantly at the margins.

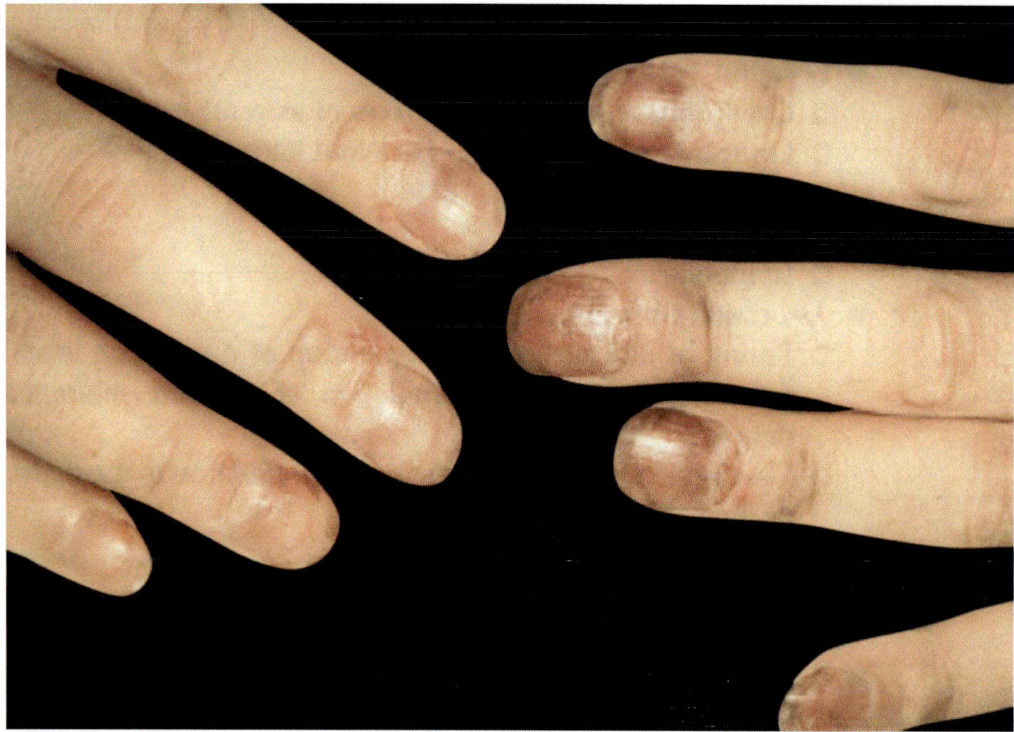

Acute psoriatic arthritis, typically affecting the distal interphalangeal joints. The nearby nails are almost always involved.

CLINICAL

- Psoriasis is often an inherited constitutional ability of skin to form psoriatic lesions.
  - Onset is usually in young adulthood, but range is from infancy to the elderly. Psoriasis starting in childhood or early teens is usually severe and is unlikely to remit. Adult-onset disease is usually milder and may wax and wane or even remit for long periods.
  - Expression of lesions may be influenced by environmental factors.
    - Sun and humidity suppress lesions.
    - Injury to skin can induce lesions at the site of injury (Koebner reaction).
    - Streptococcal pharyngitis may trigger a flare.
    - In some patients, emotional upset triggers a flare.
  - Pathophysiology
    - Epidermal cells proliferate too fast and pile up.
    - Abnormal keratin is produced, which forms loosely adherent scales.
    - Dermal inflammation occurs.
    - Cell-mediated immunity plays a pivotal role (cyclosporine administration causes a prompt and dramatic benefit).
- The condition appears as widespread, bright pink plaques surmounted by loose, and silvery scale.
  - Location:
    - Over joints and extensor surfaces of extremities
    - On trunk, especially lower back and buttocks
    - On palms and soles (*See* page 81)
    - On scalp (*See* page 5)
    - In umbilicus
  - Associated clinical signs:
    - Pitting of nail surface and separation of distal edge of nail from nail bed with accumulation of crumbly subungual debris
    - "Intergluteal pinking": Almost eroded pinkness in the depths of the intergluteal crease
    - Pink macules or plaques on penis
    - Hyperkeratosis over elbows, knees, and ankles
    - Geographic tongue (rarely)
  - Itching ranges from mild to severe but may be absent

- Uncommon clinical variants
  - Guttate (droplike):
    - Many small lesions scattered profusely over trunk and extremities
    - Scalp and nails often spared
    - Often follows streptococcal pharyngitis
    - Quite responsive to therapy and often resolves completely in a few months
  - Inverse (flexural)
    - Occurs in fold areas such as axillae, groin, and under breasts
    - Because of moist occlusion usually has no scale
  - Pustular
    - Almost eroded, bright red areas with scattered superficial pustules
    - Not infected; pustules are sterile.
    - Painful or burning discomfort
    - Often accompanied by fever and malaise; may lead to cachexia and death
    - Responds poorly to therapy and signals low likelihood of future mild psoriasis.
  - Erythroderma
    - Bright erythema of most or all of skin surface
    - Disturbs temperature regulation (hypothermia) and doubles or triples demand on cardiac output
    - Responds poorly to therapy and signals low likelihood of future mild psoriasis
- Systemic signs and symptoms
  - Psoriatic arthritis
    - Destructive arthritis of distal interphalangeal joints, spine, and large joints
    - Rheumatoid factor negative
    - May occur with no or only subtle skin signs, but nail changes often present
  - In severe widespread psoriasis it is possible to see
    - Benign lymphadenopathy
    - Fever, chills, and hypothermia
    - Increased cardiac demand and high-output heart failure
    - Increased erythrocyte sedimentation rate and uric acid, decreased serum albumin and iron, and anemia

TREATMENT

Because psoriasis is inborn, it can be suppressed but not cured. It may stay in spontaneous or induced remission for weeks, months, or years.

Agents used to treat psoriasis

- Topical corticosteroids
- Calcipotriene or calcipotriol
- Topical salicylic acid
- Tar
- Ultraviolet B (UVB)
- Tar and UVB
- Topical or oral psoralen and UVA (PUVA)
- Parenterals and oral biologics

Therapies are many and attack the disease in different ways. A summary of the agents and their effects appears in the **Box** above.

- Complete clearing of psoriasis may be achieved with the newer biologic agents.
- *See* pages 5 and 81 for treatment of scalp and palmar psoriasis.
- *See* Patient Guides, page 254.
- Mild-to-moderate psoriasis
  - Topical corticosteroids (*See* page 237)
    - Potent ones usually necessary
    - Mild ones for face and genitals, and for maintenance
    - Occlusion (*See* page 238) (shower cap, plastic wrap, vinyl suit, corticoid-impregnated tape) for stubborn areas
  - Calcipotriene or calcipotriol
    - In ointment base is applied twice daily, but once daily is fairly effective.

        - Begin to see benefit in 2 weeks; maximum benefit in 6–8 weeks.
        - 10% of patients clear, 20% do not improve at all, and the rest see moderate improvement.
        - May be irritating, more so in fold areas; commonly irritates the face (do not use there).
        - Vitamin D analog may induce hypercalcemia, so use is restricted to 100 g per week.
        - Useful adjunct with PUVA [oral psoralen and long-wave ultraviolet light (UVA)] to reduce total required ultraviolet dose.
        - Expensive.
    - Tars (*See* page 244)
        - Usually as adjunct to corticosteroid
        - Judicious exposure to sunlight: Enhances effect
        - Do not occlude—may induce irritant and microbial folliculitis
- Severe plaque psoriasis
    - The treatments discussed previously for milder forms may be effective, especially if occlusion is used. If they are not, then much more complex, expensive, time-consuming, or risky therapy must be attempted-refer to a dermatologist, if possible.
    - Artificial UVL in sunburn wavelengths [mainly narrow-band ultraviolet B (UVB)]
        - Used in conjunction with tar
        - Total-body "light box" most convenient
        - Two- or three-times weekly treatments in office
        - Home use: Patient may construct or purchase box
        - Maintenance treatment: Should be performed a few times a month of intensive treatment
    - Admission to a hospital or a psoriasis day care center—but not widely available
        - Goeckerman treatment of twice daily tar baths, tar ointments, and UVB is advised.
        - Remission is often achieved in 2–3 weeks and lasts 2–6 months or longer.
    - PUVA
        - Should be administered only by highly trained individuals in offices.
        - Excellent response but quick relapse if not given one to four times a month.
        - Long-term safety unknown; may cause an increase in skin carcinomas.
    - Antimetabolites
        - Are used less and less due to better safety and efficacy of biologic agents
        - Methotrexate is effective and requires careful clinical and laboratory monitoring.
        - Should be administered only by experienced practitioner.
        - Perform physical examination, routine laboratory screen, and consider liver biopsy. Give 5 mg methotrexate orally or intramuscularly; check white blood cell response in 7 days. If white cell count remains normal, then give 15–30 mg methotrexate orally or intramuscularly weekly. Psoriasis begins to improve in 2–4 weeks and the maximum benefit is reached in 6–10 weeks. Taper off by 2.5- or 5-mg doses to find the lowest effective maintenance dose (often 10–15 mg). Settle for less than total eradication of lesions. Check white cell count weekly or biweekly until maintenance dose is reached, then check monthly for white cell count drop. Every 4–6 months, check liver enzyme levels. A repeat liver biopsy should be repeated after total dosage of about 2 g. Patient should stop alcohol consumption during therapy to minimize risk of cirrhosis. Do not use methotrexate in an alcoholic patient or in a patient with liver disease. *Note:* See Guidelines of American Academy of Dermatology in the Journal of the American Academy of Dermatology, July 1988, *See* page 93.
    - Acitretin
        - Benefit starts in 2–4 weeks but may take up to a few months to see maximum benefit
        - Numerous side effects including dry skin and lips, headache, painful inflammatory paronychia, liver enzyme elevations
        - Marked teratogen—**not used in fertile women**
    - Cyclosporine
        - Administration of 3–5 mg/kg/day causes dramatic benefit in almost all patients, but relapses occur promptly when discontinued. At this dosage, a majority of patients develop reversible kidney changes within a few months, but the changes can become irreversible if treatment is continued.
        - Giving 3 mg/kg/day causes benefit without detectable kidney damage in about 50% of patients and can be continued for prolonged periods, but should not be administered longer than 12 months.
        - Risk of lymphoma or other consequences of prolonged immunosuppression unknown.

- Can quickly control refractory psoriasis, then discontinued as other treatments are initiated and become effective.
- Apremilast
  - Phosphodiesterase-4 enzyme inhibitor
  - A titrating dose is given for days 1–5, followed by 30 mg twice daily starting on day 6
  - Some patients do not tolerate apremilast due to diarrhea, nausea, or headaches.
- Biologic agents
  - Tumor necrosis factor (TNF)-α inhibitors and interleukin (IL)—12/23, 17, and 23-inhibitors have revolutionized the treatment of psoriasis. A multitude of other agents (e.g., oral small molecule inhibitors) are being investigated.

- Pustular psoriasis and erythroderma require immediate referral to a dermatologist. Admission to hospital and intensive topical therapy are usually required.
- Psoriatic arthritis
  - Standard disease-modifying therapies often of benefit in mild-to-moderate disease
  - In severe disease, biologic agents are preferred.

Pityriasis Rosea

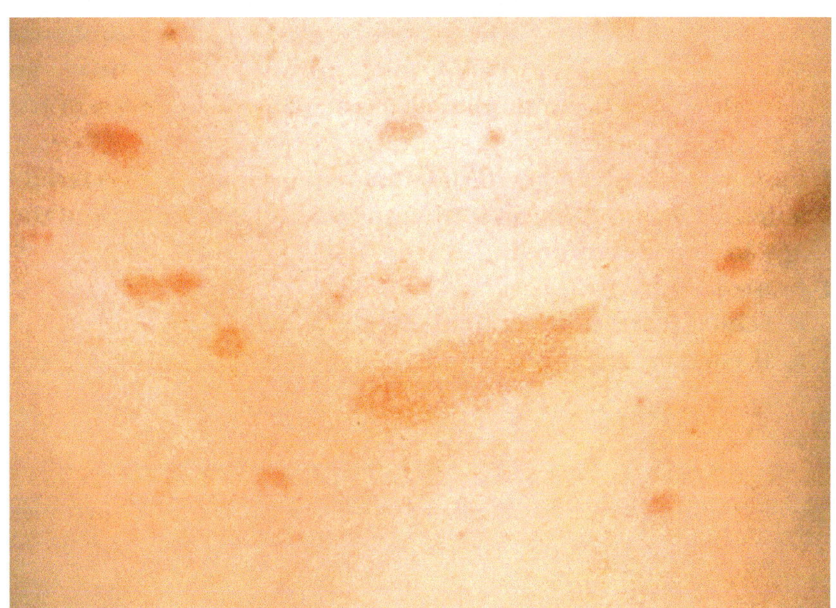

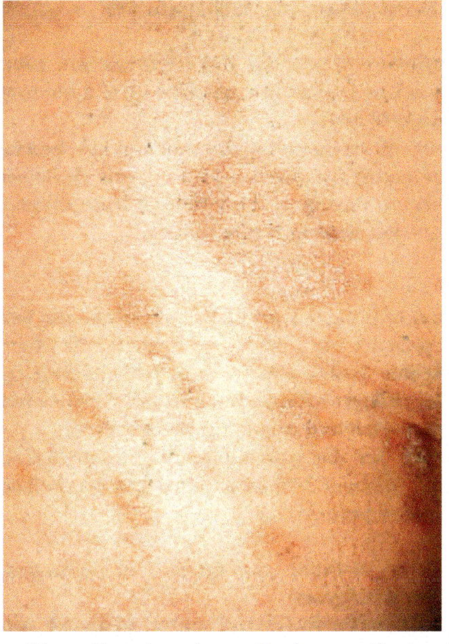

Two typical cases of pityriasis rosea, with scattered, scaly, oval lesions on the trunk. Large lesion is the "herald patch."

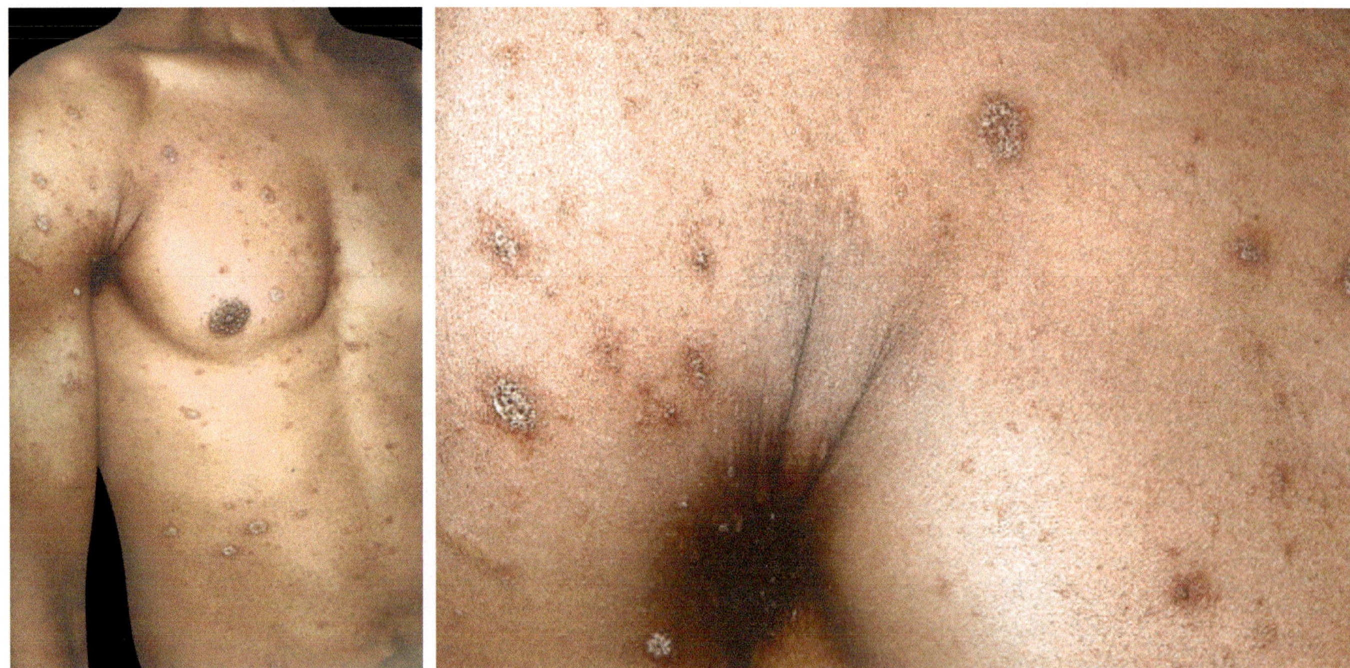

Quite inflamed and scaly lesions. The axis of the ovals is along fold lines radiating from the axilla.

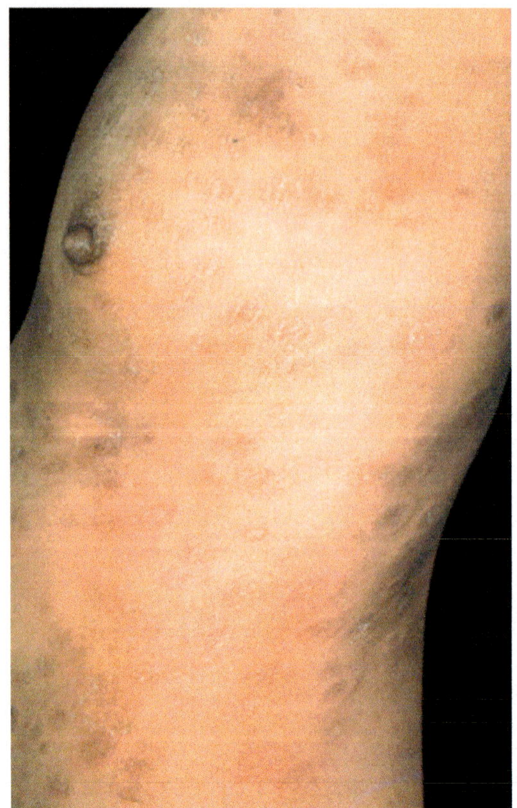

Large annular lesions are somewhat unusual in pityriasis rosea.

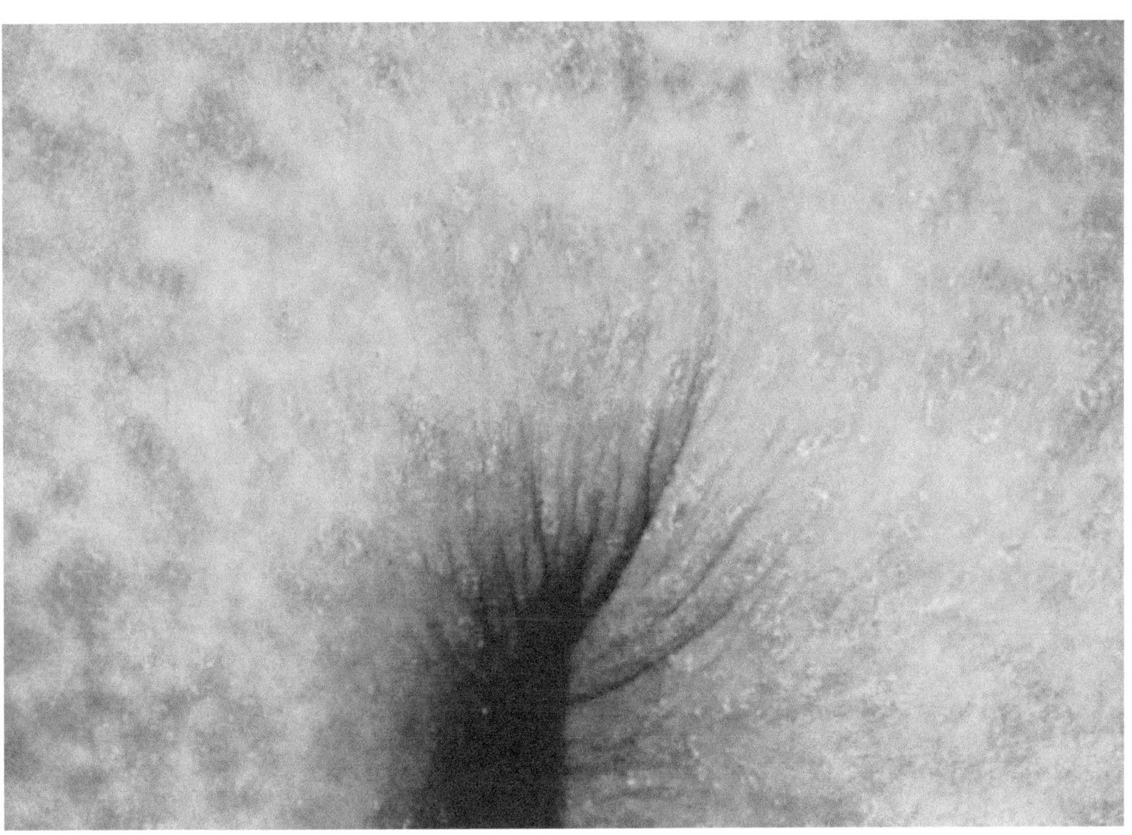

Markedly inflamed and scaly lesions, again showing radiation along fold lines from axilla.

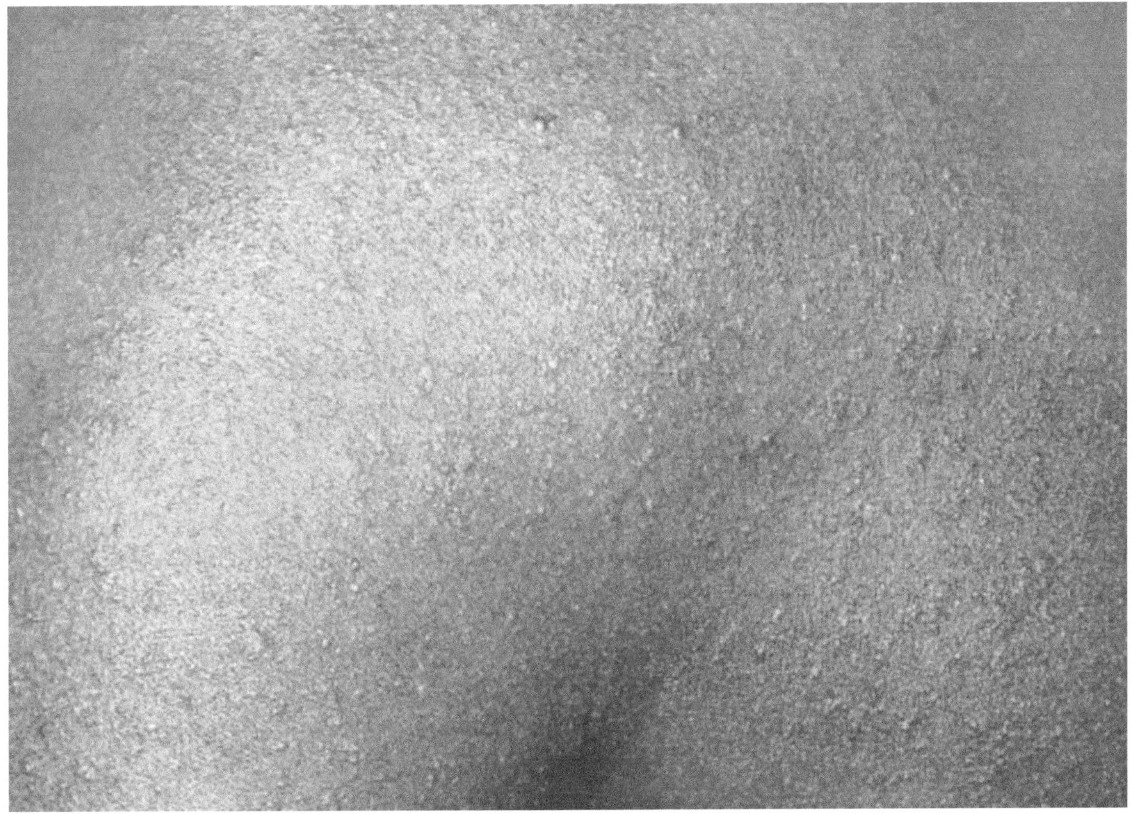

In dark-skinned persons, pityriasis rosea is often not red and is composed of small papules. Patterning along fold lines is still evident.

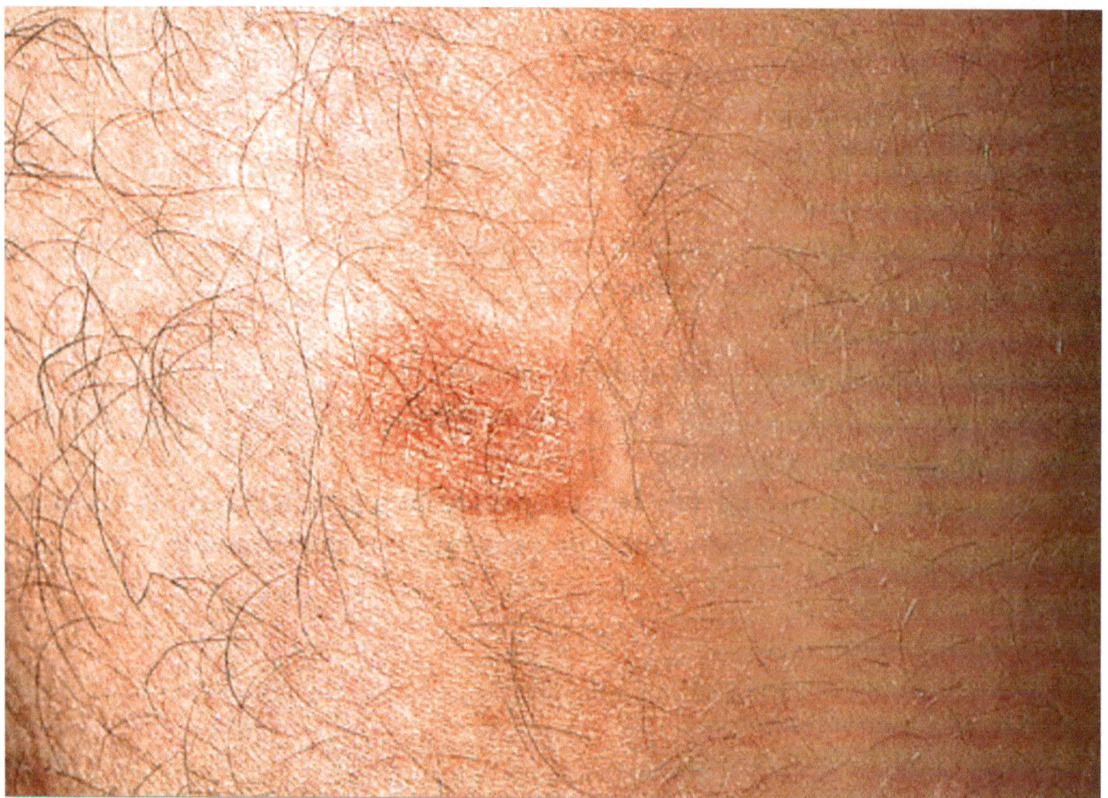

Typical lesion is a faint pink oval with a collarette of scale well inside the border. This patient had only three lesions.

CLINICAL

This disease has a typical age group, lesion appearance, and pattern, but atypical cases are common. Experience teaches the broad range of possibilities.

- A large (1- to 10-cm) "herald patch" occurs first in 50% of patients.
- Numerous smaller patches appear over the next few days.
  - Lesions
    - Oval, fawn-colored (pink-tan) with lighter or darker centers
    - Macular to slightly elevated to quite papular (especially in the dark skinned)

Characteristically, a fine collarette of scale exists inside the pink border. Scale is peripherally attached and pointing inward; to lift scale with a fingernail, one must scratch from the center of the lesion outward to get under the free edge. This is in contrast to tinea and other annular eruptions, in which the scale is at the advancing edge, not behind it, and is randomly attached.

  - Location
    - Usually on trunk and proximal parts of extremities
    - Spares face, hands, and feet
    - Atypical patterns: Flexural areas (axillae, groin, neck), face, and acral areas (hands and feet)
  - Pattern
    - Oval patches oriented on lines radiating from flexures and in "Christmas tree" pattern from spine
  - Duration
    - Typically 6 weeks but may last 8–10 weeks and, rarely, 3 months
    - Spreads and increases markedly the first 2 or 3 weeks and more slowly thereafter
  - Itching
    - Usually mild and intermittent
    - Occasionally severe, especially in the more papular cases
- Systemic symptoms
  - Mild malaise has been reported as a prodrome of or accompanying the rash, but true association is questionable.

- Associated with reactivation of human herpesvirus (HHV) 6 and/or 7, and possibly other viruses
    - Characteristic age group (young adults usually but seen also in children and the middle-aged)
    - Seasonal and temporal "epidemics" in large populations
    - Remission after set course
    - Rare recurrence
- Secondary syphilis may mimic pityriasis rosea. Consider serum laboratory testing.

TREATMENT

- General.
    - **Lesions resolve spontaneously**
    - Patients require education (*See* Patient Guides, page 251) and reassurance.
        - Disease will go away by itself.
        - The face and arms are usually not affected.
        - The disease will not leave scars.
        - It is not contagious.
        - Internal organs are not affected.
        - The condition rarely recurs.
- Itching may be treated by:
    - First-generation (sedating) antihistamines (*See* page 243)
        - At bedtime to allow sleep
        - Often too sedating for daytime use
    - Baths (colloidal oatmeal) may be somewhat soothing
    - Topical corticosteroids
        - Potent ones may relieve itching of individual patches.
    - Ultraviolet light (or sunlight)
        - An erythema (peeling) dose often relieves itching for a few days and may hasten resolution of lesions.
        - Repeated treatments are often required.

Lichen Planus

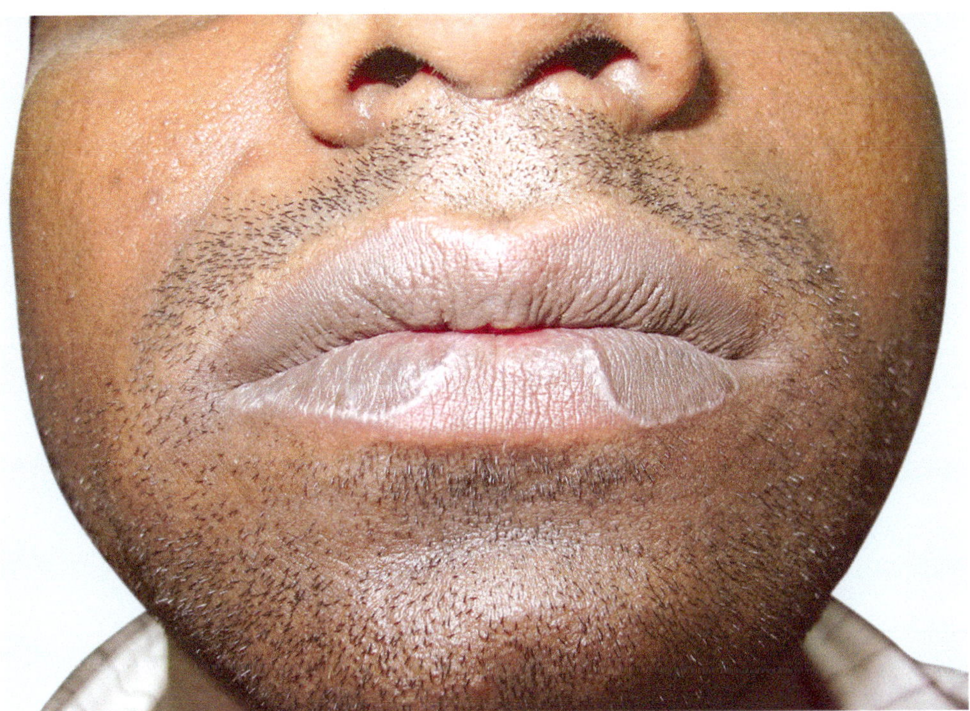

Annular LP over the lips with central resolution, subtle atrophy and a well-defined raised violaceous border

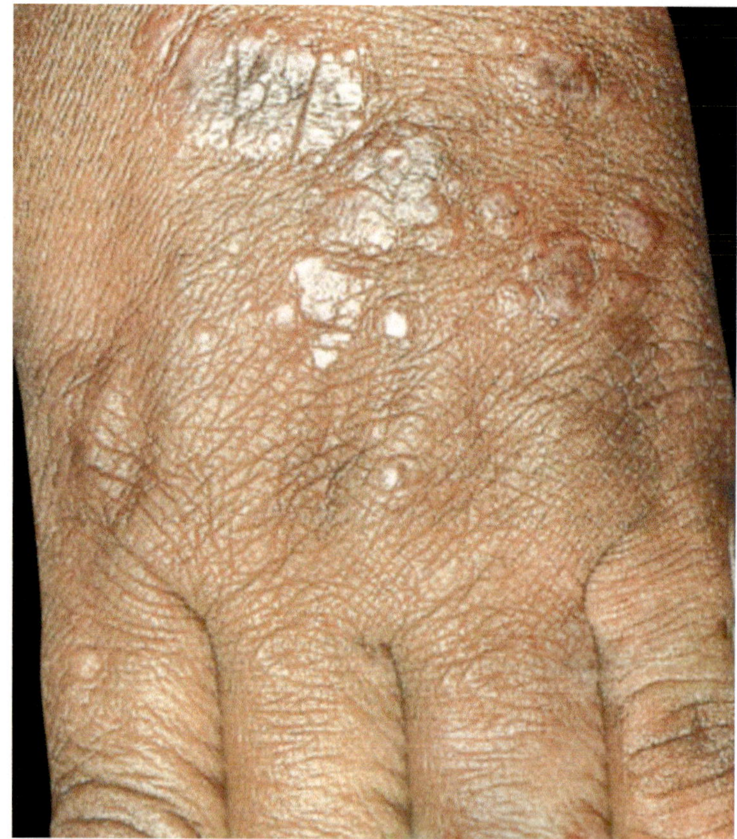

Typical lichen planus lesions: polygonal, scaly, flat-topped, and violaceous.

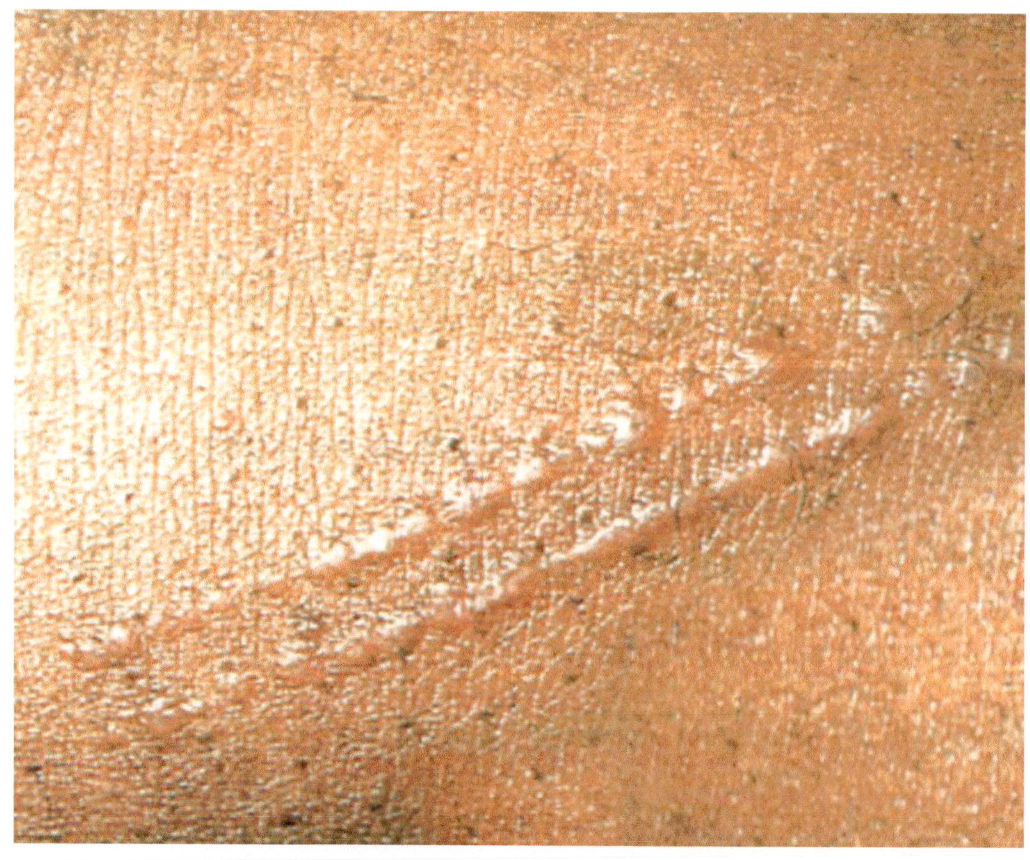

Koebner phenomenon, or development of lesions in areas of trauma.

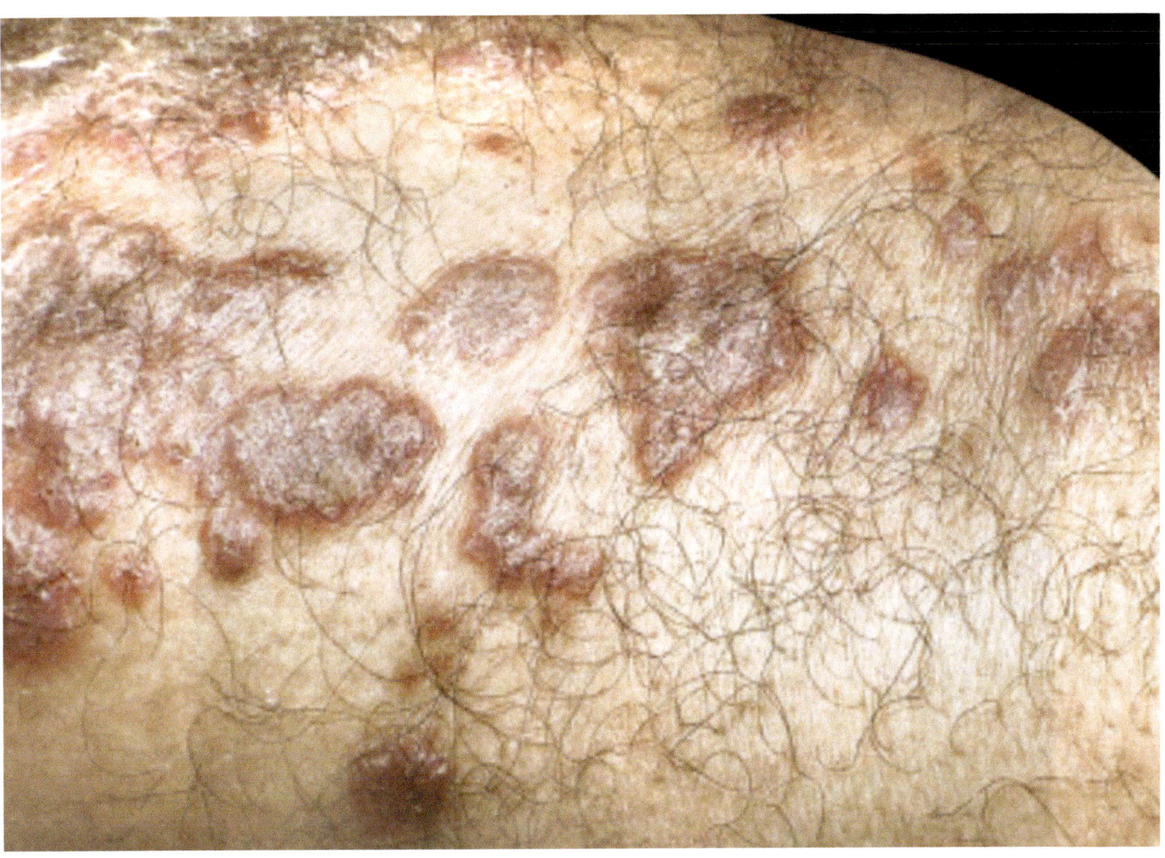

Early hypertrophic or thick lesions on the leg. Fine, white-etched lines of the surface are Wickham's striae.

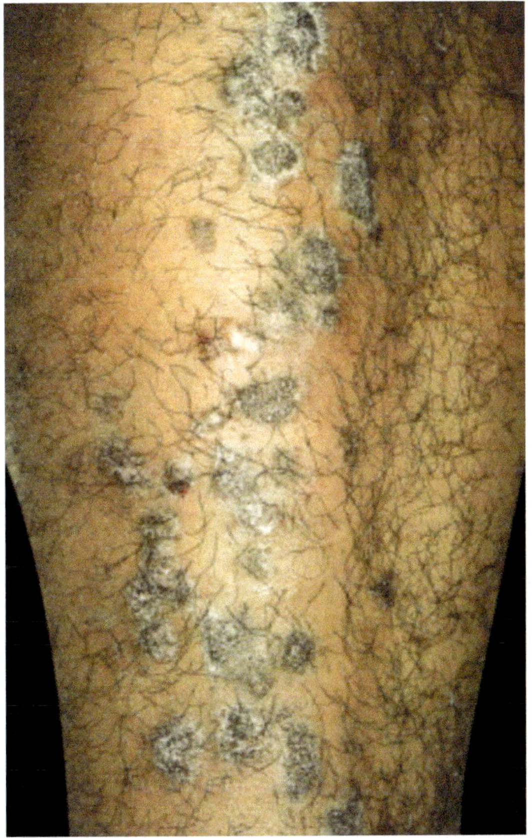

Dry, chronic, hypertrophic lesions, present 2 years.

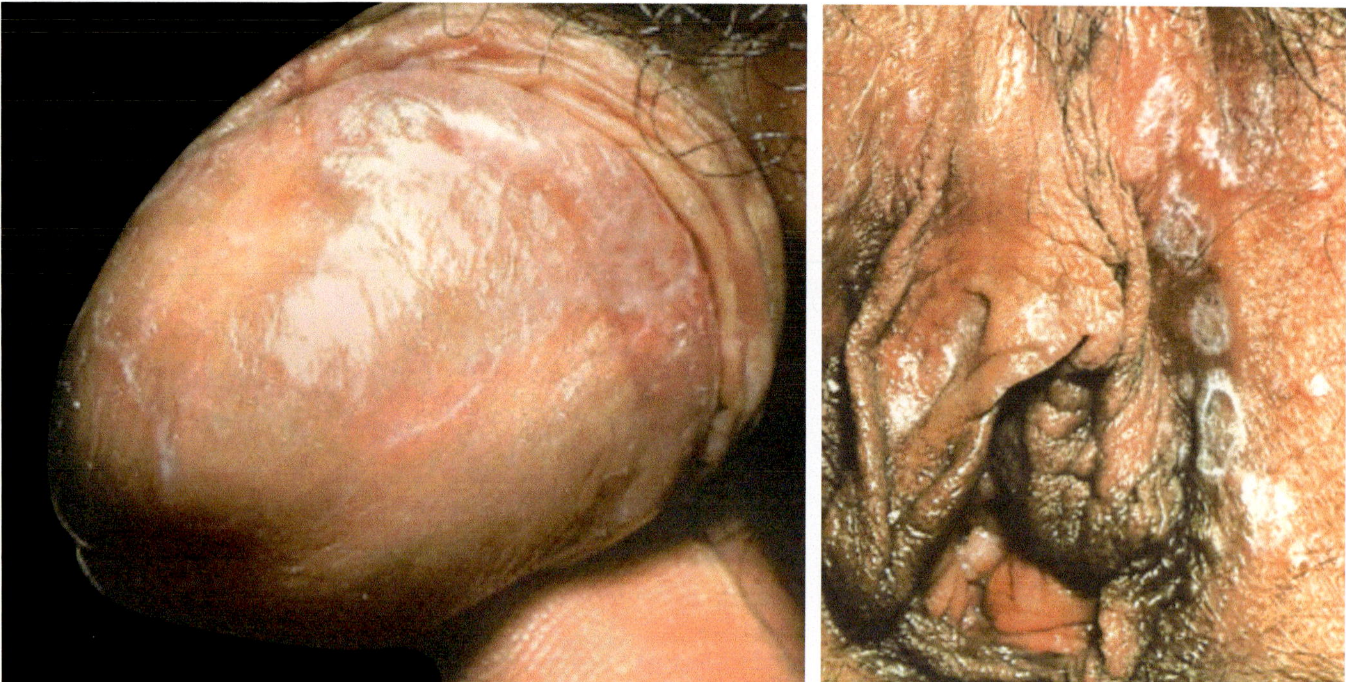

The genitals are a common site of lichen planus. The lesions are usually annular with a light-colored border.

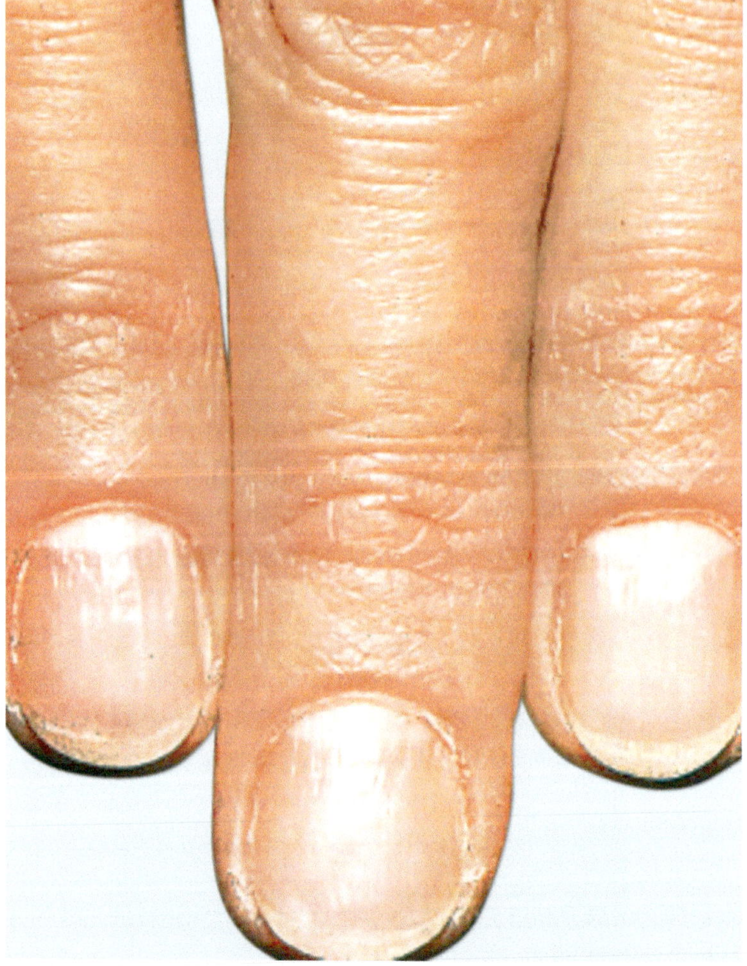

Nail involvement is not uncommon. The nail plate is thinned and has longitudinal striations.

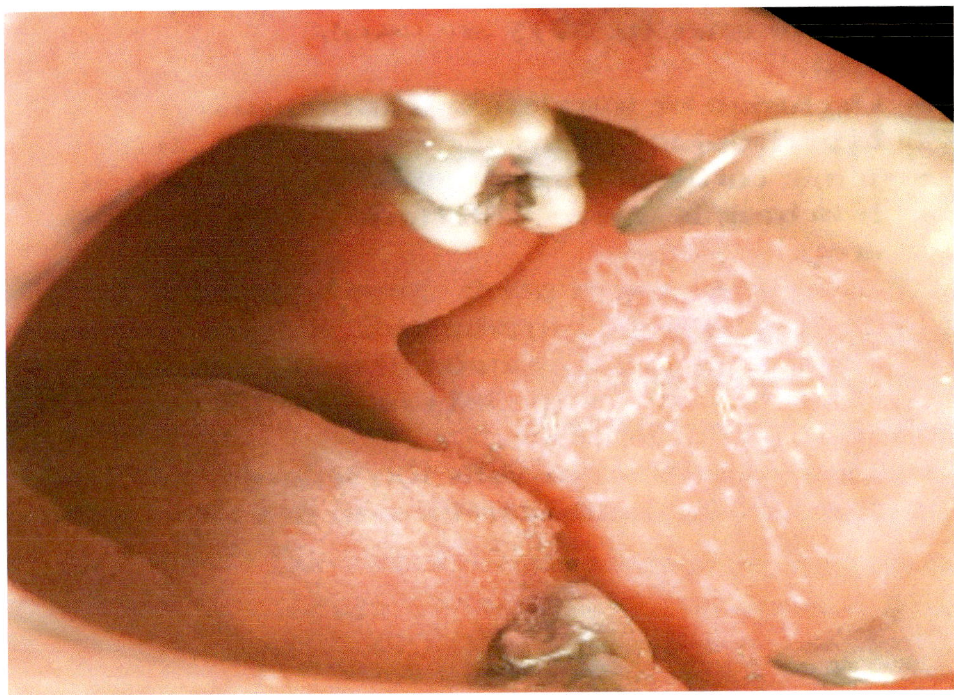

Oral lesions are usually on the buccal mucosa and are lacelike.

CLINICAL

- Lichen planus is an eruption of small, polygonal, flat-topped, and violet papules.
  - Often confined to wrists, ankles, and groin but may be generalized.
    - Genitals commonly involved
  - Papules 2–15 mm, usually with a shiny surface due to slight scale
    - On shins may be hypertrophic with thick, verrucous scale
    - Quickly become hyperpigmented and leave a deep pigment when healed
- Oral involvement is common and sometimes the only manifestation.
  - Lacy white or light gray reticulate pattern occurs on buccal mucosa. Vermilion of lips may be involved.
  - Erosions are occasionally persistent and painful.
- Idiopathic
- The condition usually lasts 6–24 months, except hypertrophic and oral lesions, which may last longer.
- Itching ranges in intensity from absent to severe.
  - Itching is usually at its worst during first few weeks when erupting, then milder after the condition is stabilized.

TREATMENT

- No treatment shortens the course of the disease; it just relieves itching or improves the cosmetic appearance.
- Topical corticosteroids are the most common treatment.
  - Potent ones (*See* page 238) are usually required (except for the genitals).
  - Occlusion or intralesional corticosteroids are often needed for hypertrophic lesions.
- Narrow-band UVB or PUVA for widespread cases
- First-generation oral antihistamines (*See* page 243) may be administered as sedatives and antipruritics at bedtime.
  - These agents are usually too sedating for daytime use.
  - Nonsedative antihistamines do not affect itching.
- Oral lichen planus
  - No treatment if asymptomatic
  - Corticosteroid in carboxymethylcellulose, gelatin, and pectin (Orabase) twice daily
  - Intralesional corticosteroid (*See* page 240) if stubborn
  - Repeated short course (5–15 days) of oral corticosteroid is effective. Dose is prednisone 40–60 mg every morning (or other corticoid equivalent) with rapid taper.
  - Tacrolimus 0.1% ointment twice daily is sometimes effective.

Urticaria (Hives)

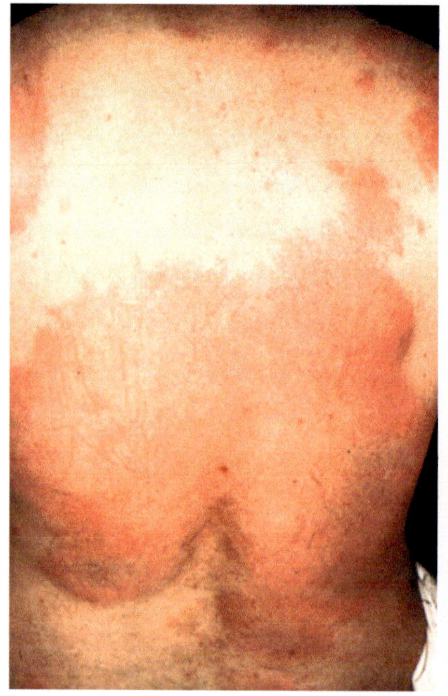

Huge wheals in a patient allergic to penicillin.

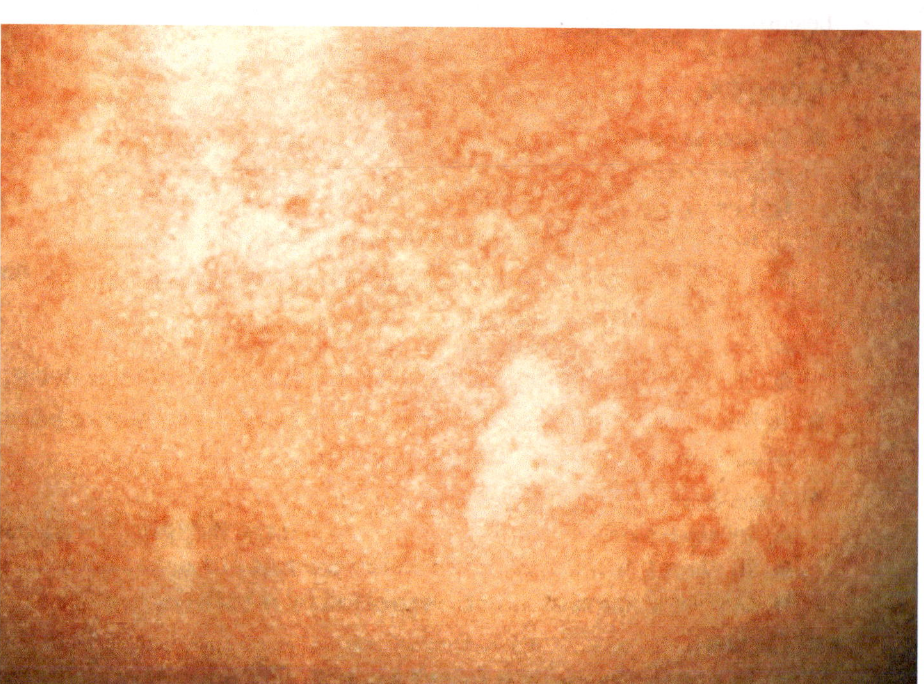

Small, confluent hives in a person reacting to an unknown illicit drug. The light area is normal skin.

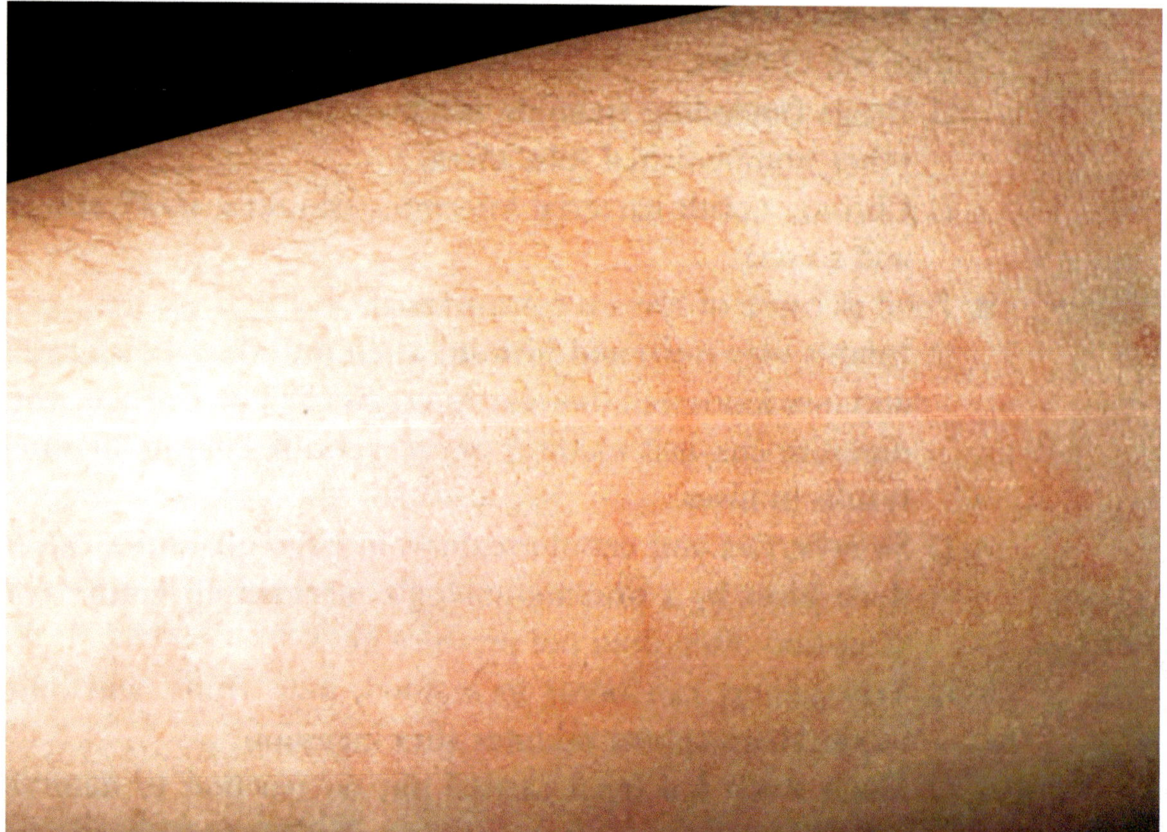

Wheal induced in a clinic with artificial ultraviolet light in a person with solar urticaria.

CLINICAL

- Urticaria consists of pink edematous papules and plaques with normal overlying epidermis.
  - Lesions may have blanched halos or be so tensely edematous as to be blanched themselves.
  - Lesions are randomly scattered over body, including the face and scalp.
  - Edema of lips, hands, and feet is common.
  - No lesion lasts >24 hours, but new ones may occur.
- Itching is usually severe but may be mild or absent. Severe edema of face, hands, or feet may be painful.
- Usually the condition is of abrupt onset.
  - In *acute* hives, reaches peak in 1–3 days, fades in 7–21 days
  - In *chronic* hives, waxes and wanes for months or years
  - May be recurrent attacks separated by months or years
- Causes
  - In *acute* hives, cause is found about 20% of time; most commonly
    - Drugs, inoculations, foods or food additives, intravenous radiopaque contrast medium, hymenopteran stings
    - Internal acute infections (usually bacterial) or inflammations (rheumatoid flare, inflammatory bowel disease, and so on)
    - Marked emotional tension may precipitate (cholinergic urticaria) or exacerbate hives
  - In *chronic* hives (>6 weeks), the cause is found in fewer than 5% of cases.
    - Drugs (including vitamins, laxatives, mints, toothpaste, and other nonmedicinal substances)
    - Chronic occult bacterial infections (sinusitis, tooth abscess, and so on)
  - Food as cause of hives is controversial.
    - Infants may flush and urticate when introduced to formula and new foods, but this reaction ceases by 1 year of age, when digestive enzymes mature, and re-exposure later in life rarely results in hives.
    - Strawberries and certain seafood in large quantities can induce hives by a nonimmunologic mechanism. Future consumption often does not produce hives.
    - True allergy can occur to seafood, nuts, fruits, and other foods. Hives appear minutes after ingestion.
    - Much study has been carried out on reaction to naturally occurring salicylates in food, as well as to salicylate, tartrazine, and benzoate additives, but their actual role is undetermined.
  - Certain chemicals can degranulate mast cells by nonimmunologic means and may worsen hives, so their intake during an attack of hives should be avoided.
    - Aspirin
    - Morphine, codeine
    - Reserpine, polymyxin B, alcohol
- Special clinical types of hives:
  - Cholinergic urticaria, mediated by acetylcholine, not histamine, is nonimmunologic.
    - Young adults most frequently affected
    - Evanescent papules on the upper trunk
    - Triggered by heat, exercise, emotion
  - Physical urticarias, immune reaction triggered by physical exposures-rare, familial, or sporadic
    - Cold
    - Pressure
    - Sunlight
  - Dermographia ("skin writing") is the production of hives by light rubbing or trauma: nonimmunologic, familial or sporadic, congenital or acquired and is mediated by immunoglobulin (Ig) E.

TREATMENT

- Triggering factors should be identified and removed, but the patient should be told that such identification is often impossible. Frustration and dissatisfaction commonly occur and tax the doctorpatient relationship.
  - Obtain a careful history, particularly of medications, vitamins, tonics, digestive mints, and other nonprescription cultural remedies. Ask about stings, inoculations, and radiographic tests. Inquire about diet fads (e.g., kelp, flavoring agents). Review all systems with an eye toward occult bacterial infections. Ask about emotional tension. Repeat these inquiries at each visit.
  - Laboratory tests are usually unproductive but may be indicated in recalcitrant patients. Those usually recommended are:
    - Complete blood count and sedimentation rate
    - Urinalysis
    - Liver function test
    - Ear, nose, and throat and sinus X-ray examinations
    - Dental examination, including X-ray examination
    - Stool, for ova, and parasites
- Topical therapy:
  - Cool baths or compresses often give temporary relief and reduce inflammation. Colloidal oatmeal baths are often soothing.
  - Emollients with added menthol or pramoxine may be of added benefit.
- Systemic agents are usually required.
  - Epinephrine (adrenaline) 1:1000, 0.3–0.5 mL subcutaneously for severe acute episodes gives fast relief
  - First-generation antihistamines (*See* page 243)—the drug of choice
    - Effect starts 45–60 minutes after oral dose; reaches peak in 2 hours. Response from intramuscular dose is only slightly faster.
    - Nonsedating antihistamines such as fexofenadine, and cetirizine are ideal and can be pushed to gastrointestinal tolerance. Often one morning dose is adequate, especially if hives occur mostly in the latter part of the day (as commonly occurs).
    - Traditional sedating antihistamines are practical for bedtime use, and many are considerably less expensive than the nonsedating ones.
    - Hydroxyzine seems particularly effective in cholinergic urticaria. Cetirizine is a less-sedating analog.
    - Warn patient about risk of operating automobiles or dangerous machinery while taking sedative antihistamines.
  - Corticosteroids
    - Often have little impact on acute hives but help to reduce edema of face, hands, and feet.
    - If all else fails in chronic urticaria, short-course corticosteroids may be helpful.
    - The anti-IgE monoclonal antibody omalizumab is package-labeled for urticaria lasting 6 weeks or more
- Acute anaphylactic urticaria

The treatment of acute urticaria associated with hypotension, shock, and bronchospasm is outside the scope of this book. One should start an intravenous drip, establish an airway, and administer subcutaneous or intravenous epinephrine (adrenaline) and possibly intravenous antihistamines, corticosteroids, and vasoconstrictors. This procedure should be closely monitored with blood gas determinations, cardiograms, measurement of urine output, and other procedures.

Erythema Multiforme

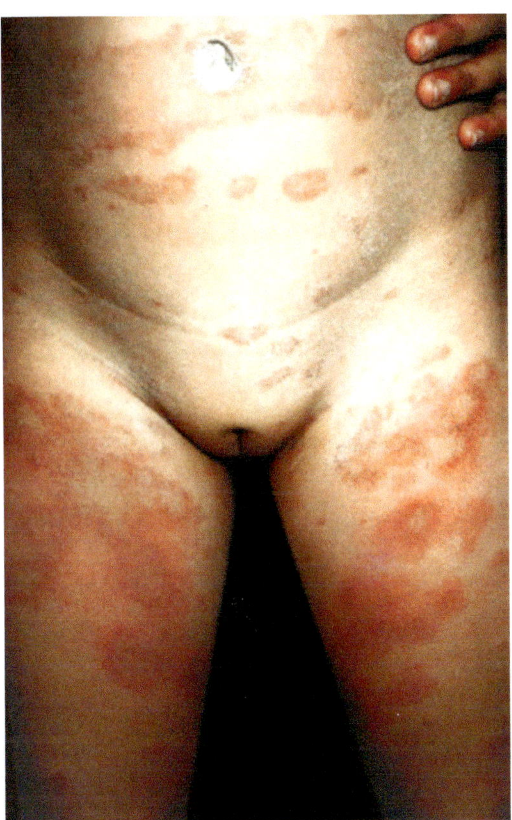

Scattered annular lesions of acute erythema multiforme in a child infected with Mycoplasma pneumoniae. Target lesions were present on the palms and soles.

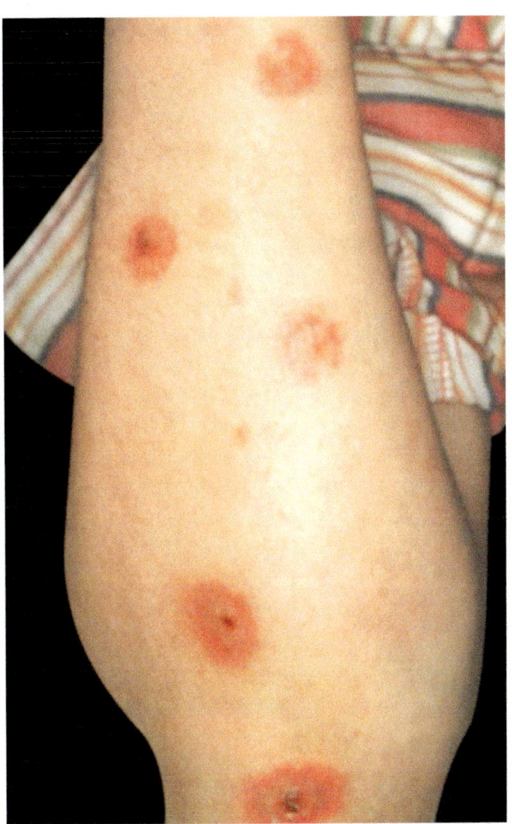

Classic iris or target lesions secondary to herpes simplex of the lips.

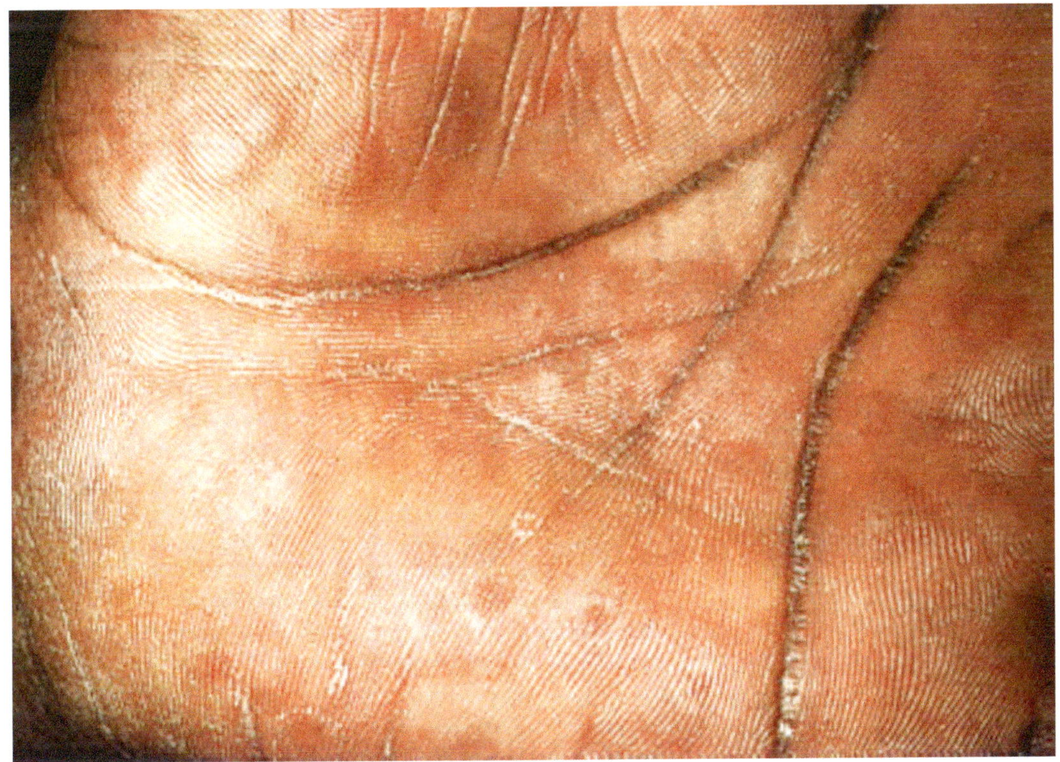

Typical annular lesions secondary to herpes simplex of the genitals.

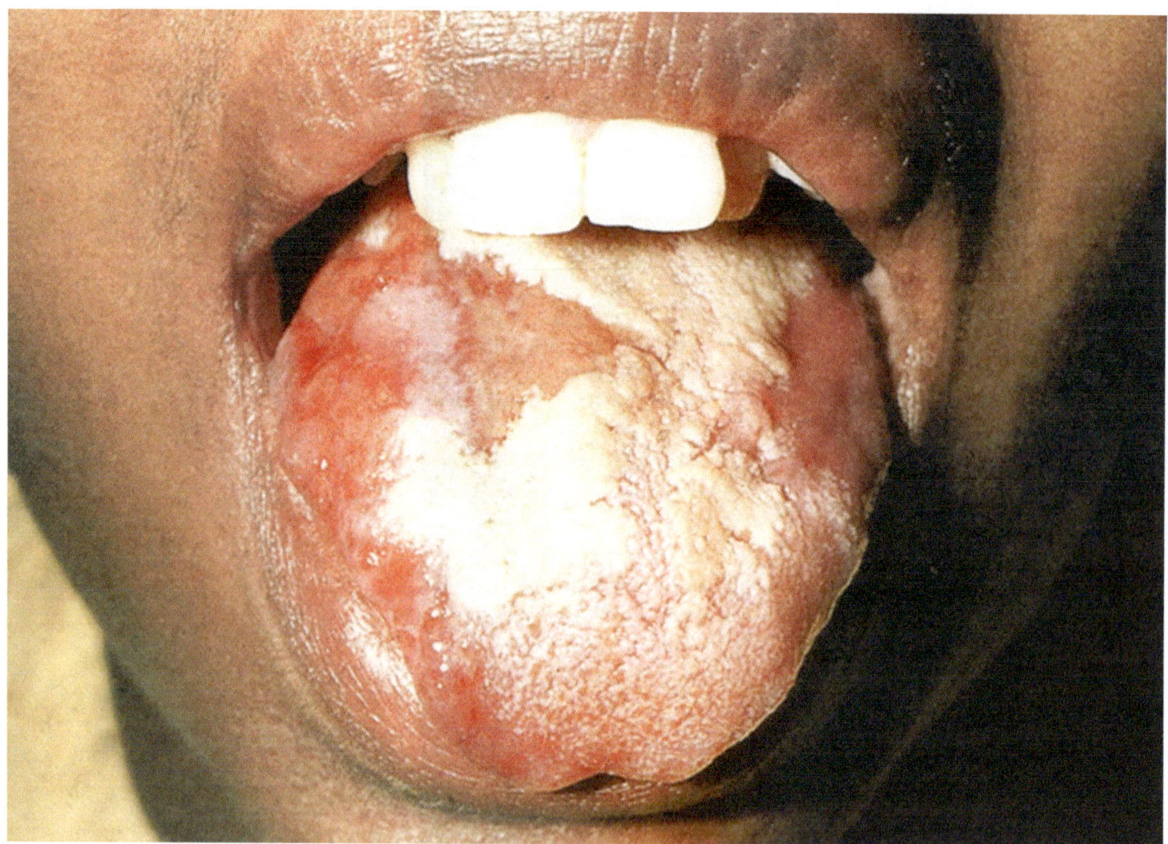

Idiopathic recurrent oral erythema multiforme.

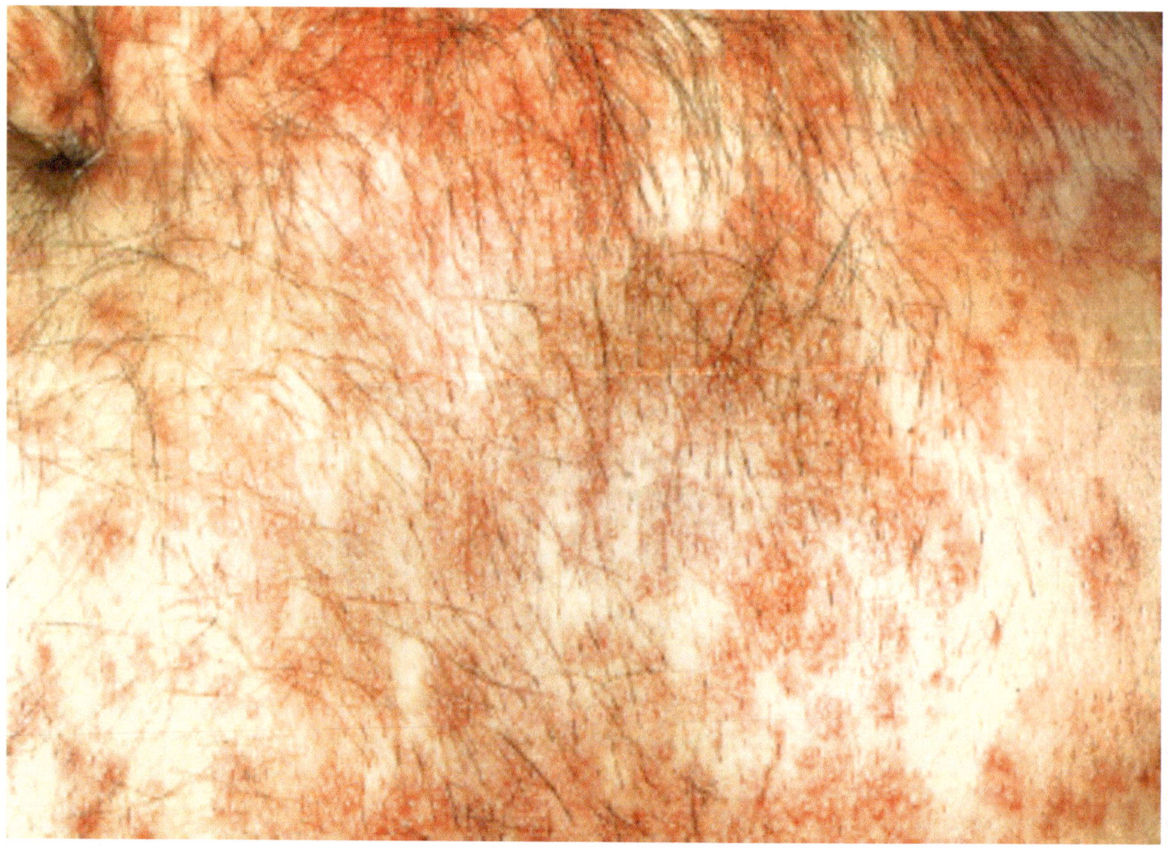

Generalized idiopathic erythema multiforme with tiny vesicles in the centers of many lesions. The patient felt well and had no mucous membrane lesions.

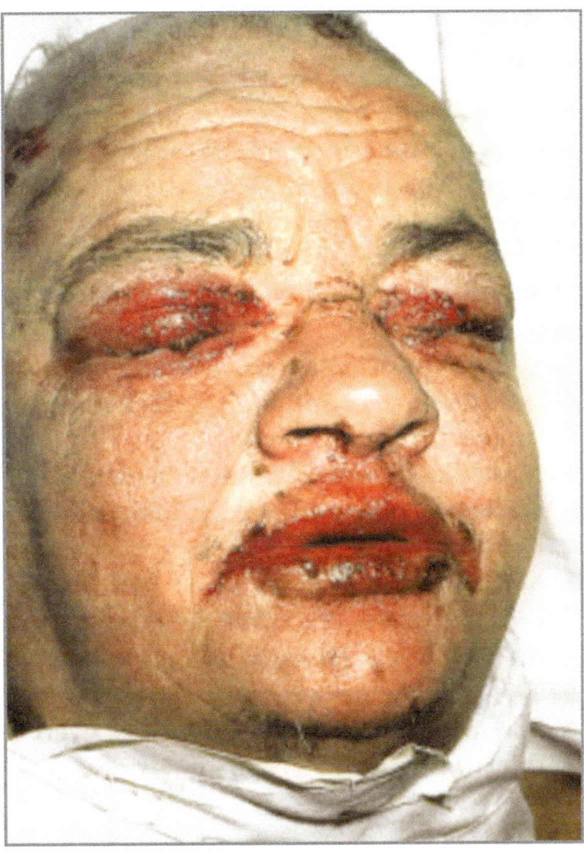

Stevens–Johnson syndrome secondary to phenytoin.
This was the patient's second episode caused by the same drug.

CLINICAL

- Classically, erythema multiforme consists of "iris" or "target" lesions (concentric rings of shades of red) on the palms, soles, genitals, mouth, and extensor surfaces of arms and legs. However, lesions can be of man types ("multiforme"), such as morbilliform, large patches of erythema, or long-lasting wheals (true hives always resolve in <24 hours). Occasionally the lesions are vesicular or bullous.
  - May be localized or widespread
  - Mild to severe itching, or tenderness
- The cause is presumed to be an immunologic or "toxic" reaction to various antigens.
  - In mild cases is almost always viral or mycobacterial
    - Most commonly herpes simplex, which may recur with each attack
    - Also atypical *(Mycoplasma)* pneumonia, and influenza viruses
  - Occasionally a reaction to drugs; nearly any type can be the culprit, but often reported with the use of sulfa drugs, thiazides, anticonvulsants, and barbiturates
  - Occasionally idiopathic
- The usual duration is from 10 to 20 days.
- Oral lesions are often bullous or eroded; may occur without cutaneous lesions.

TREATMENT

- Question and examine the patient for herpes, *Mycoplasma* pneumonia, other infections, and drugs.
- Mild-to-moderate erythema multiforme
  - Mild-to-mid-potency topical corticosteroids may relieve mild lesions.
  - The administration of oral corticosteroids (e.g., prednisone 40–60 mg) for a few days relieves severe itching and discomfort.
  - Oral antihistamines (*See* page 243) may be administered at bedtime to aid sleep if itching is severe.

Miliaria (Heat Rash)

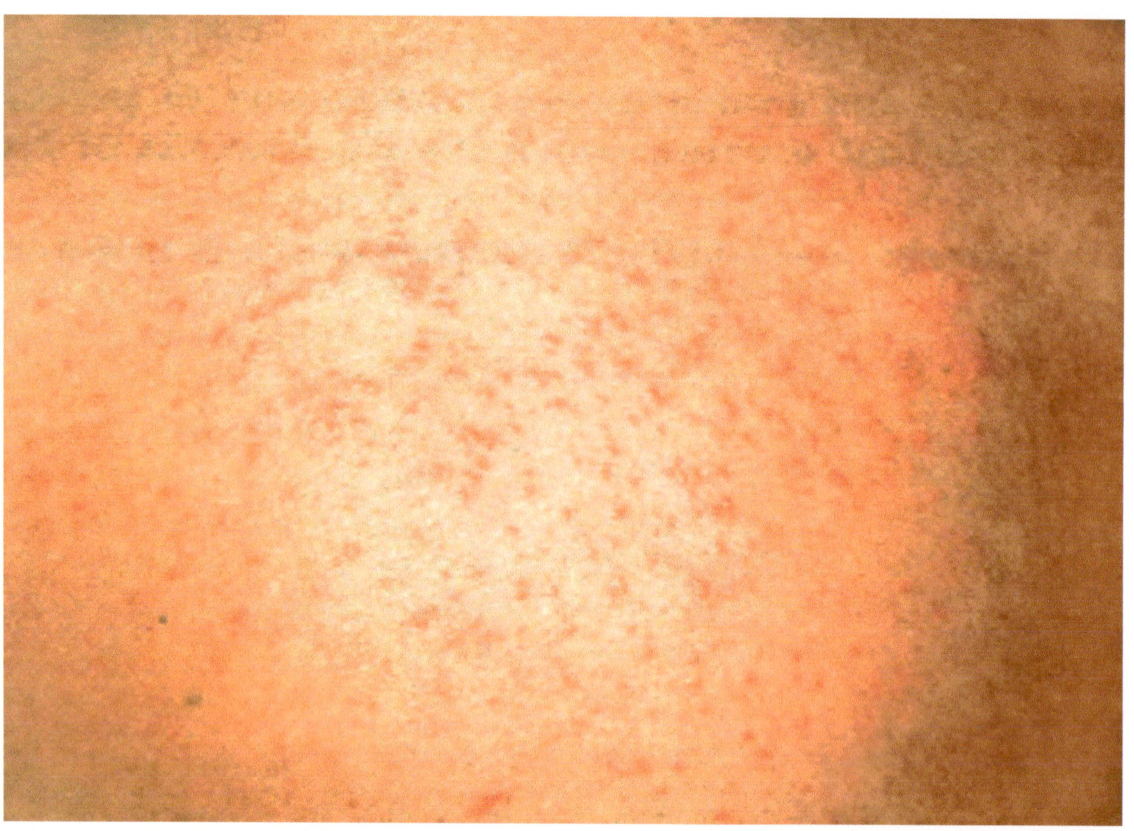

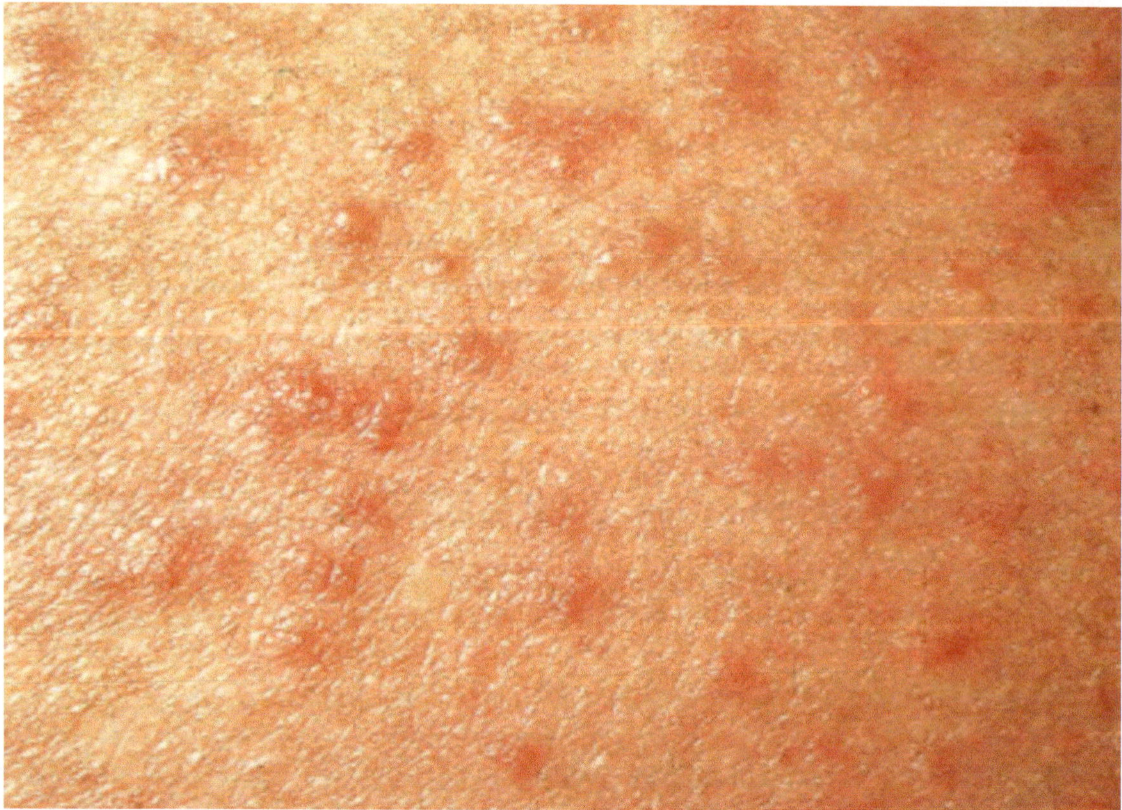

Typical miliaria rubra, or heat rash: scattered discrete, edematous, bright red papules.

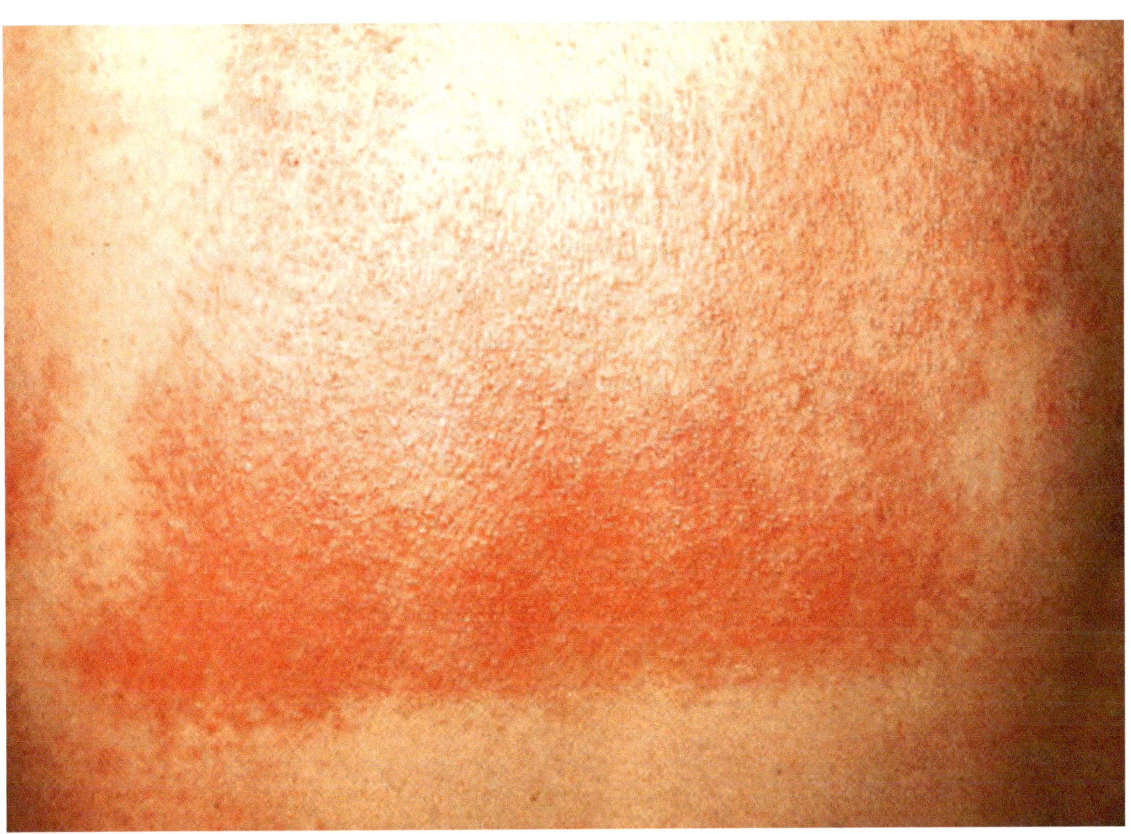

This woman sat in a chair for 3 hours. The vinyl upholstery prevented the escape of sweat, but her cotton underwear absorbed it.

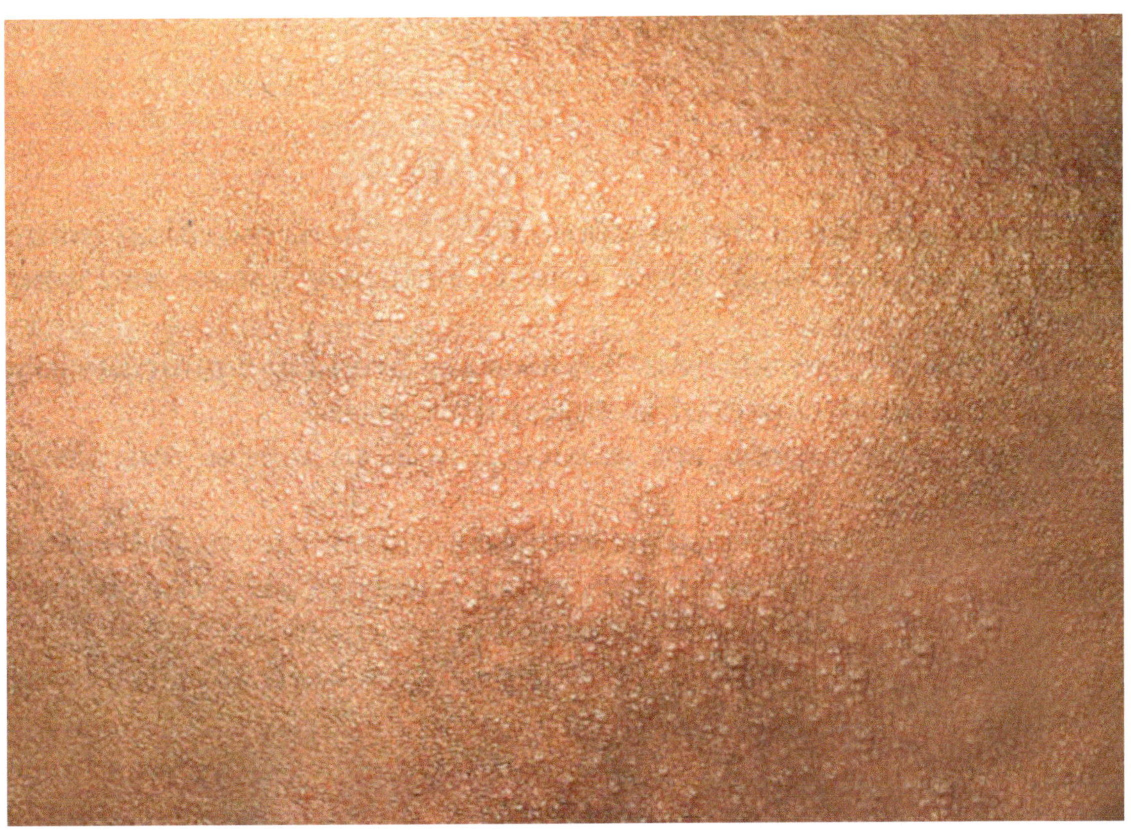

Redness may not be as evident in dark-skinned people. Papules are so edematous as to appear almost vesicular.

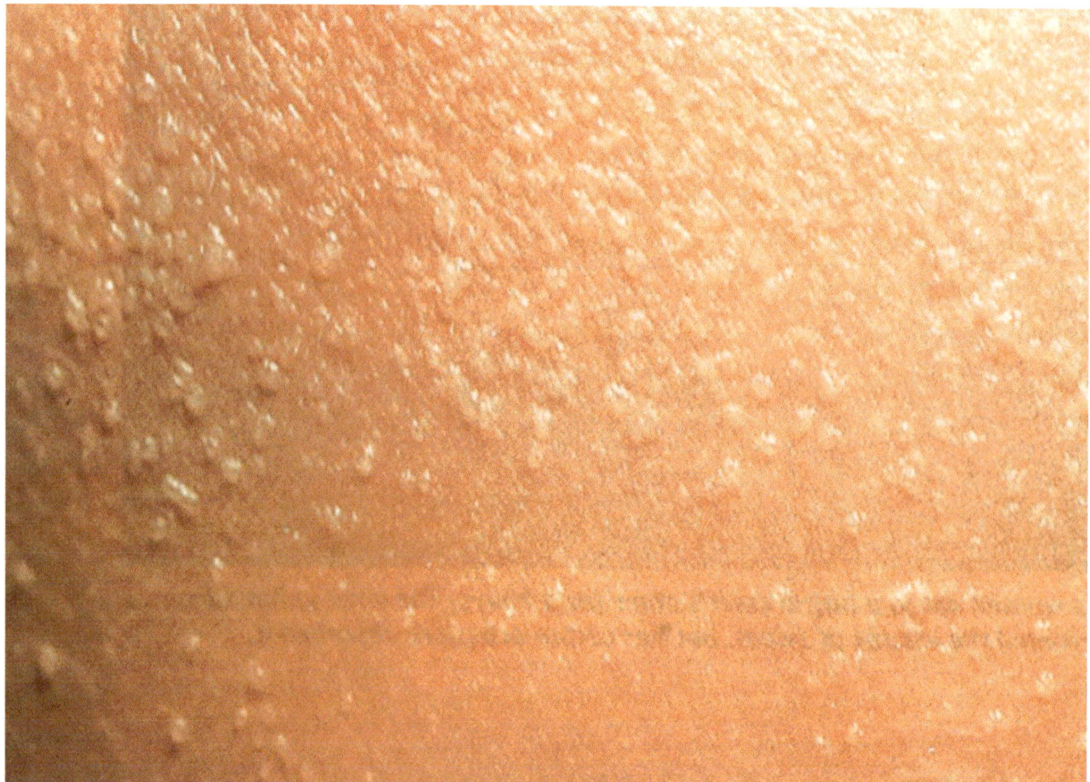

Miliaria crystallina: Tiny vesicles just under the keratin layer cause no inflammation or itching.

CLINICAL

- Miliaria results from the rupture of sweat ducts. Sweating pumps irritating sweat through these defects, inducing lesions and symptoms.
- Miliaria rubra ("prickly heat") consists of bright red punctate macules and papules clustered in susceptible areas.
  - Occasionally papules are so succulent as to appear vesicular or pustular.
  - Miliaria rubra occurs on areas of occlusion under nonabsorbent clothes, under folds of skin, or at points of skin contact with nonabsorbent upholstery. Common examples are:
    - On the faces of infants, when saliva-soaked skin is pressed against plastic mattress covers
    - On domes of buttocks and back in drivers and office workers sitting on plastic-covered seats
    - Under plastic bathing suits and nonabsorbent tight clothing
  - The condition is more common in humid weather, not just hot weather.
    - New residents may acclimatize after several days.
  - In patients in whom the condition is widespread, sweating may be so disrupted as to produce heat stroke.
  - Itching is often prominent.
    - An insistent prickling occurs when sweating is induced and stops when skin cools.
  - Healing occurs in a few days if sweating is minimized, and acclimatization occurs.
    - For a few weeks thereafter, the affected sites may relapse upon exposure to mildly provoking conditions.
- Miliaria crystallina consists of tiny (1-mm), thin-roofed, clear, droplike vesicles. Sweat duct rupture and sweat accumulation are just under keratin layer.
  - The vesicles are not inflamed or red.
  - They rupture easily because of the thin roof.
  - They are not symptomatic.

TREATMENT

- Inactivity of sweat glands removes all symptoms and allows healing.
  - Only environmental control achieves this.
  - No medication stops sweat gland activity (antiperspirants work by blocking sweat ducts).
  - Absorption or removal of sweat from the surface of the skin is of no benefit.

- Healing occurs if sweating is avoided for several days.
  - This is best done in a cool and dry environment.
    - 8 hours of each 24 hours often adequate
  - Reduce physical activity.
  - Avoid occlusive clothing and sitting on nonporous upholstery.
- Topical corticosteroids
  - These agents may reduce inflammation and itching.
  - Use nonocclusive lotion base, not ointment.

Secondary Syphilis

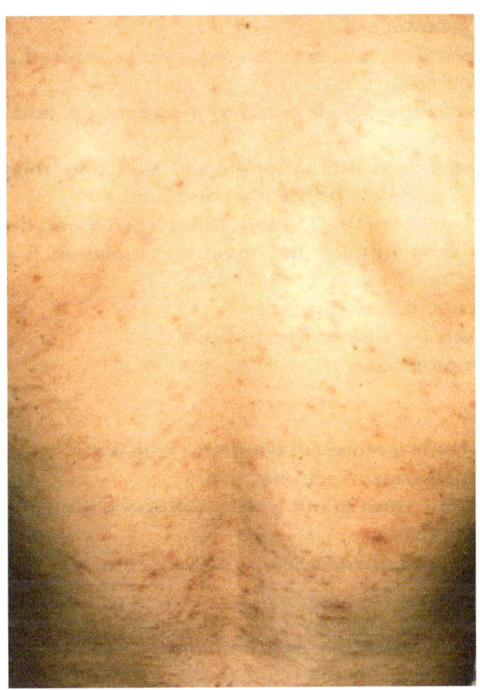

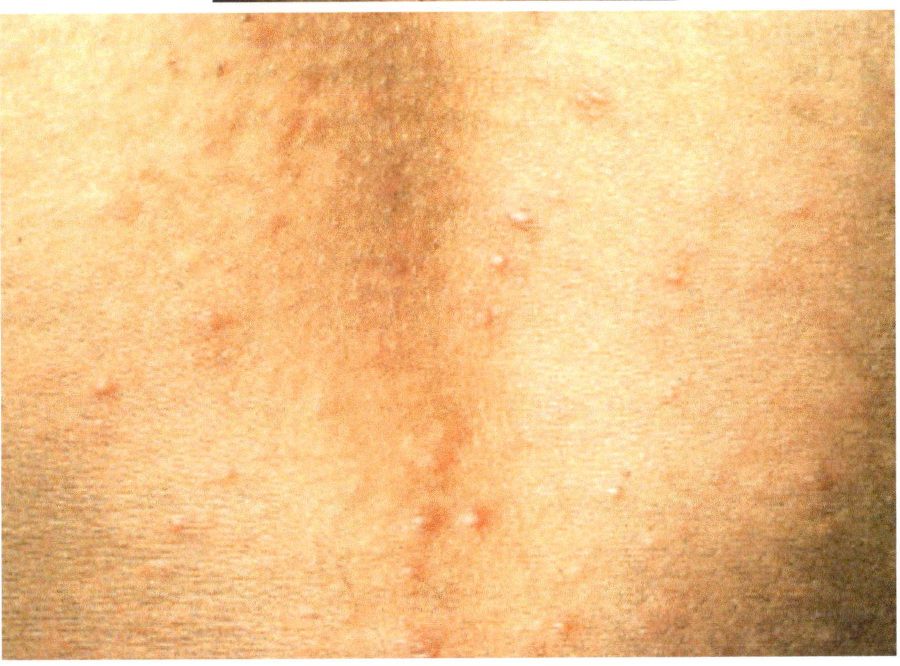

Generalized rash of secondary syphilis. VDRL (Venereal Disease Research Laboratory test) was 1:512. Often the lesions are fewer, larger, flatter, and scaly.

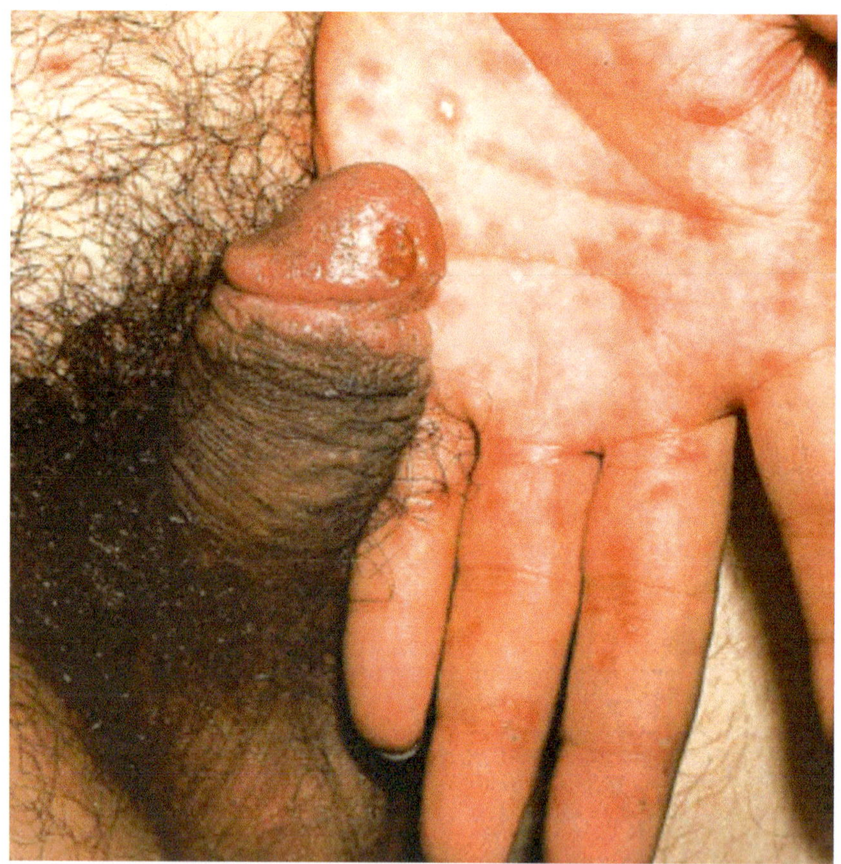

"Copper-colored" macules of the palm. A primary chancre is still present.

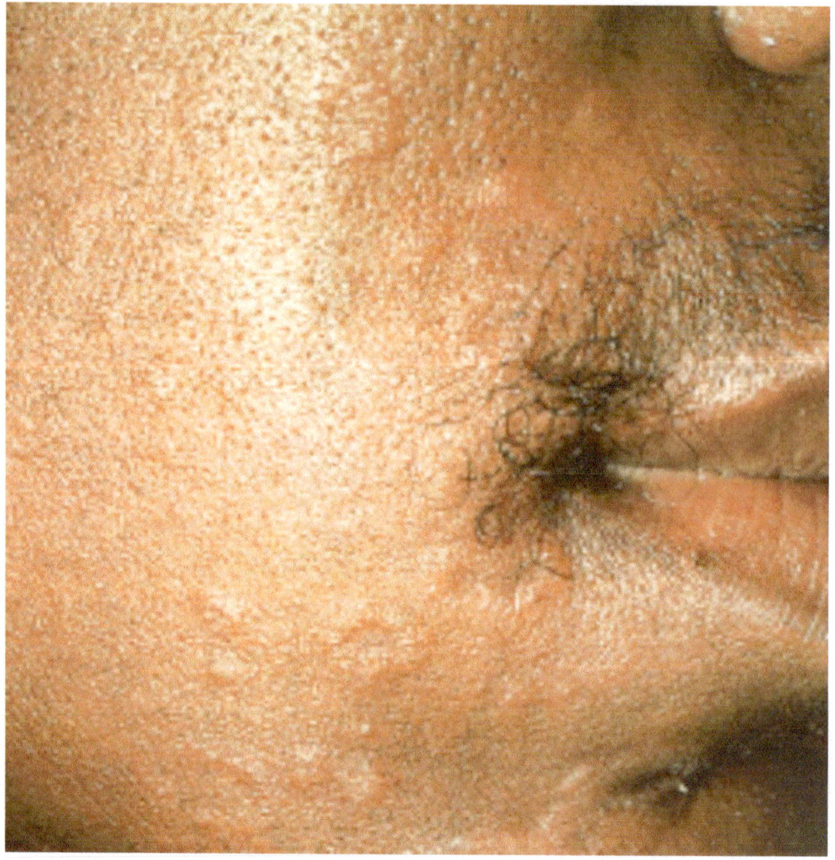

Facial lesions are often round ("nickel and dime lesions") and grouped around orifices.

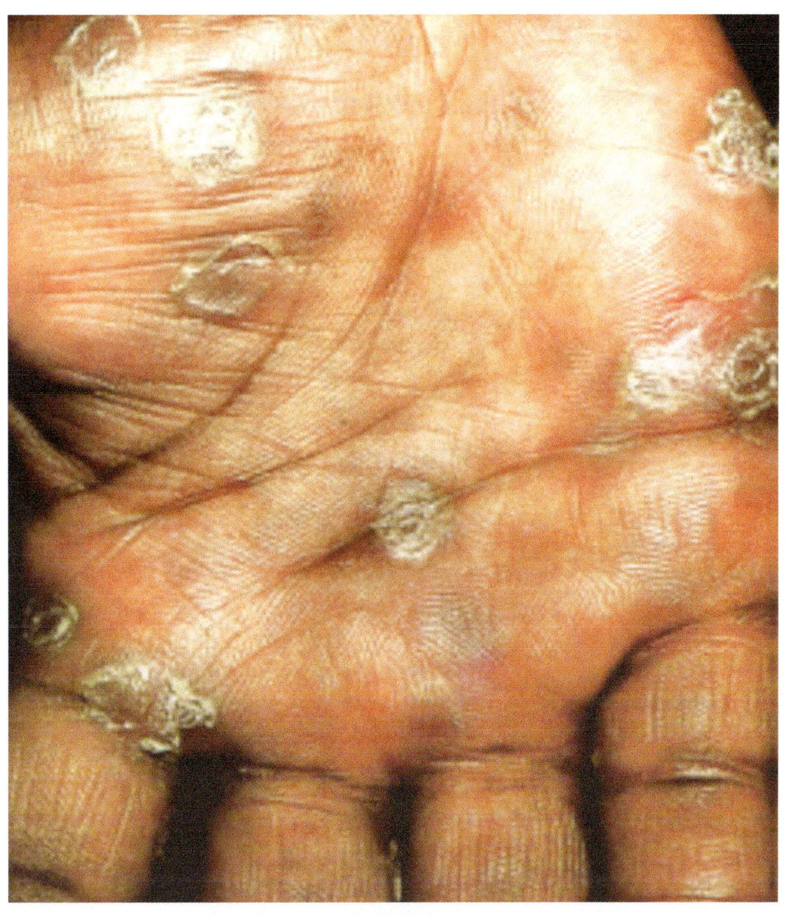

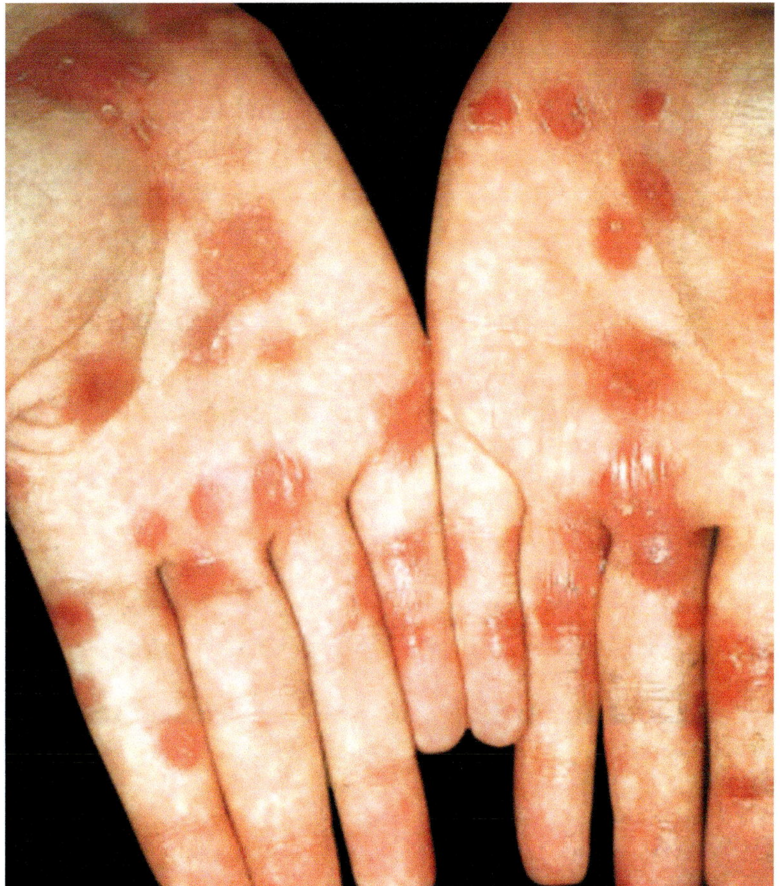

Palmar lesions may be markedly inflamed but often are dry and keratotic.

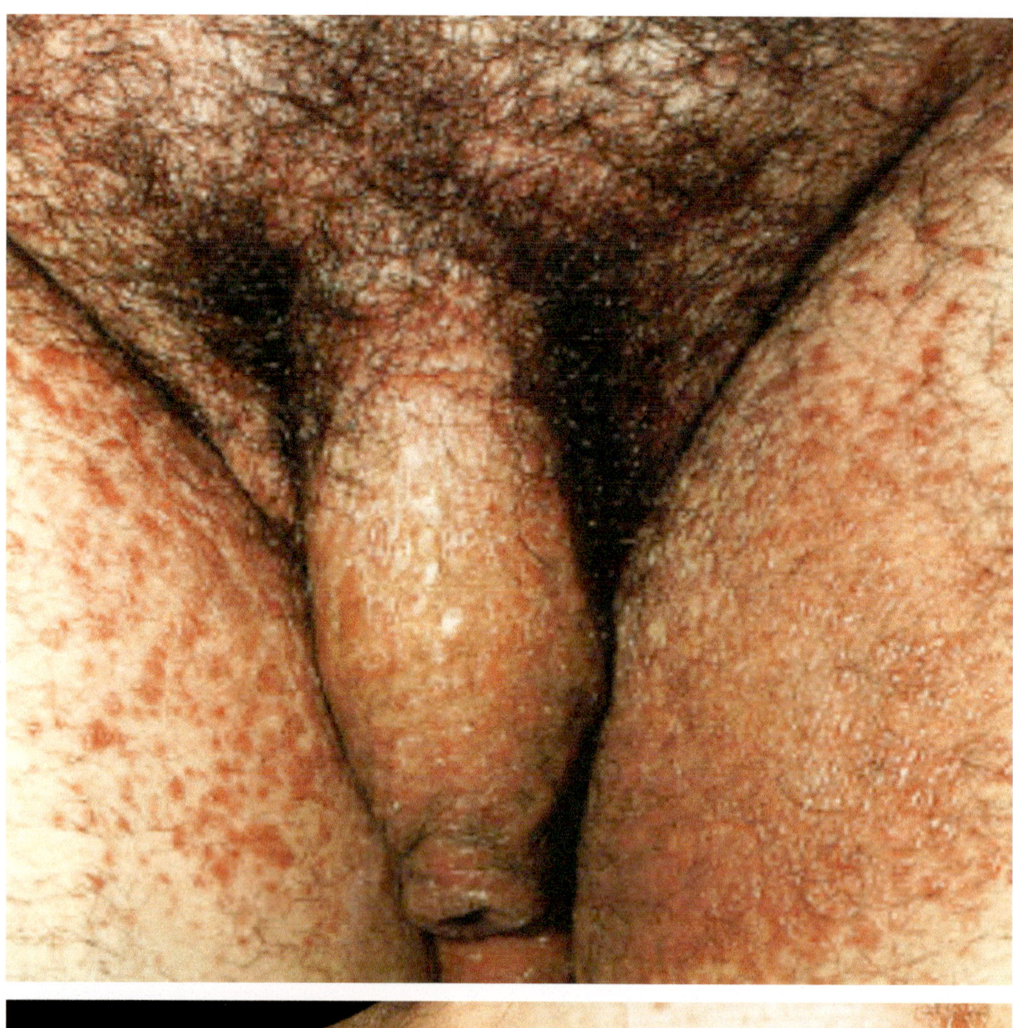

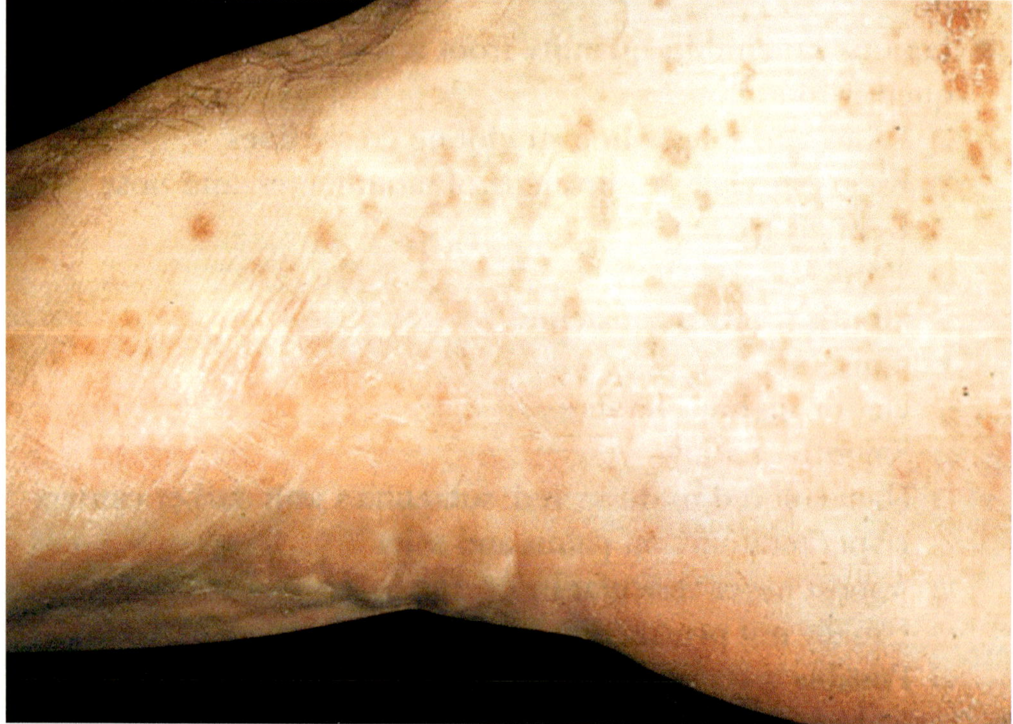

The genitals and fold areas are common sites of secondary syphilis, as in this case in which the soles were also involved. The VDRL was 1:128.

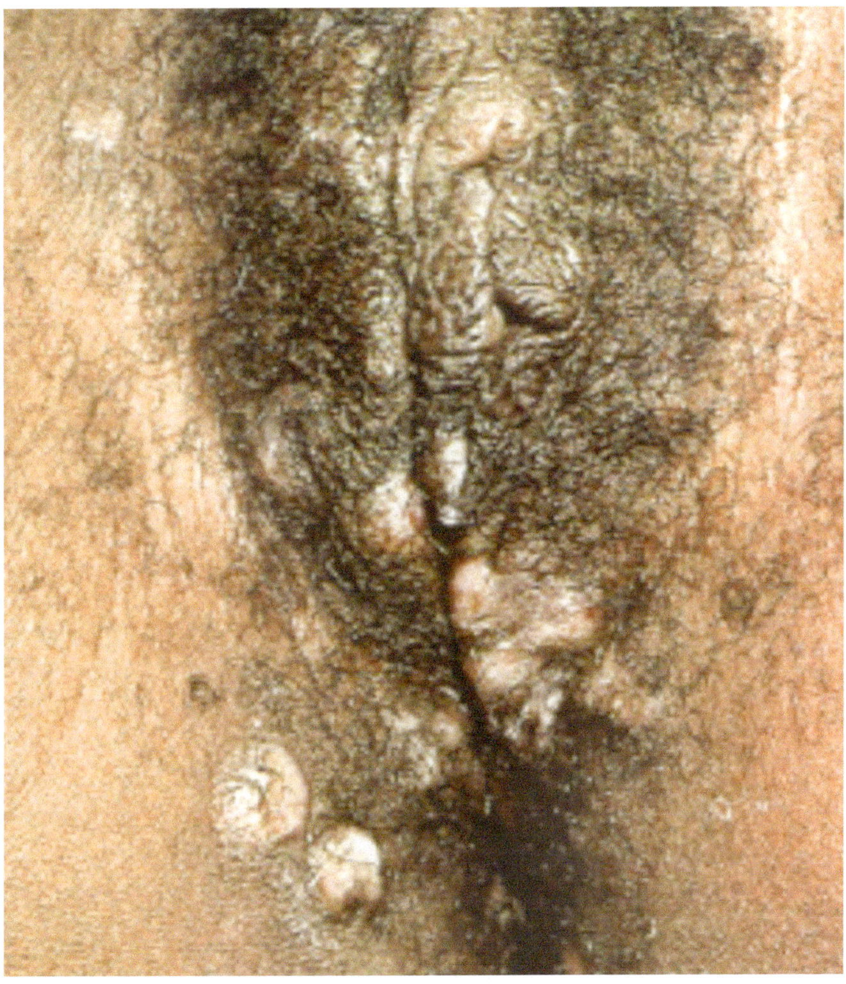

Soft, whitish, moist plaques of condylomata lata.

CLINICAL

- Rash
  - Lesions ranging in quantity from a few to many are most frequently found on:
    - Palms and soles, often straddling crease lines
    - Face, especially at the angle of mouth, eyes, and nose
    - Genitals (*See* page 59)
    - Trunk
    - Mouth ("mucous patches")
  - Lesions are:
    - Flat or slightly elevated
    - Smooth or scaly
    - Copper-colored to dusky red, sometimes with darker centers
    - Hyperkeratotic, on palms and soles
    - Almost never vesicular or oozing
    - Usually not pruritic but may itch severely
    - Possibly associated with a patchy "moth-eaten" alopecia of scalp and beard
- Systemic symptoms
  - Fever and malaise
  - Sore throat
  - Nonpainful (usually), generalized adenopathy
  - Rarely
    - Syphilitic hepatitis
    - Bone and joint pain

- Secondary syphilis: occurs 6 to 12 weeks after contact
  - Primary chancre may still be present.
  - Rash lasts 4–6 weeks without treatment.
    - May recur two to three times over the next 2 years
  - Syphilis is highly contagious in the secondary form.

Examiner should wear gloves.

- *Serologic tests:* Nonspecific serologic test for syphilis (STS) and fluorescent treponemal antibody (FTA)
  - In *secondary* syphilis, the results of both tests should be positive.
  - Titer is high (over 1:8) in nonspecific test.

If the nonspecific test result is negative, the cause is the *prozone phenomenon:* the titer is so high that it will not precipitate in test plates at low dilutions, which are the only ones used in screening tests. If secondary syphilis is strongly suspected, send another blood sample and ask for "prozone test" or examination at higher dilutions.

- Dark-field examination result is positive for primary and secondary lesions.
  - **Training and skill are required for successful examination.**
    - Squeeze fluid from lesions with firm pressure, even using the jaws of a hemostat.
    - Keep the organisms alive in a saline drop on the microscope slide; do not allow to dry out.
    - Examine immediately under a well-calibrated dark-field microscope.
- Examine and test for other sexually transmitted disease.
- Caution the patient to abstain from intimate contact until 24 hours after treatment.
- Report to public health authorities.

TREATMENT

- Be aware of updated national and local treatment recommendations. Current Public Health Service recommendations for *primary* and *secondary* syphilis are:
  - Benzathine penicillin G 2.4 million units intramuscularly once.
  - If the patient is unable to take penicillin, then give **doxycycline 100 mg bid for 14 days or tetracycline** 500 mg four times a day for 14 days.
  - Persons with HIV infection who have primary or secondary syphilis should be treated similarly to those without HIV
- Local soaks or compresses (*See* page 241) may be applied for a few days if ulcer is painful, infected, or oozing copiously.
- Follow-up serologic testing is advised.
  - Result of FIA remains positive indefinitely—do not retest.
  - Nonspecific STS
    - Check titers at 6 and 12 months after treatment
    - Titers usually decrease fourfold in 6–12 months after treatment for primary and secondary syphilis. About 10–20% of patients may not achieve a fourfold reduction in titers within 12 months after treatment. This may be associated with multiple factors and the patient should be examined by a specialist.
    - If titers rise at least fourfold and persist for over 2 weeks, assume new infection, and treat again.

For retreatment, weekly injections of benzathine penicillin G 2.4 million units intramuscularly for 3 weeks are recommended.

Scabies

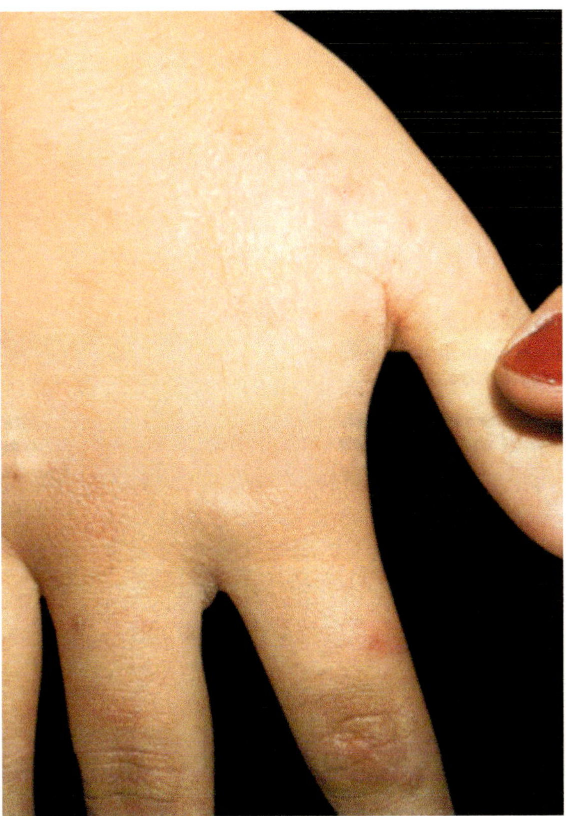

Severe itching but only scattered fine papules typify scabies. Fingerweb involvement is very common.

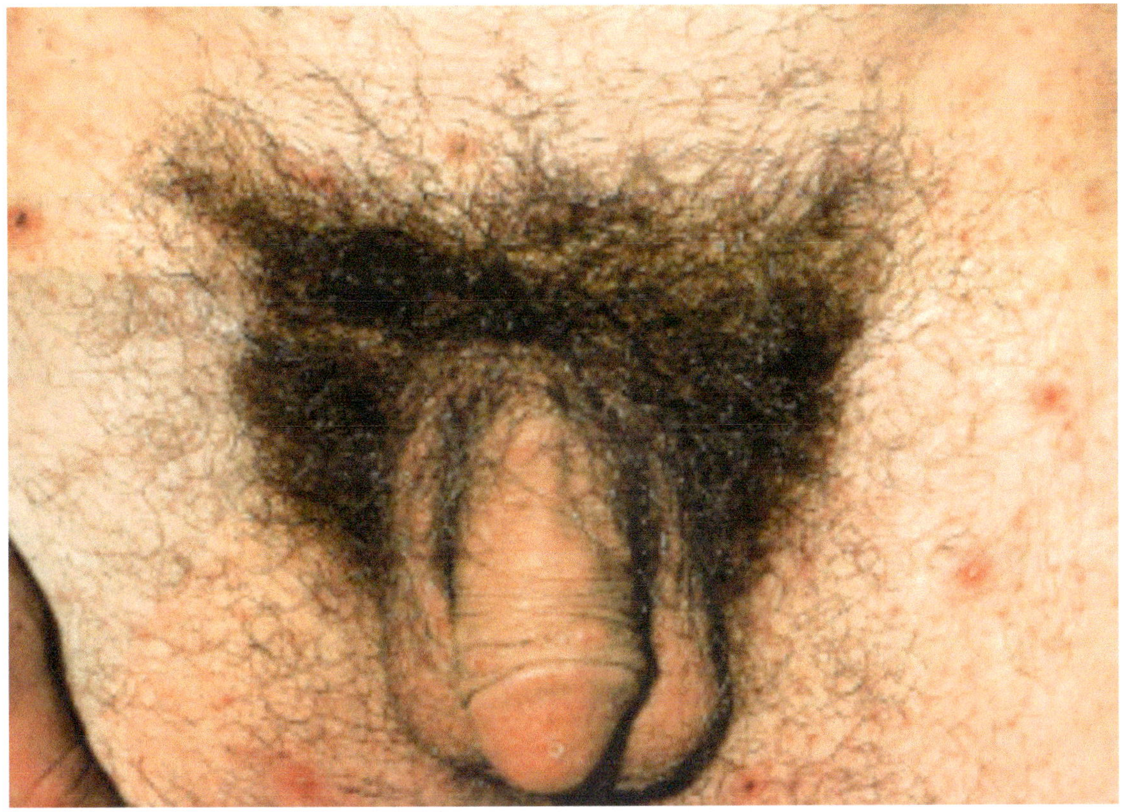

Typical excoriated papular eruption of scabies. Penile papules are characteristic.

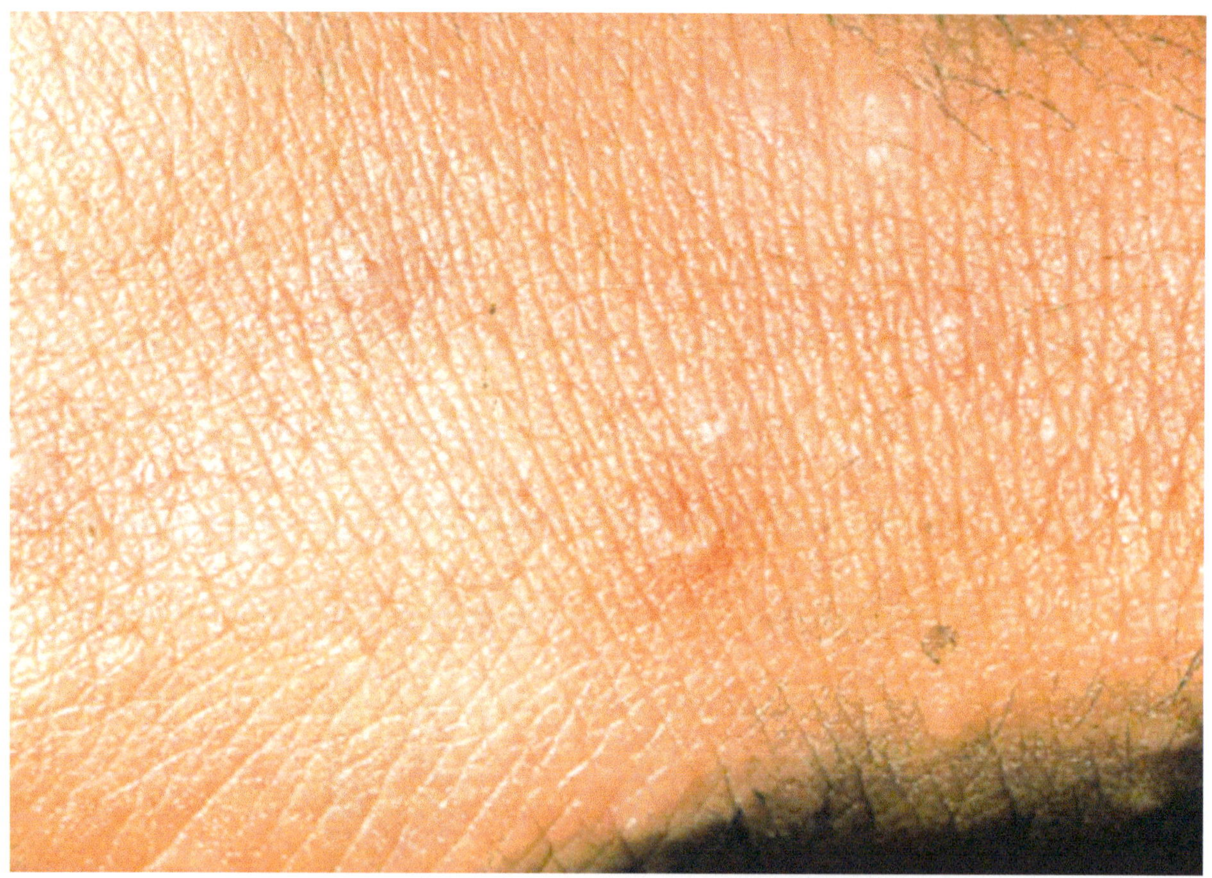

Most of the rash is an allergic reaction. The J-shaped white lesion in the center of the photograph is a burrow that contains an organism.

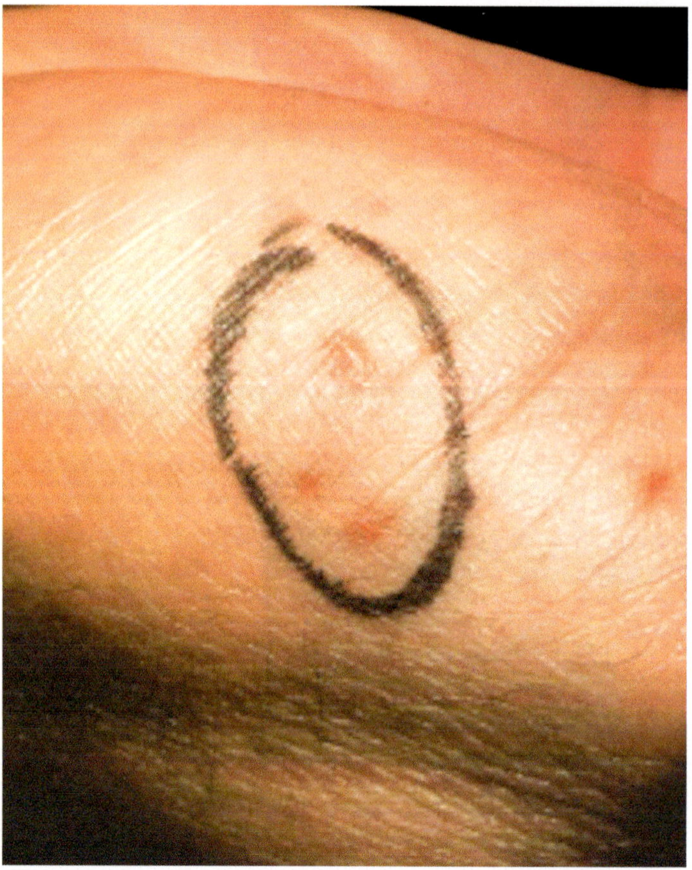

A linear burrow on a typical location, the margin of the palm.

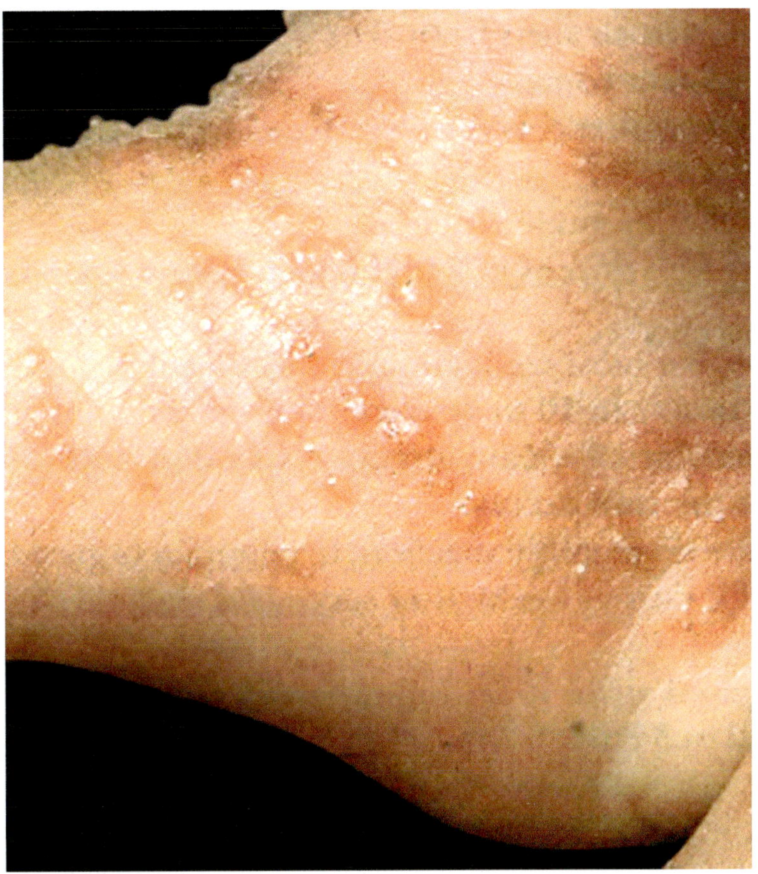

Scabies in infants is often vesicular and affects the palms, soles, and face.

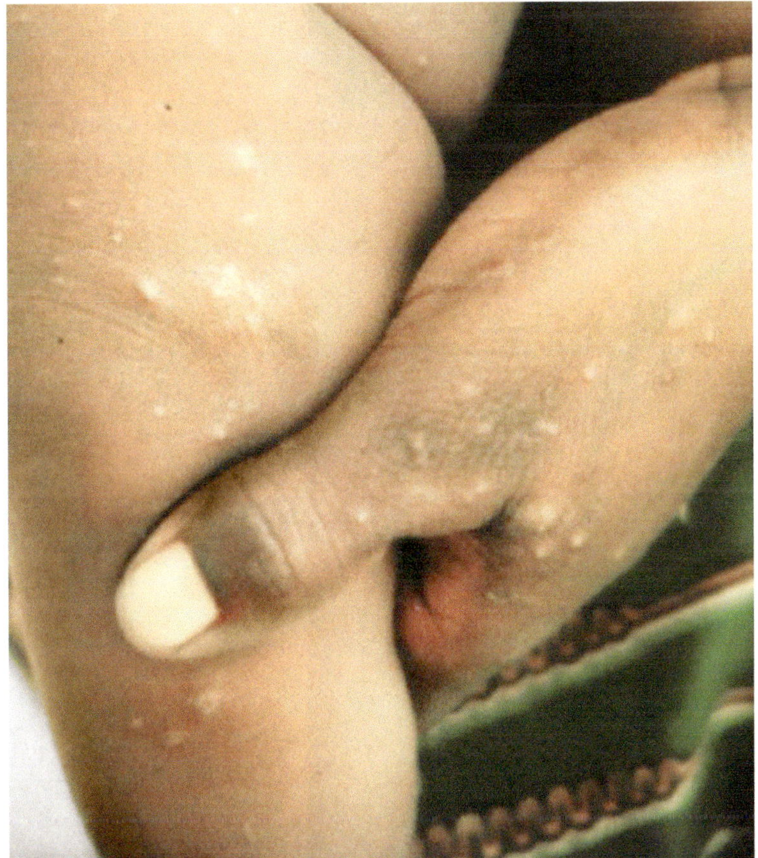

Secondarily infected scabies in a mother and child.

CLINICAL

- Condition is caused by the mite *Sarcoptes scabiei.*
  - Usually requires prolonged contact with the exception of the heavily infested patient.
  - Barely visible to the naked eye
  - Human parasite that burrows into keratin layer
    - Little inclination to be shed from skin
  - Passed by intimate skin contact
    - Rarely spread by casual contact (e.g., handshake or medical examination)
- Itching and rash are an immune reaction.
  - Organisms multiply to dozens in 2–3 weeks, but no symptoms are present.
    - The organisms are most contagious at this time.
  - Hypersensitivity occurs in 10–20 days; then the rash appears.
  - The immune reaction kills many organisms so that only a few are present after the rash occurs.
    - Most lesions are an immune reaction; few contain organisms.
  - Itching persists for days to weeks after successful scabicide therapy.
  - If scabies is acquired again in an immune individual, then the rash appears in 2–3 days.
- Rash
  - Typically in sexually active young adults
    - Very itchy, especially at night
    - Concentrated in fingerwebs, wrist folds, axillae, umbilicus, groin, and genitals
    - Spares the face and scalp
    - More prominent on dorsal hands and feet
    - Fine, excoriated papules
    - Often a few papules surmounted by a 1- to 4-mm fine, white-etched *burrow*
  - In infants
    - Face, palms, and soles may be involved.
    - Lesions may be vesicular, especially on palms and soles.
  - In the elderly
    - Itching may be intense but rash may be absent or may consist of only a few papules in atypical locations.
- Diagnosis may be confirmed by shave and microscope examination of appropriate lesions. The presence of mites, eggs, or feces confirms the diagnosis, but their absence does not exclude it (*See* page 229 for technique).
- Secondary staphylococcal pyoderma may occur.
  - The lesions become painful.
  - Oozing and yellow crust formation occur.

TREATMENT

Patients should be educated about the characteristics of the disease so that they can understand the possible sources, the contagiousness during the incubation period, and the persistent itching after treatment (*See* Patient Guides, page 252).

- Scabicides (*See* page 237)
  - A cream or lotion should be applied to the entire body from neck to feet, being sure to treat the genitals, umbilicus, and all body folds. It is left on overnight and washed off in the morning.

- Permethrin 5% cream is applied from the neck down to the feet and washed off after 8–14 hours. It is the treatment of choice in young children and pregnant women.
    - Benzyl benzoate is applied daily for 3 days. It is not readily available in the United States.
- An alternative scabicide is sulfur 5–10% in petrolatum.
    - Apply twice daily for 3 days.
    - This product may be irritating.
    - A topical corticosteroid is often added.
    - Ivermectin 200 mcg/kg orally as a single dose, repeated in 2 weeks.

Note: Pyrethrins (*See* page 237) are effective against lice but *not* against scabies.

- Treatment of itching
    - The worst itching fades in 1–2 days, so treatment may not be necessary.
    - Sedating antihistamines given at bedtime aid sleep.
    - Baths (*See* page 241) are mildly soothing.
    - Corticosteroids
        - Potent topical corticosteroids are occasionally used and may relieve itching.
        - A high dose of systemic corticosteroid (40–60 mg prednisone) may be administered for a few days to relieve severe itching in heavily infested patients.

Persistent itching and rash may be due to:
- Guilt-ridden and disgusted patients greatly irritating skin by repeated application of scabicides and/or compulsive frequent bathing, often with strong soaps.
- Failure to apply scabicide to *entire* body surface (below neck) (typically patient skips areas that do not itch)
- Washing hands after applying scabicide, thus removing effective treatment to that site
- Reacquisition of scabies from untreated contacts and family members

Treatment failure is rare. But permethrin-resistant organisms have been reported.

- Treatment of contacts
    - Should include:
        - All bed partners for 1 month before onset of rash
        - Children and family members in the household with whom there is intimate contact
    - May exclude:
        - Roommates or housemates with whom there is no intimate skin contact
        - Casual acquaintances
- Environmental treatment

Remember that the organism is not easily shed from the skin, and it usually lives off the human for only 12–24 hours.

- Upon arising from overnight scabicide treatment
    - Wash bed linen, pajamas.
    - Don clean clothes or clothes not worn during the preceding 2 days.
    - Wash clothes worn during preceding day, or set aside for several days.
- *Do not*
    - Wash or dry-clean entire wardrobe.
    - Fumigate house or try to clean mattress and furniture.

- Scabies is often sexually transmitted. Look for signs of other sexually transmitted diseases and perform a serologic test for syphilis at the time of diagnosis and again in 6 weeks.

Tinea Versicolor (Pityriasis Versicolor)

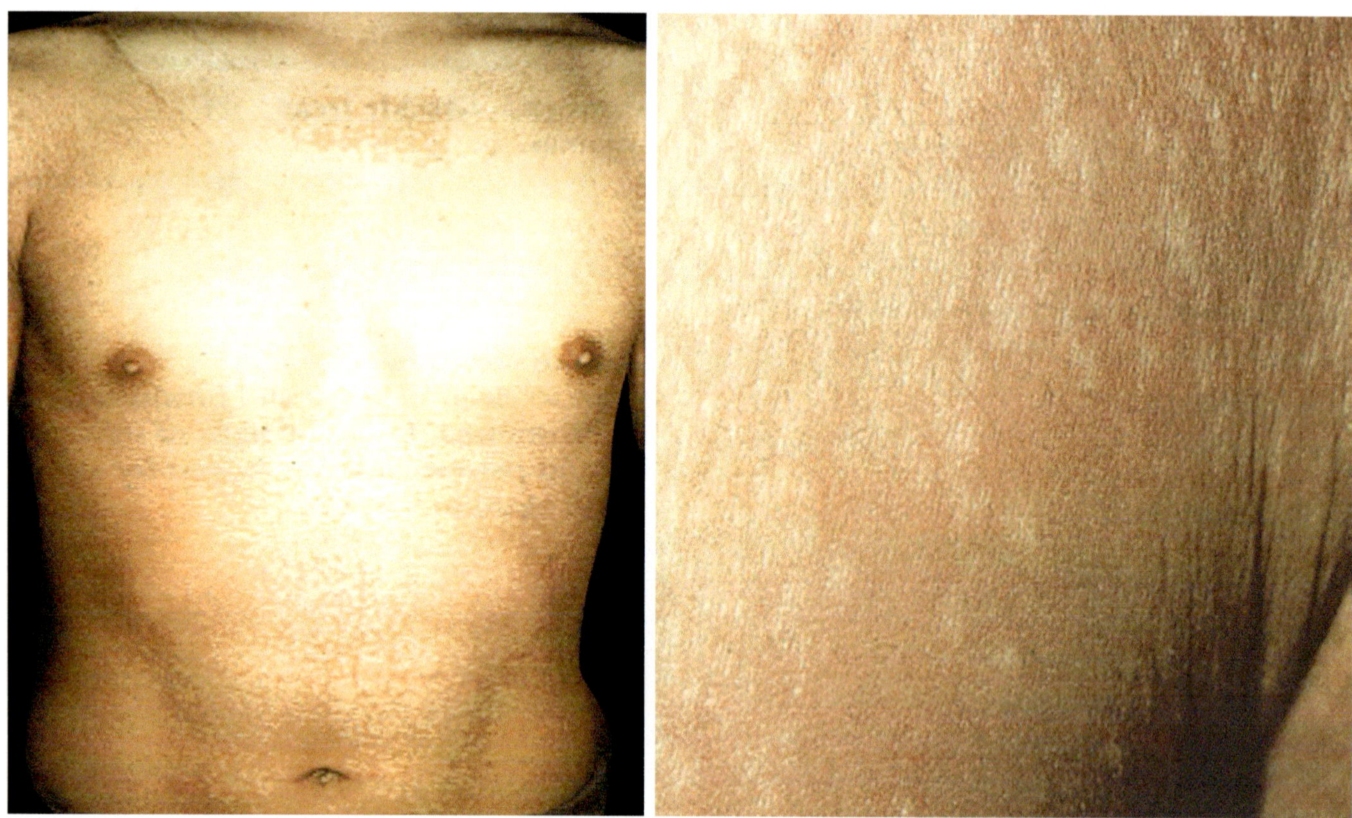

Diffuse hypopigmenting tinea versicolor in a fair-skinned person. Distributed as if "paint poured from above." Close-up shows typical scaly satellite lesions.

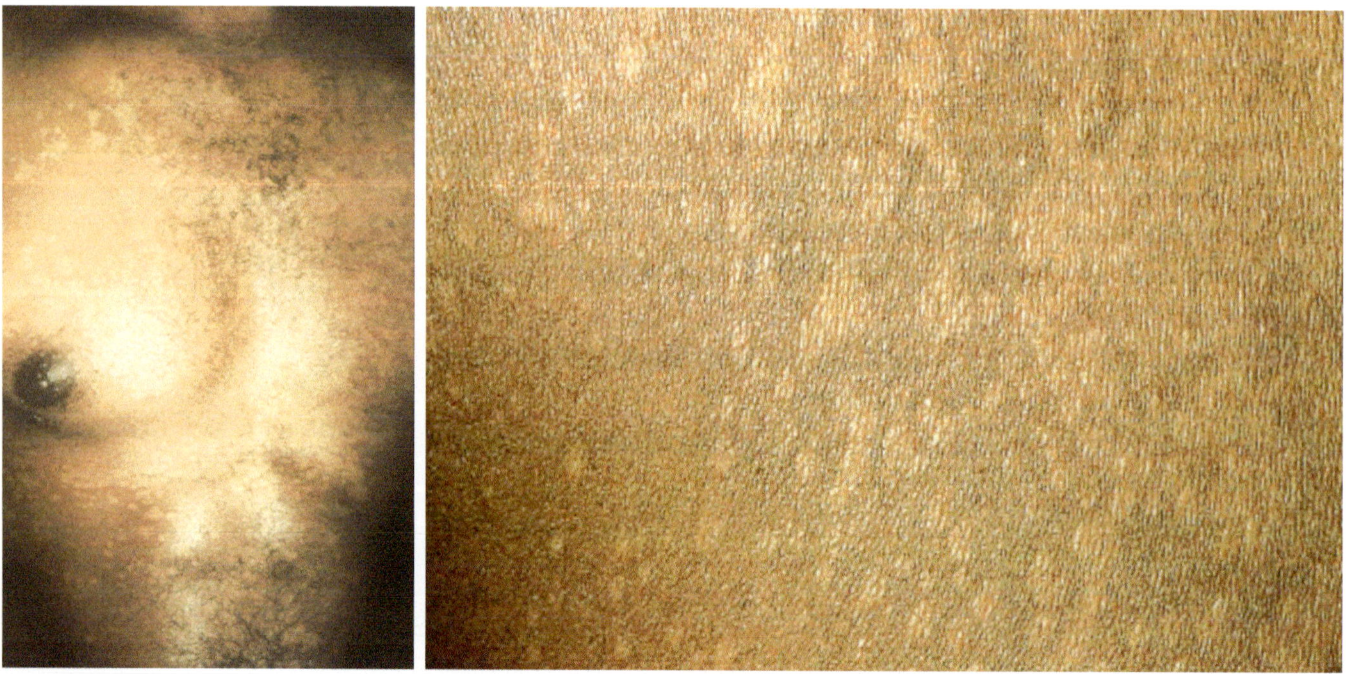

Two shades of hypopigmenting tinea versicolor in dark-skinned individuals.

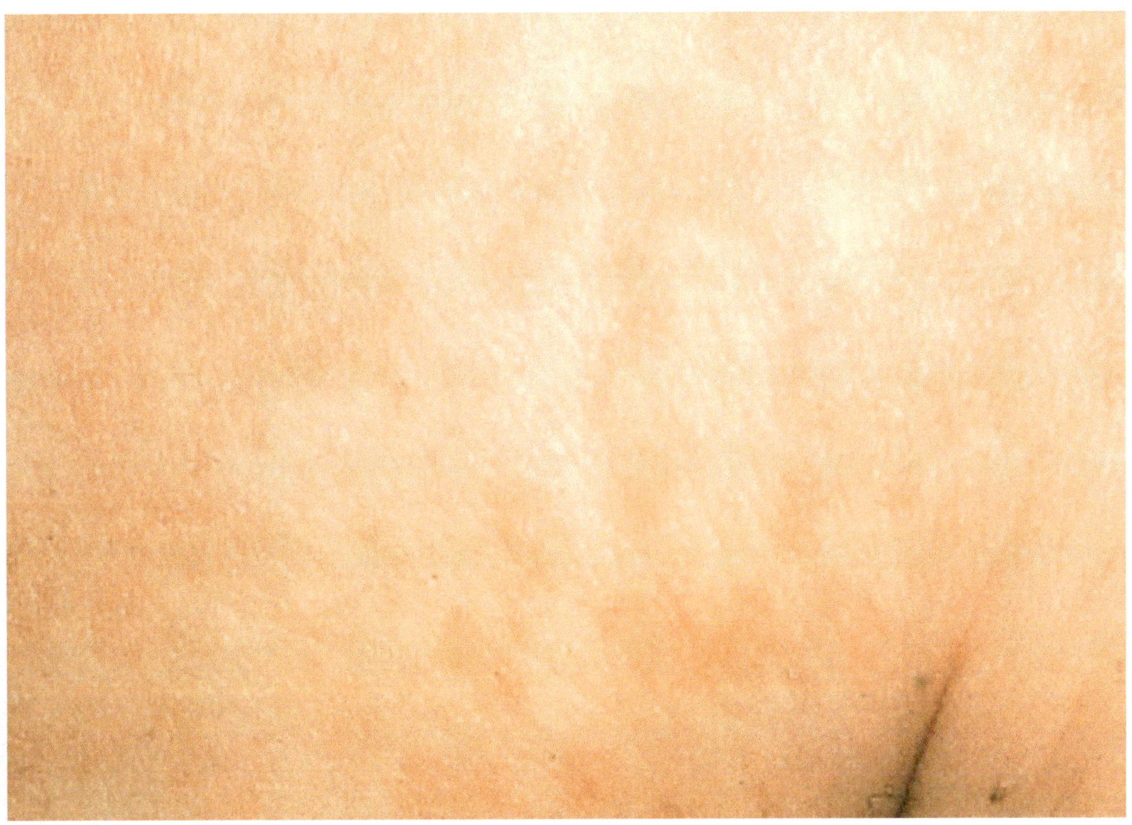

Tinea versicolor in this fair-skinned person is pink-tan.

CLINICAL

- This condition appears as a discolored scaly eruption in young adults.
  - The eruption consists of sharply demarcated discrete and confluent macules with a fine, cigarette-ash scale.
    - The scale is absent for a few hours after bathing.
  - Eruptions are distributed over the shoulders and upper trunk ("as though paint were poured from above"). Occasionally they occur in isolated patches.
  - Ranges from fawn-tan hypopigmentation to dark-brown hyperpigmentation, depending on skin color ("versicolor" means changing colors).
  - This condition occurs more frequently in summer and in hot, humid climates; it almost never occurs in prepubescent patients and is rare in patients over 40 years of age.
  - Tinea versicolor is occasionally mildly itchy.
- The condition is caused by proliferation of a yeast-like organism *(Malassezia furfur)*.
  - It is not known why this normal skin inhabitant proliferates in some individuals and not in others.
  - Condition is not "contagious," as all adults carry the organism.
  - Potassium hydroxide (KOH) examination (*See* page 226) reveals the organism as "spaghetti and meatballs" with short, curly hyphae and clusters of spores. These will not grow on standard culture media. Scale may be absent for a few hours after bathing and positive KOH identification is then impossible. If clinical diagnosis is in question, have patient return without bathing for KOH examination the next day.

TREATMENT

- General
  - The organism is not harmful or contagious.
  - The organism is a normal skin inhabitant, so the clinical relapse rate is high. Inform patient of its benign nature. Treatment clears *scaling* quickly, but *color* does not return to normal for 2–3 months.
  - Because various therapies work and relapse is common, treatment is one of the least standardized in dermatology.

- Keratolytics. The organism lives *on* the keratin layer (not *in* it, as do ringworm fungi), so removal of a superficial layer of keratin is therapeutic.

Dandruff shampoo is most commonly used. Selenium sulfide 2.5% shampoo is applied thinly to the entire trunk with a generous margin of normal skin. Leave on from 15 minutes to overnight, depending on patient tolerance; wash off using more shampoo as soap, and scrub briskly with a facecloth. Repeat this procedure daily for 1–2 weeks. Relapses occur months later in one-third of cases, requiring a repeat course (Patient Guides, *See* page 251). *Note:* Other dandruff shampoos are probably equally effective as selenium sulfide, but controlled studies are lacking.

- Antifungal agents
  - All topical antifungal agents (*See* page 235) are effective but must be applied to the entire trunk twice daily for 2 weeks.
    - Somewhat inconvenient to use
    - Appropriate for a patient on whom a few localized lesions are present
    - Oral antifungal agents are reserved for widespread or recalcitrant cases
    - Fluconazole is usually given as 300 mg once weekly for 2 weeks, but a single dose of 400 mg may be effective in some patients.
    - Itraconazole can be given as 200 mg per day for 5 days.

Tinea Corporis

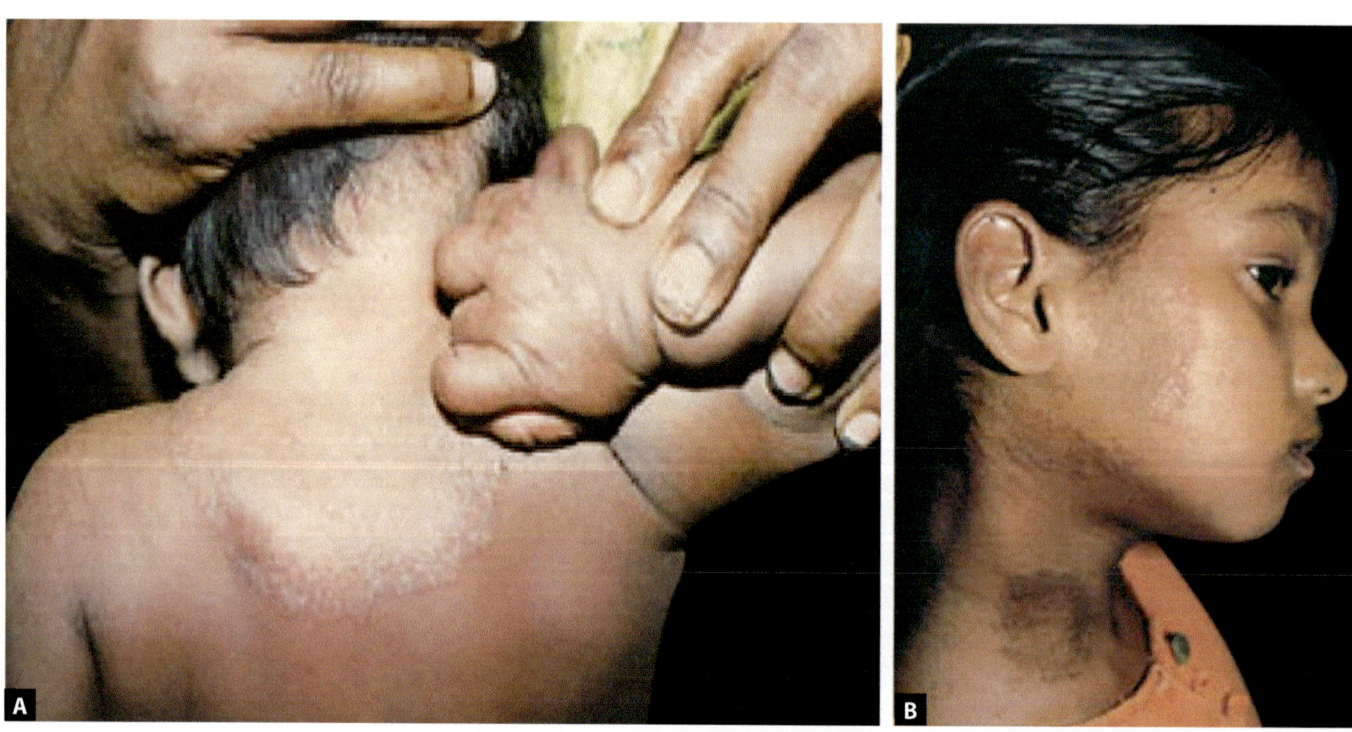

Ring-shaped lesion with peripheral scales over the back. The picture shows the child scratching—typical tinea corporis (A). Similar morphological pattern over the face—tinea faciei (B).

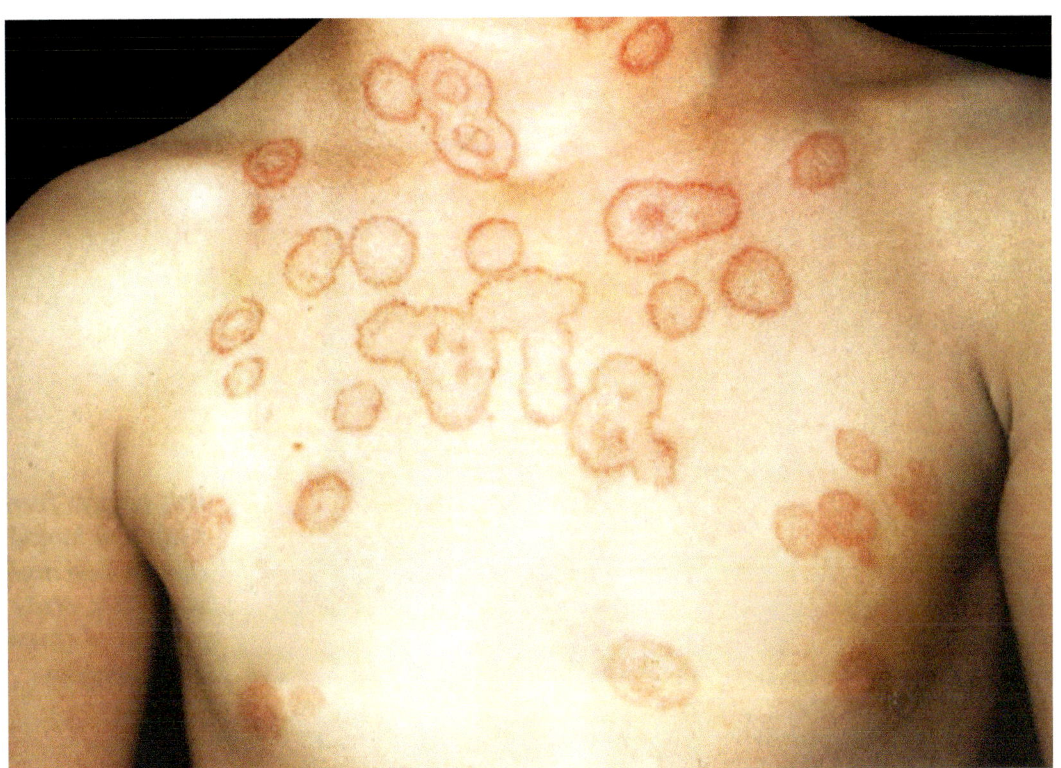

Dramatic widespread tinea corporis in a child.

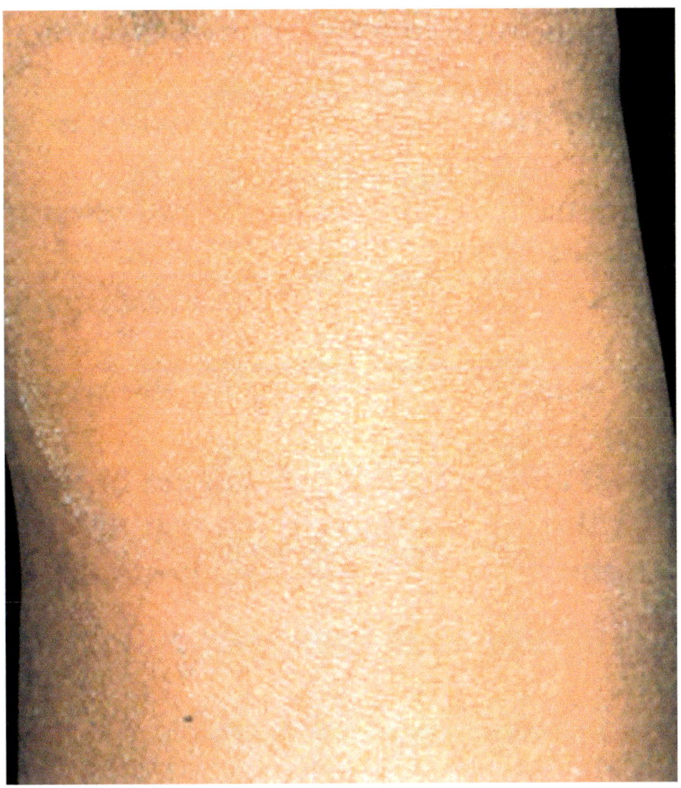

Subtle expanding ring lesion in an adult.

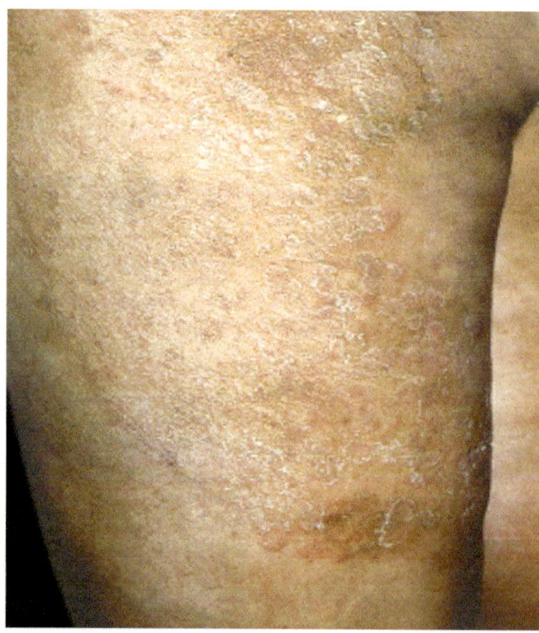

This patient from a hot and humid climate had many large, dry, scaly plaques of chronic tinea corporis.

CLINICAL

- Consists of dull red, scaly patches on the trunk or extremities
  - Usually annular or arcuate, with red, scaly border and clearing center
    - More common in children
  - May be uniformly red scaly patch
    - More common in adults living in warm, humid climates
  - Usually moderately itchy
- In children, the condition is often acquired from dogs or cats, and lesions are inflammatory.
- In adults, the lesions are usually less inflammatory and often preceded by tinea cruris or tinea pedis.
- Both types are fairly rare in temperate climates and more common in hot, humid climates.
  - Tinea survives best on moist skin, accounting for the common occurrence in the groin and on feet.
- Occasionally the lesion will appear as dull red papules in the red patches or separate from them (especially from shaving on the legs). In this form it is a *follicular* infection.

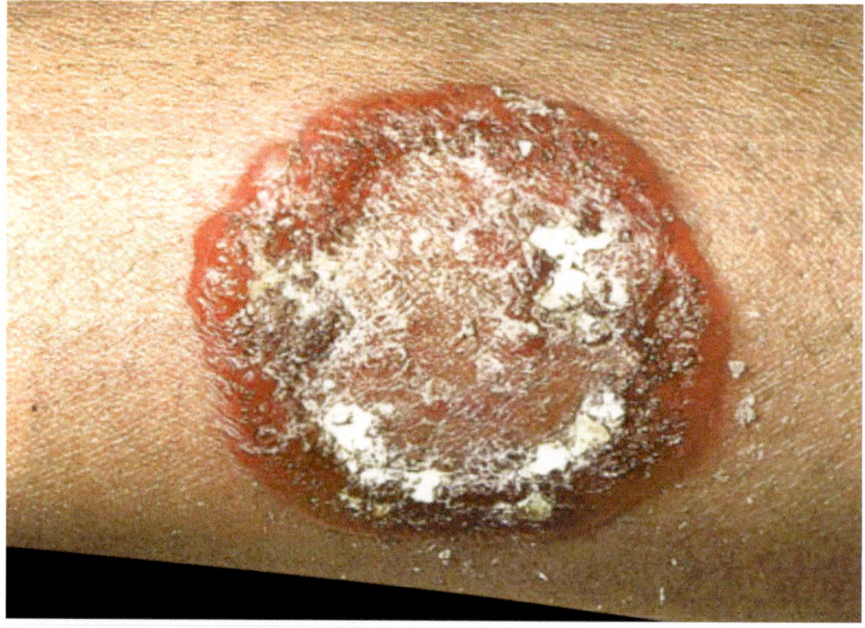

This woman worked in a school in which many children had scalp ringworm.

TREATMENT

- If small and localized the lesions will respond to topical antifungal therapy (*See* page 235) applied twice daily for 10–20 days.
  - Ciclopirox, clotrimazole, econazole, ketoconazole, miconazole, naftifine, and tolnaftate are probably equally effective.
  - Undecylenic acid and iodoquinol are also effective.
- If severe, widespread, follicular, or resistant to topical agents, give oral antifungal drugs (*See* page 235).
  - Itraconazole 200 mg bid for 7 days (not approved in the United States for tineas)
  - Fluconazole 150–200 mg once weekly for 2–4 weeks
  - Micronized griseofulvin 250–500 mg twice daily for 2–4 weeks is less commonly used.
- *See* also tinea capitis (*See* page 5), tinea faciei (*See* page 23), tinea cruris (*See* page 68), tinea pedis (*See* page 82), and onychomycosis (*See* page 86).

Impetigo and Bacterial Pyoderma

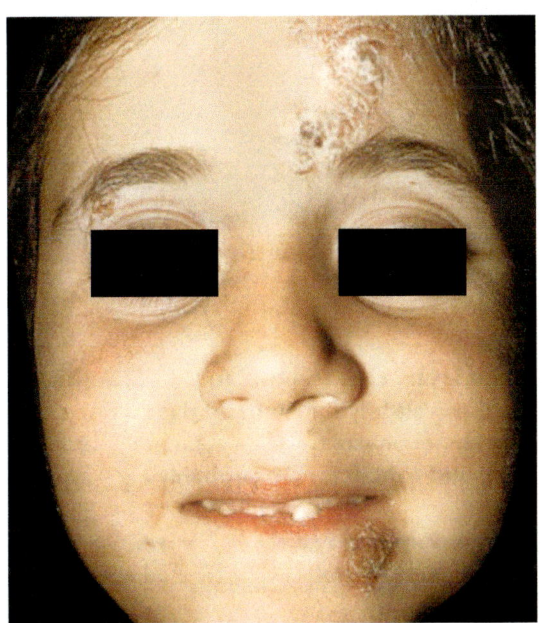

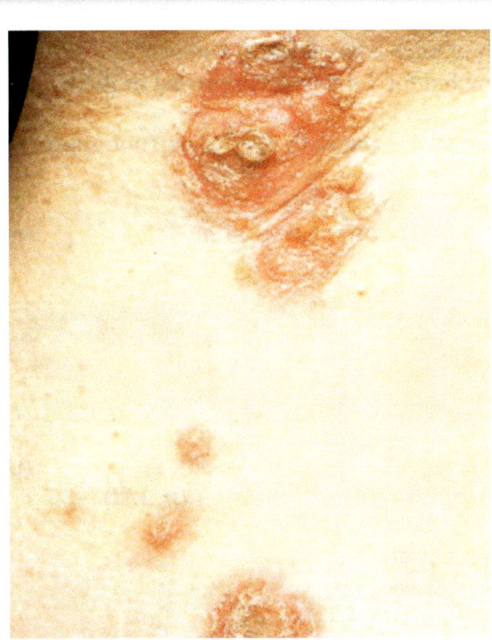

Typical impetigo contagiosa: honey-colored crusts on red erosions, on the face and in a fold area (axilla).

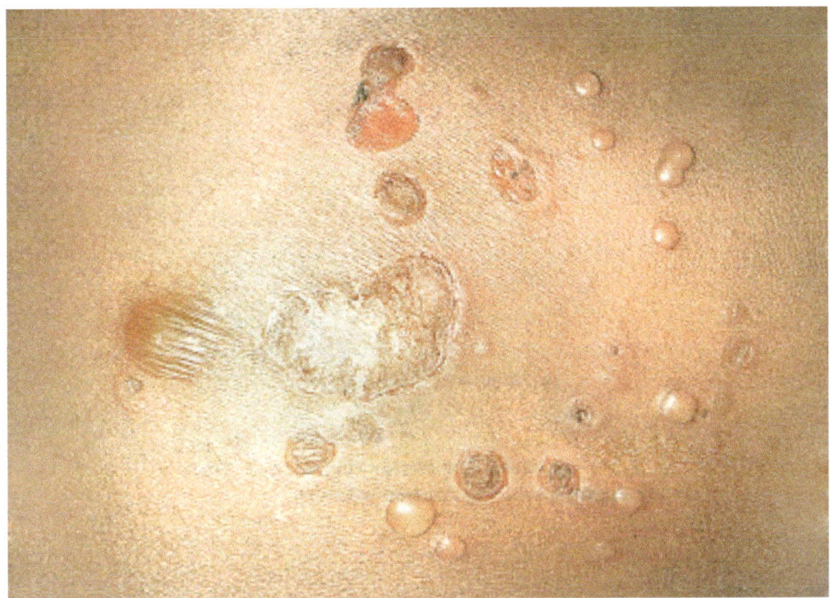

Early localized bullous impetigo in an infant. The absence of inflammation in this infection is striking.

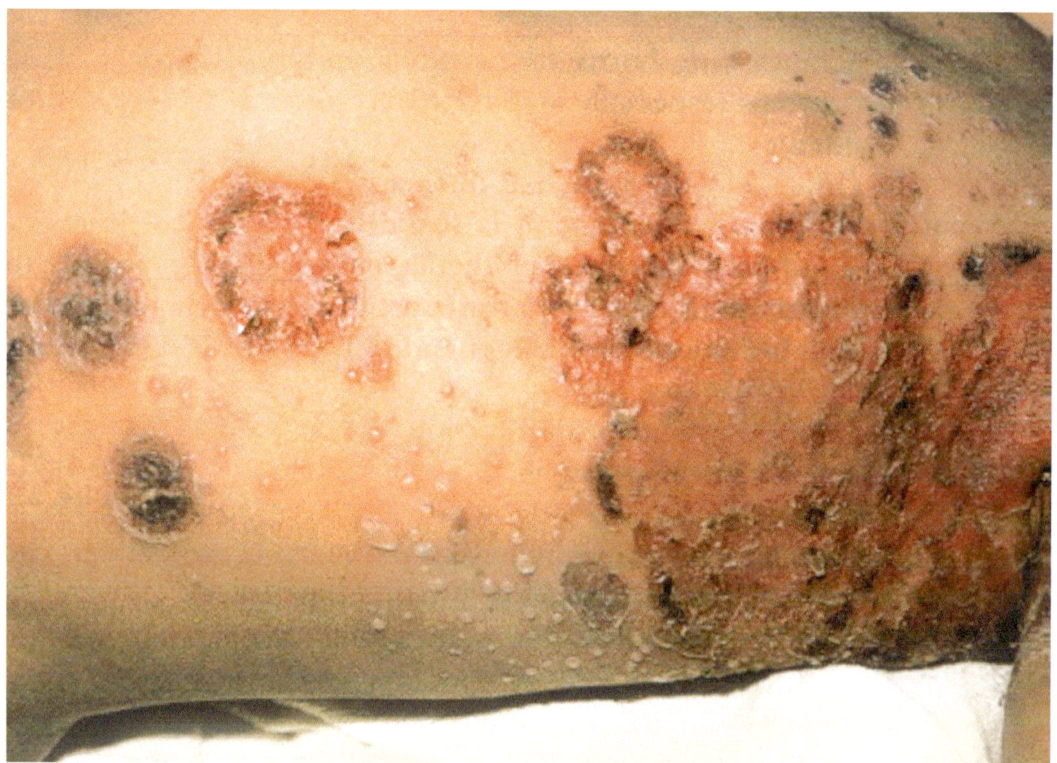

Extensive bullous impetigo in a 9-month-old.

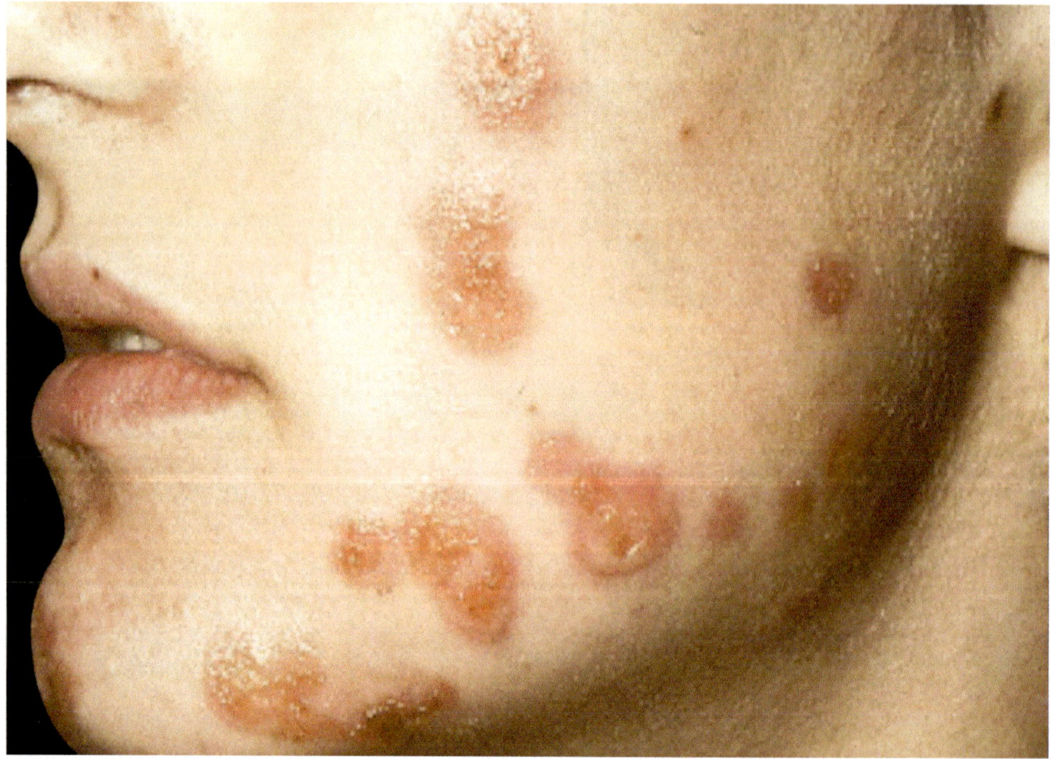

Bullous impetigo in an adult. The blister roofs are so thin and fragile that they often are ruptured during routine washing.

CLINICAL

- Secondary bacterial infection
  - The infective organism is usually *Staphylococcus aureus.*
    - Occasionally *Streptococcus*

- Any spontaneous or induced lesion may become infected. Common ones are:
  - Scrapes, cuts, burns, excoriations, and insect bites
  - Eczemas (especially atopic, *See* page 103), stasis dermatitis, bullous diseases
  - Other infections, such as tinea and candidiasis
- Development of infection is signaled clinically by the occurrence of pain, increased erythema, increased weeping, and the formulation of thick, yellowish crust. In dermatitis, particularly, itching becomes more insistent and the lesions become tender.

- Impetigo contagiosa
  - A common primary skin infection
  - A typical clinical setting is:
    - Children
    - Hot, humid environment (southeastern United States, Central America, or summers in temperate zones)
    - Crowded, poor socioeconomic conditions
  - Typical lesions
    - Are located on face, fold areas (neck, axillae)
    - Start as oozing erosion or transient thin-roofed blister, grow rapidly (1–3 days), develop honey-colored granular crust. Often, after 1–2 weeks, they dry up. In temperate climates the lesions often heal spontaneously, especially as the weather cools. In tropical climates, lesions may persist for weeks and new ones may develop.
    - May be asymptomatic, itchy, or tender
  - In the United States the most common organism is *S. aureus,* but group A streptococci may cause impetigo and in endemic areas may be the most common organism.
    - Cultures may show streptococci, staphylococci, or both
  - These conditions are a major cause of streptococcal-induced glomerulonephritis in endemic circumstances.
    - In the United States more glomerulonephritis is secondary to impetigo than to pharyngitis.
- Bullous impetigo
  - A sporadic and rare primary infection of skin
  - Typically occurs in infants, often in nursery epidemics
    - Occasionally in adults, especially on face
  - Lesions are vesicles and bullae on bland, noninflamed skin. In a few days dried, collapsed blister roofs cover very superficial erosions, which often heal in a few weeks.
  - Infecting agent is *S. aureus.*
    - Occurs only in uncommon instance when the strain of *Staphylococcus* produces an epidermolytic toxin that chemically splits the epidermis, causing blister formation.

A related condition is staphylococcal scalded skin syndrome, in which a toxin-producing organism inhabits the nose or other internal site, and the toxin is bloodborne, causing lysis and denudation of large areas of skin or of the entire body. The mortality rate is up to 25% in the absence of appropriate medical care.

TREATMENT

- Secondary pyodermas
  - Keeping an injury clean, especially with the use of antibacterial soap, minimizes the likelihood of infection. Also preventive is the use of petrolatum.
  - The prescription-requiring antibiotic ointment mupirocin cures many superficial infections. Treatment should be preceded by gentle washing or soaking [water, astringent (*See* page 241) or antibiotic soap] twice a day and gentle debridement with fingers or gauze during soaks. Protection between treatments with dressings probably speeds healing, compared with leaving the wound open.
- Impetigo contagiosa

A major controversy exists in the treatment of streptococcal impetigo because of its high contagiousness and the possibility of glomerulonephritis. Neither systemic nor topical care will prevent glomerulonephritis in a person with established infection. Systemic administration of antibiotics causes lesions to be "sterile" of *Streptococcus* in 24 hours. Conscientious *topical* treatment stops the shedding of organisms in only 65% of patients after 5 days. Impetigo often occurs in crowded, poor socioeconomic conditions, in which contagion is high and likelihood of rigorous topical care is low. Oral erythromycin can be used in reliable patients; it avoids the risk of penicillin allergy. For localized disease, topical care may be satisfactory.

- Topical care is the same as for secondary pyoderma.
- Systemic antibiotics
  - Dicloxacillin 25–50 mg/kg/day divided every 6 hours or 250–500 mg by mouth four times daily for 7 days
  - Cephalexin 25–50 mg/kg/day divided every 6–8 hours or 250–500 mg by mouth four times daily for 7 days
  - For penicillin-sensitive patients: erythromycin 30–50 mg/kg per day in divided doses or 250–500 mg every 6–12 hours daily for 7 days
  - If methicillin-resistant *Staphylococcus aureus* (MRSA) is suspected, treatment with sulfamethoxazole-trimethoprim, clindamycin, or doxycycline is recommended.

- Bullous impetigo
  - For small, isolated lesions, topical care (as earlier) is adequate.
  - For resistant or widespread cases, systemic antistaphylococcal treatment is necessary.
  - If the patient is in a nursery or with other infants, isolate and check contacts for infection.

Staphylococcal scalded skin syndrome must be treated by admission to hospital, systemic antibiotics, and close attention to fluid and electrolyte status.

Herpes Zoster (Shingles)

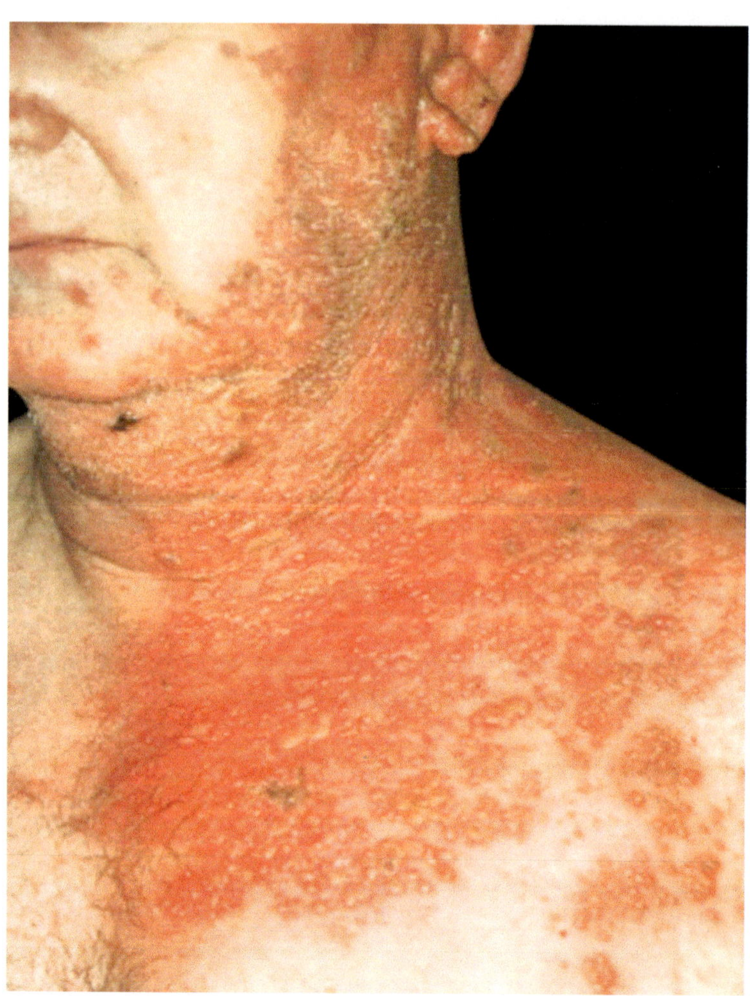

Widespread zoster.

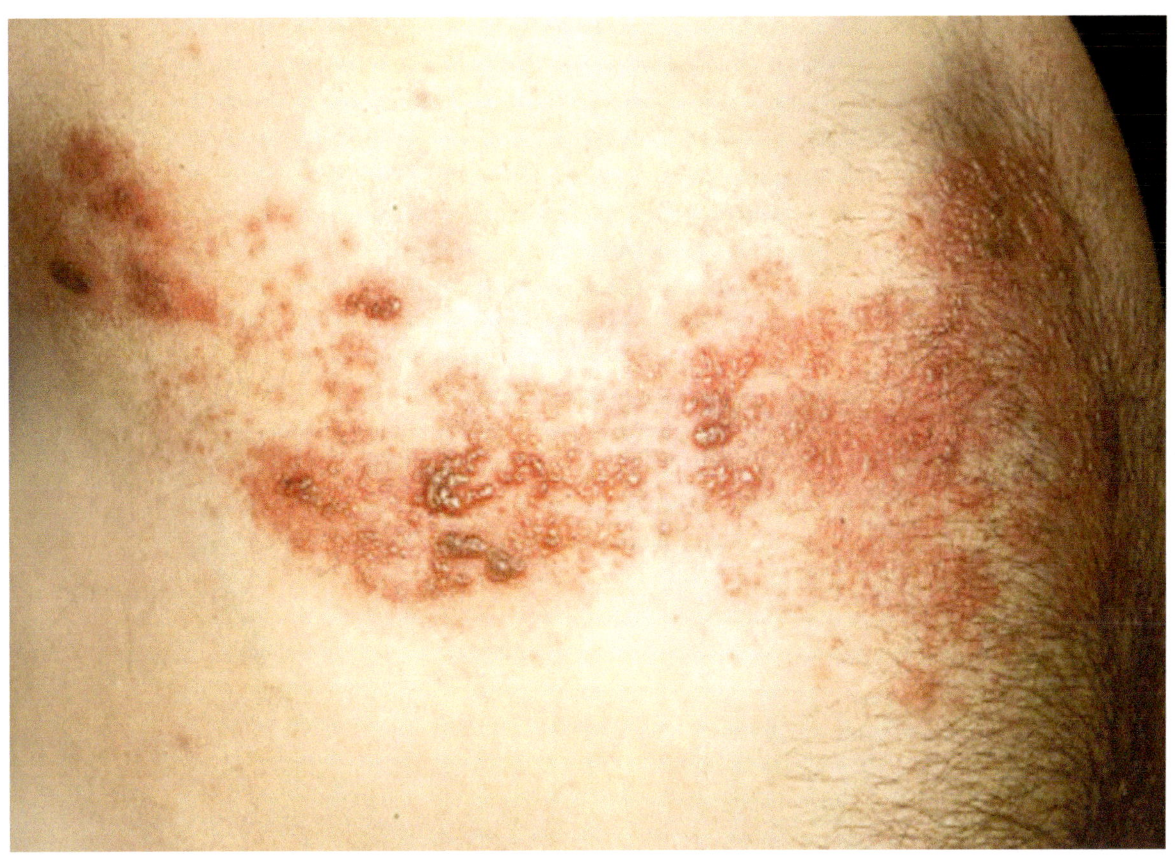

A belt of "shingles" (from Latin: cingulus, a girdle), vesicles on an inflamed base. Hemorrhage into vesicles is common.

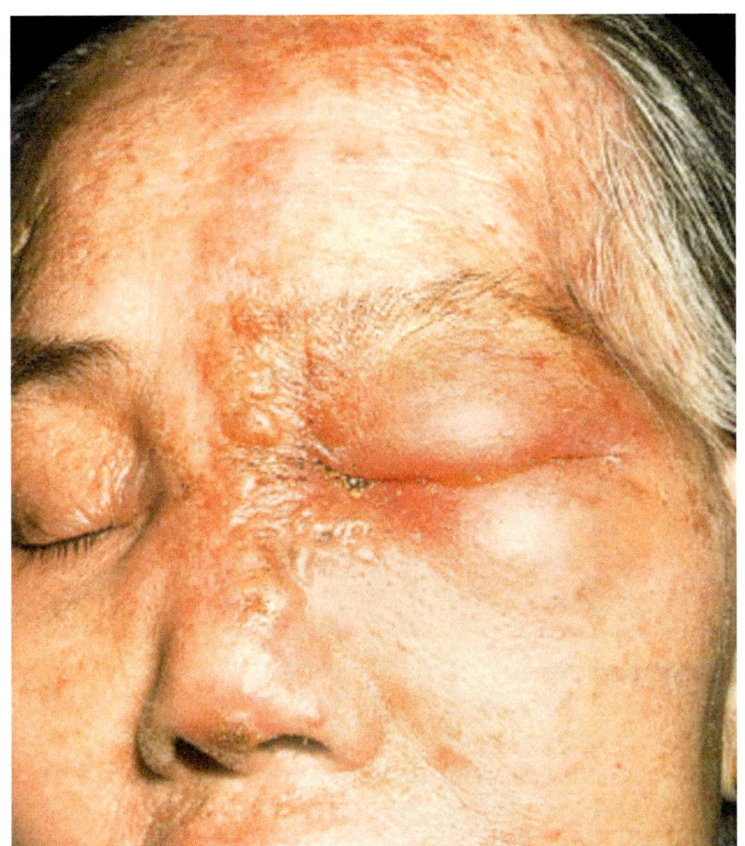

When the tip of the nose is affected, the eye is usually involved, as in this case.

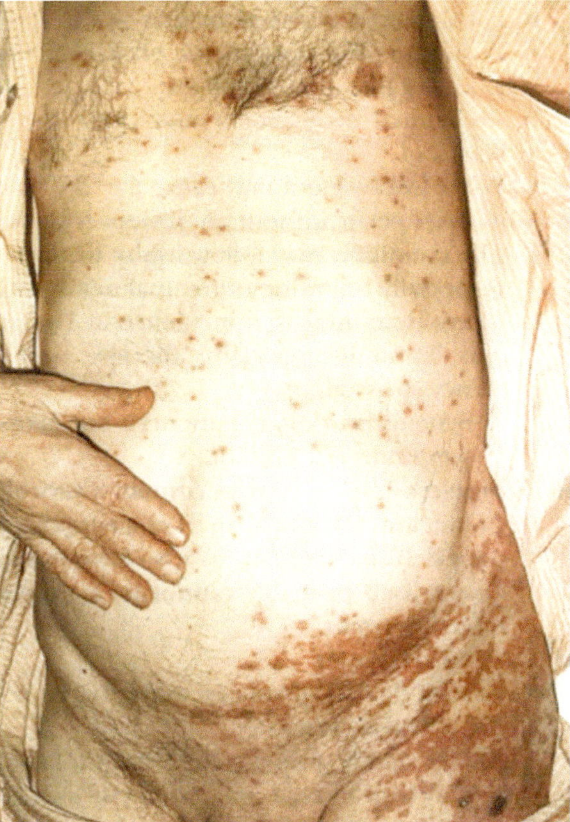

Disseminated zoster in an immunosuppressed person.

CLINICAL

- Rash
  - Shingles appear as grouped vesicles on bright red, edematous plaques.
    - These are sometimes pustular or hemorrhagic.
    - Often the vesicles have ruptured, leaving only punctate scabs or erosions on a pink plaque.
    - Sometimes plaques appear without vesicles.
  - The plaques are distributed unilaterally along the dermatome.
    - The entire eruption may be only one small plaque or dozens of large, confluent plaques.
  - It ranges from being asymptomatic to very painful.
    - The likelihood of pain increases with age.
    - Hemorrhagic vesicles are often associated with severe pain.
    - The affected dermatome may be hyperesthetic.
- Systemic symptoms
  - Local painful adenopathy may occur.
  - Involvement of ophthalmic branch of the facial nerve may include an infection of the eye.
  - Abdominal involvement may cause 2 or 3 days of hypotonic bowel.
  - Pelvic involvement may cause 2–3 days of hypotonic bladder.
- Most cases occur without an obvious triggering stimulus.
  - The condition may follow injury to the spinal or cranial nerve (especially following trigeminal nerve surgery).
  - There is an increased incidence in Hodgkin's disease, lymphomas, immunosuppressive therapy, and human immunodeficiency virus (HIV).
    - Systemic workup of patients is not necessary unless suggestive symptoms are present.
- Oozing erosions or vesicles contain a varicella-zoster virus.
  - Contagious (in the form of chickenpox) by direct contact with people (usually children) who have not had chickenpox.
  - Zoster itself probably cannot be acquired by contact with the infecting agent but a nonimmune person may contract varicella from contact with a zoster blister
- Generalized zoster
  - At least dozens of vesicles more than a few centimeters beyond the affected dermatome.
    - May signify immune suppression; look for the cause
    - May lead to fatal pneumonia or encephalitis
- Postzoster neuralgia
  - Consists of dermatomal pain and hyperesthesia lasting weeks to months after a 2-week course of acute eruption and pain.
  - The incidence, severity, and duration increase with age.
- Recurrence rarely seen in the immunocompetent but may be seen in the immunosuppressed.

TREATMENT

- Antiviral therapy is recommended if started within 72 hours of symptom begin, or if new lesions are appearing.
- These agents can shorten zoster-associated pain but there is conflicting evidence regarding reduction of postherpetic neuralgia.
- Immunosuppressed patients may require hospitalization for intravenous acyclovir.
- Valacyclovir (*See* page 237) may be the drug of choice. One gram three times per day given orally for 7 days is completely absorbed and is converted to the active form internally.
- Famciclovir (*See* page 237) is as effective as oral acyclovir but requires dosing only three times daily (500 mg/dose) instead of five times daily. This agent is given for 1 week.
- The dose for oral acyclovir is 800 mg five times daily for 7 days.

- Eruption
  - Cool compresses or soaks three times a day to wash off serum and dry up erosions, if present
- Acute pain
  - Appropriate oral analgesics
  - For mild pain, acetaminophen or nonsteroidal anti-inflammatory agents may be sufficient
  - Oral corticosteroids in high doses (50–60 mg of prednisone) with tapering over 10–14 days may help relieve acute pain, if moderate or severe.
    - Does not decrease incidence of postherpetic neuralgia
    - Does *not* increase likelihood of viral dissemination but may potentially increase the risk of secondary bacterial infection
- Postherpetic neuralgia
  - Oral tricyclic antidepressants may be of benefit.
    - Refer the patient to a neurologist for therapy.
- Hyperesthesia

Frequently a very annoying, persistent symptom.

  - A tight T-shirt, elasticized underwear or stockings, or wrap provides continuous, firm pressure, which suppresses hyperesthesia.

Molluscum Contagiosum

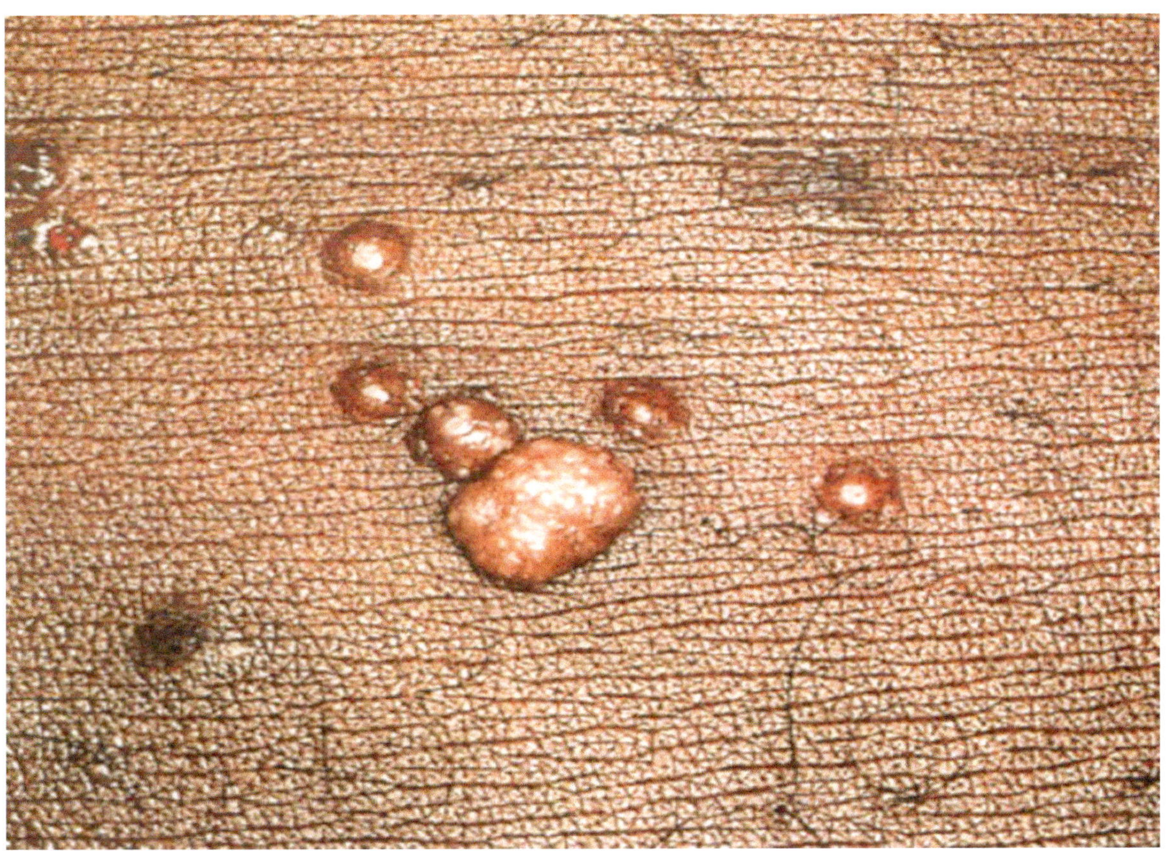

Note multiple cores in a large lesion of molluscum contagiosum.

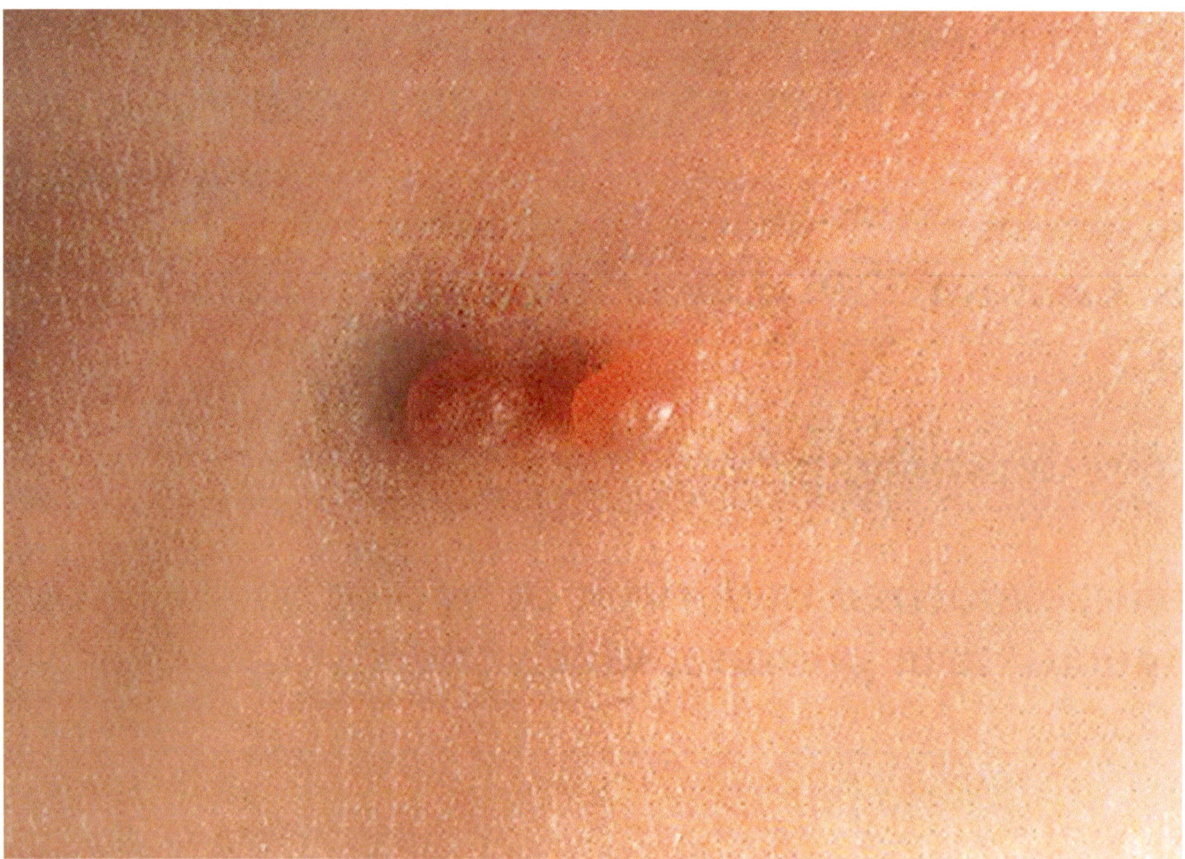

Side light highlights the cores of the papules, confirming the diagnosis.

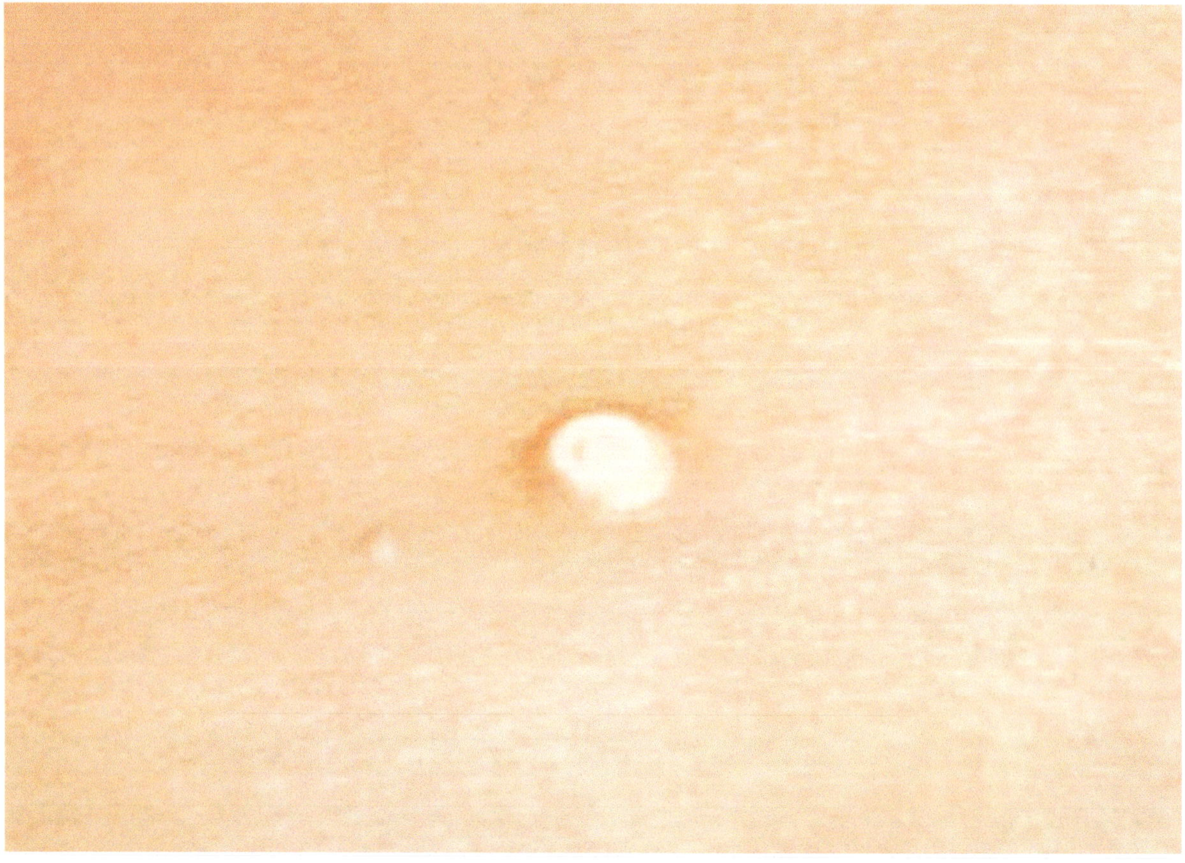

Freezing accentuates the central cores of the papules.

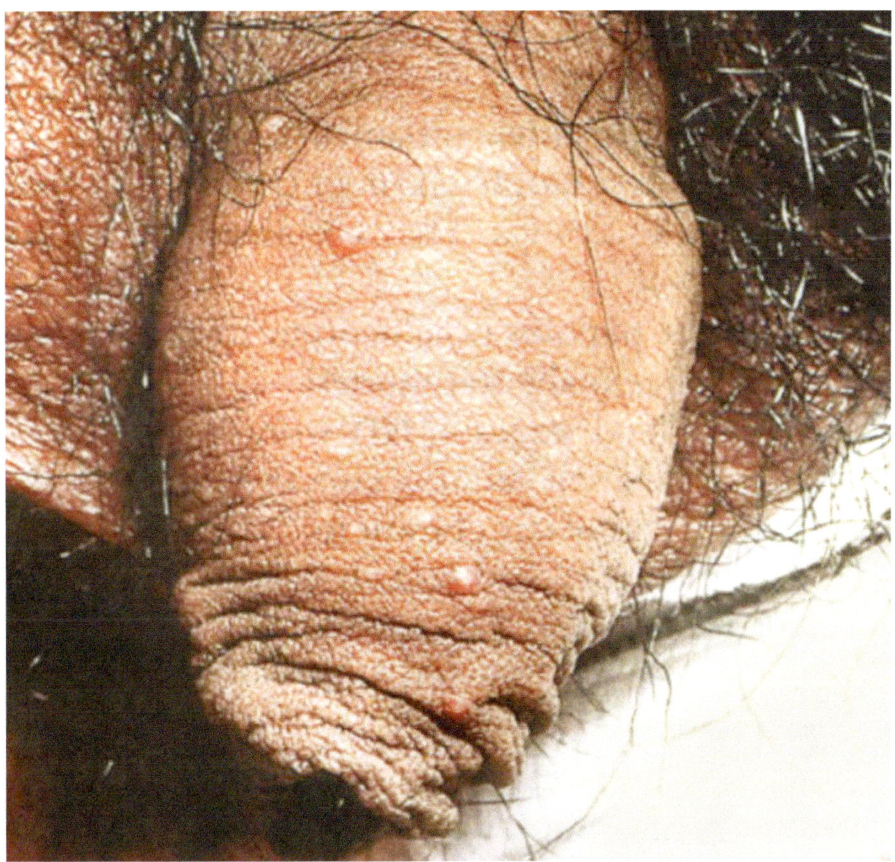

The pubic area is most commonly affected in adults.

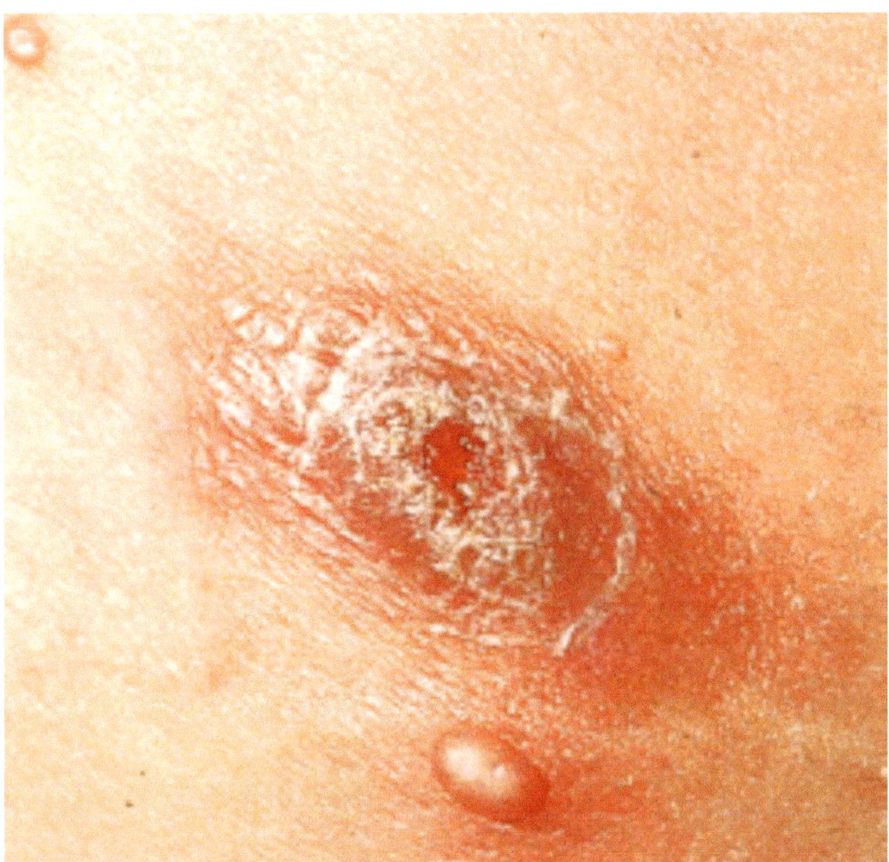

Spontaneous inflammation ("molluscum dermatitis") and resolution may occur.

CLINICAL

- The condition consists of 1- to 4-mm flesh-colored, hemispherical papules with a central white core or dimple.
  - Occasionally up to 15-mm nodule with multiple cores
  - Occasionally inflamed, with halo of erythema ("molluscum dermatitis")
  - Asymptomatic unless inflamed
- The papules commonly occur in children on the face, arms, and trunk, often in groups. They are acquired by direct contact with other children.
- In adults, the papules usually occur in the pubis and lower abdomen and are sexually transmitted.
- Common in later stages of HIV infection, when CD4 cell count is <200. Then often occurs as multiple lesions primarily on the face but can occur elsewhere.
- The condition is caused by a virus implanted into the skin.
  - Incubation period 2–3 weeks
  - Spreads on an individual by autoinoculation, especially by scratching
  - Spontaneously resolves in 6–12 months (in children) when immunity develops; may last longer in adults. Involution may be accompanied by inflammation.

TREATMENT

- General
  - Treatment is not medically necessary unless the affected area is very inflamed, but treatment might be preferred for cosmetic reasons or because a school or preschool objects to a contagious disease.
  - Minimize scratching and direct skin contact with others.
- Destructive treatments must be gentle and not cause scarring, as the lesions will resolve without scarring if untreated.
  - Light liquid nitrogen cryotherapy (cotton swab for 10–20 seconds) is usually effective.
    - Cryotherapy is of diagnostic help in early papules (in which cores are not evident). Freezing greatly enhances the appearance of core.
    - Avoid excessive freezing, which causes scarring.
    - Cryotherapy is often impossible in young children with multiple lesions, because of pain. Pretreatment with topical anesthetic [eutectic mixture of local anesthetics (EMLA), *See* page 231] may allow cryotherapy.
  - An effective treatment is to gently pick out the core with a needle or curette.
    - A light anesthetic spray (ethylchloride or benzocaine) minimizes pain and hardens the core for easier removal.
    - This method may be difficult in children because it is slightly painful and requires a steady target.

Vitiligo

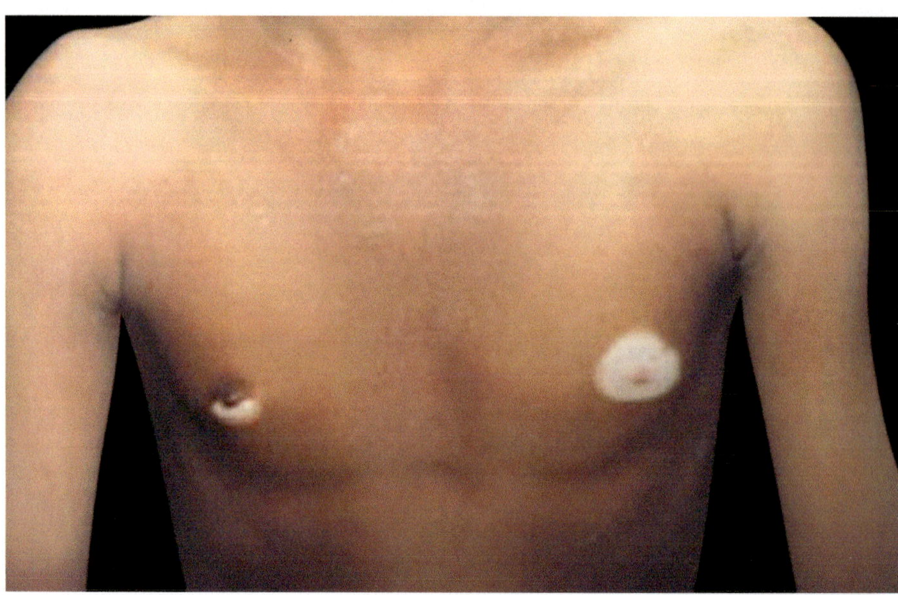

Vitiligo around both nipples.

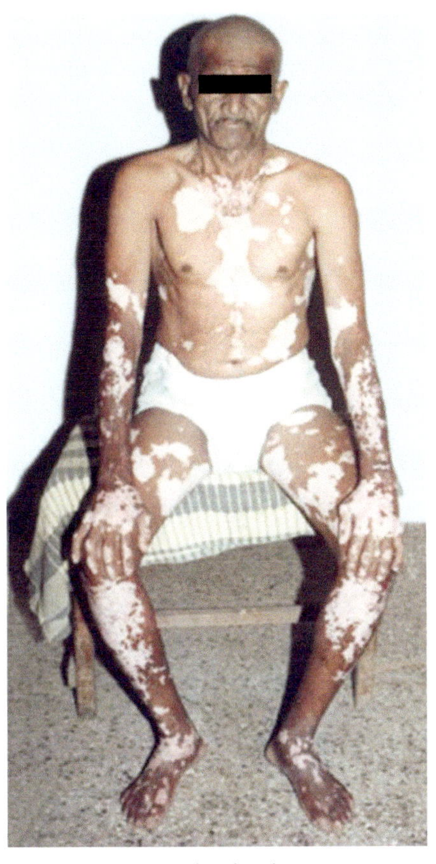
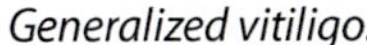

Generalized vitiligo.

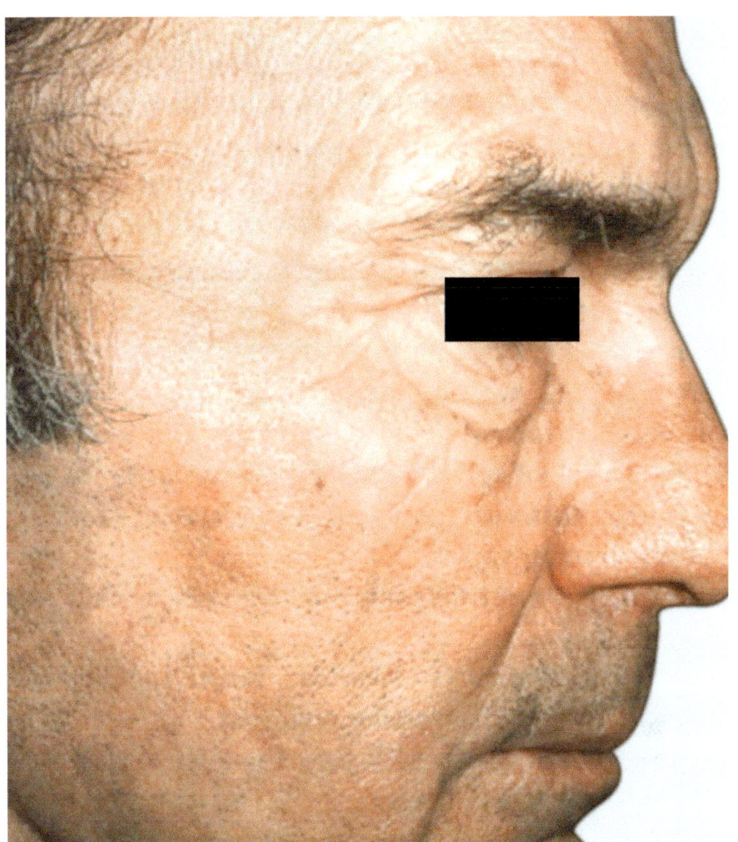

Pigment absence may be subtle in the fair skinned.

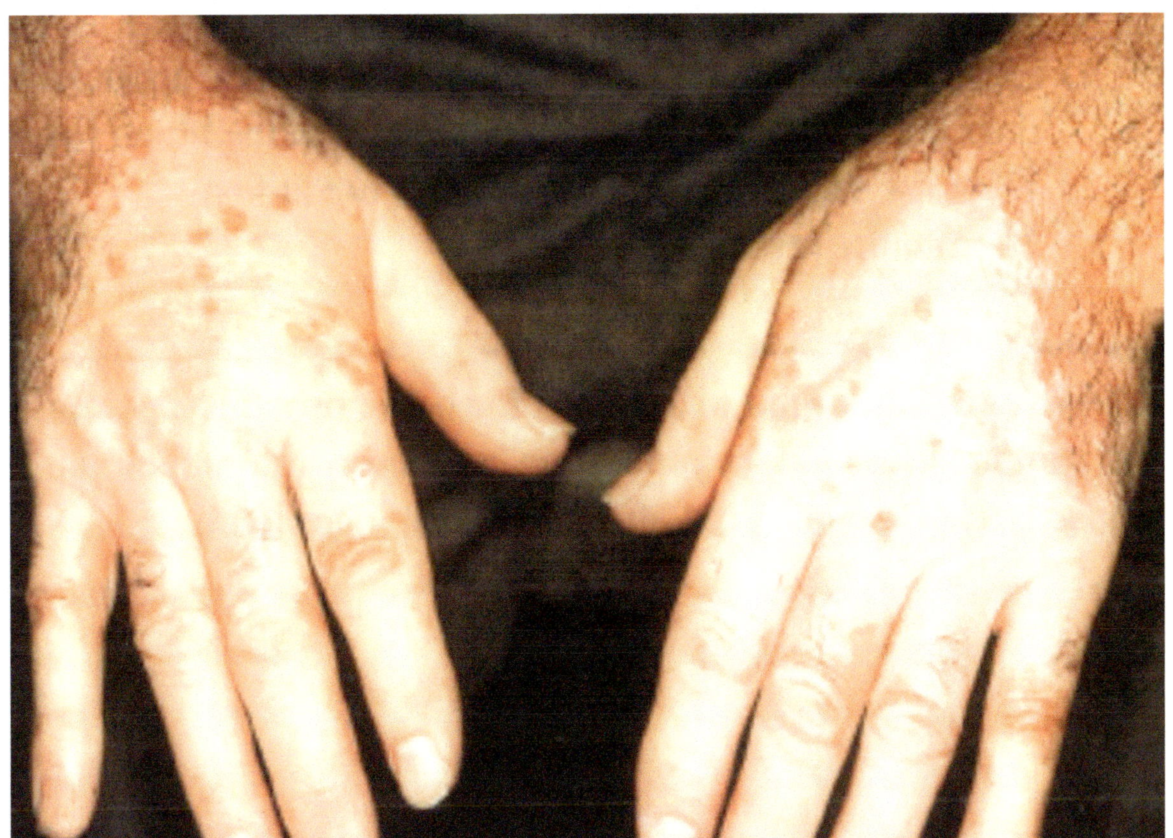

Typical vitiligo with symmetric, sharply demarcated areas of complete depigmentation.

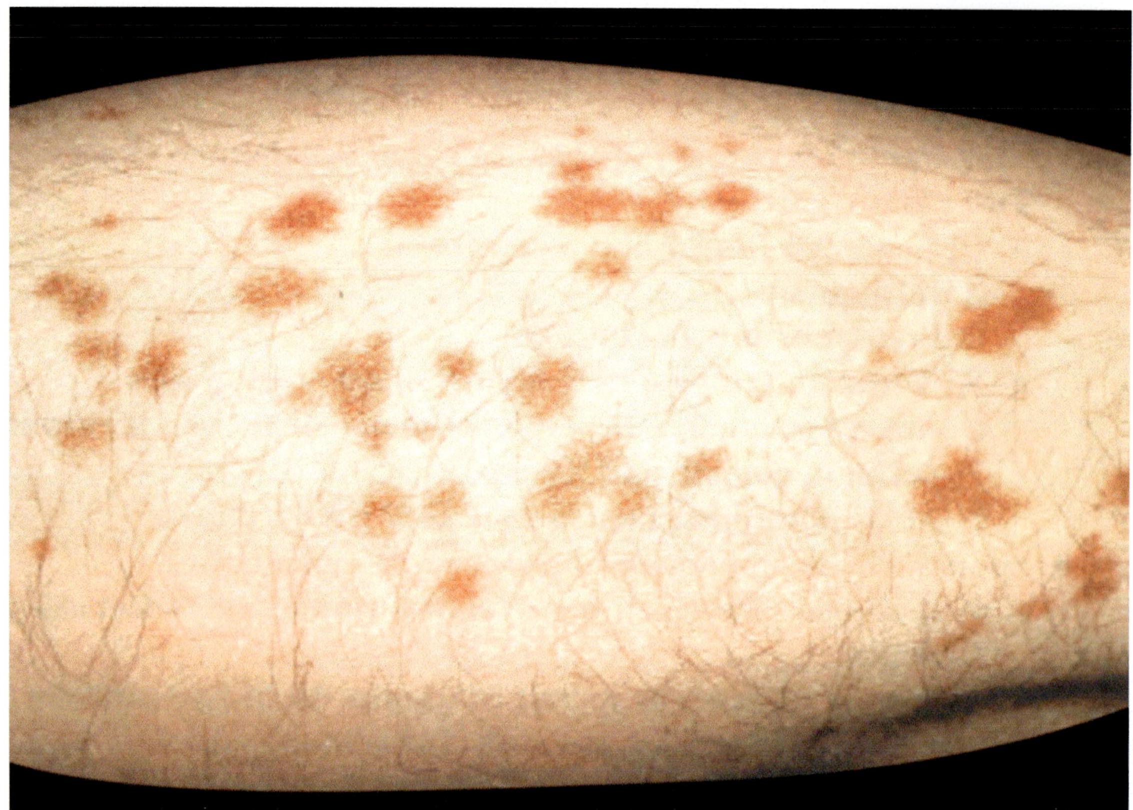

Repigmentation is spreading from follicles.

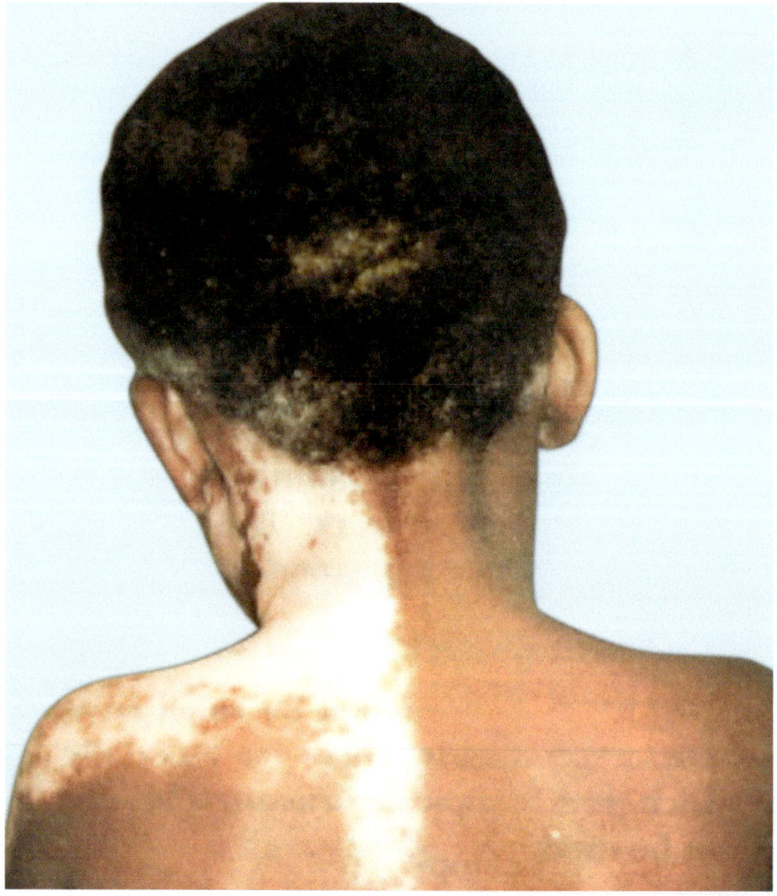

Dermatomal vitiligo. Note "trichrome" quality of inferior margin.

CLINICAL

- This condition consists of areas of complete absence of pigment.
  Two patterns are seen
  - Segmental (typically only on one side of the body)
    - Infrequent
    - Predominantly in children
  - Widespread, can affect any site but generally occurs in two types of sites:
    i. Areas normally hyperpigmented, such as periorbital, perioral, genital, and flexural
    ii. Areas of trauma, such as knuckles, elbows, knees
- Spontaneous complete disappearance of melanocytes
  - Widespread pattern on biopsy shows lymphocytes attacking melanocytes
    - Can be induced or spread by trauma, including sunburn
    - Occasionally associated with autoimmune diseases such as thyroiditis, pernicious anemia, and diabetes
  - The dermatomal type is probably not associated with autoimmune lymphocyte attack.
    - Affected area shows sympathetic nerve dysfunction.
    - Catechol neurotransmitters probably destroy melanocytes.

TREATMENT

Treatments for vitiligo are **unreliable, difficult, and time consuming**. Complete repigmentation can be expected in only 15–20% of cases, with 75% repigmentation in perhaps another 15%. There is no response in at least 20% of cases. Response is manifested by the development of enlarging pigmented spots (follicular) in the center of the lesions or as irregular encroachments of pigment at the margins. Facial and genital lesions are the most responsive; lesions over joints are the least. If there is no response after 3 months of treatment, then continuation of it is unlikely to work. The most recent lesions tend to respond best. Once repigmentation occurs, it usually persists.

- Skin dyes and cosmetics are recommended for small areas, especially in very dark-skinned individuals. These are especially useful on the eyelids, on which potent topical corticosteroids and ultraviolet light should not be used.
  - An individually prepared cosmetic to match skin color (Covermark, Dermablend)
  - Temporary water-washable dye (Vitidye) or dihydroxyacetone
- Topical corticosteroids
  - Potent corticosteroids should be applied twice daily for months.
    - Examine the patient every 1–2 months for signs of cutaneous atrophy from the treatment.
  - This treatment works only in the widespread pattern, not in segmental areas.
- Ultraviolet light

These treatments should be performed only by those experienced in their use. Referral to a dermatologist is recommended.

  - Narrow-band UVB two to three times weekly is the preferred method.
  - Photochemotherapy with oral 8-methoxypsoralen (PUVA) is occasionally used for generalized cases.

Skin Findings in HIV Infection

In HIV infections, there is primarily infection of and eventual disappearance of T-helper (CD4) lymphocytes. This leads to increased frequency and severity of infections but also to general dysregulation of inflammation with subsequent hypersensitivity and worsening of inflammatory skin diseases such as dermatitis, drug eruptions, and psoriasis. The following is a brief outline of associated conditions, with some discussion of the more characteristic ones.

- Infections
  - *Acute exanthem.* Similar to any acute viral syndrome with fever, malaise, sore throat, and lymphadenopathy. Seen in perhaps half of newly infected persons about 2–8 weeks after exposure. The exanthem is indistinguishable from other viral exanthems.
  - *Herpes simplex* (*See* pages 44 and 54). Early in course of HIV is similar to "fever blisters" in the immunocompetent but often more frequent and slightly more severe. Late in HIV may form chronic and nonhealing ulcers. Acyclovir resistance is increasing in this population.
  - *Herpes zoster* (*See* page 162). Typical zoster may be an early sign of HIV infection. As the CD4 count falls, there may be recurrence (rarely seen in the immunocompetent). Late, one may see a chronic and inflamed hyperkeratotic form.
  - *Oral hairy leukoplakia.* This is an asymptomatic white plaque usually seen on the lateral sides of the tongue. Usually seen after moderate drop of CD4 cell counts. Probably mostly caused by Epstein–Barr virus but has been attributed to human papillomavirus.
  - *Warts.* Late in HIV infections, warts may be widespread and very refractory to therapy, especially on the face. May occur frequently on the genitals or in anal area and sometimes eventuate in squamous cell carcinoma.
  - *Molluscum contagiosum.* Usually seen after the CD4 count is below 200, frequently on the face but possibly anywhere. May be large (4–10 mm) with multiple "cores" in one nodule. Much more likely to recur after destructive therapy than in the nonimmunosuppressed (*See* page 165).
  - *Candidiasis.* Most frequently oral (thrush), but intertriginous (*See* page 70) chronic and recurrent infections are also common.

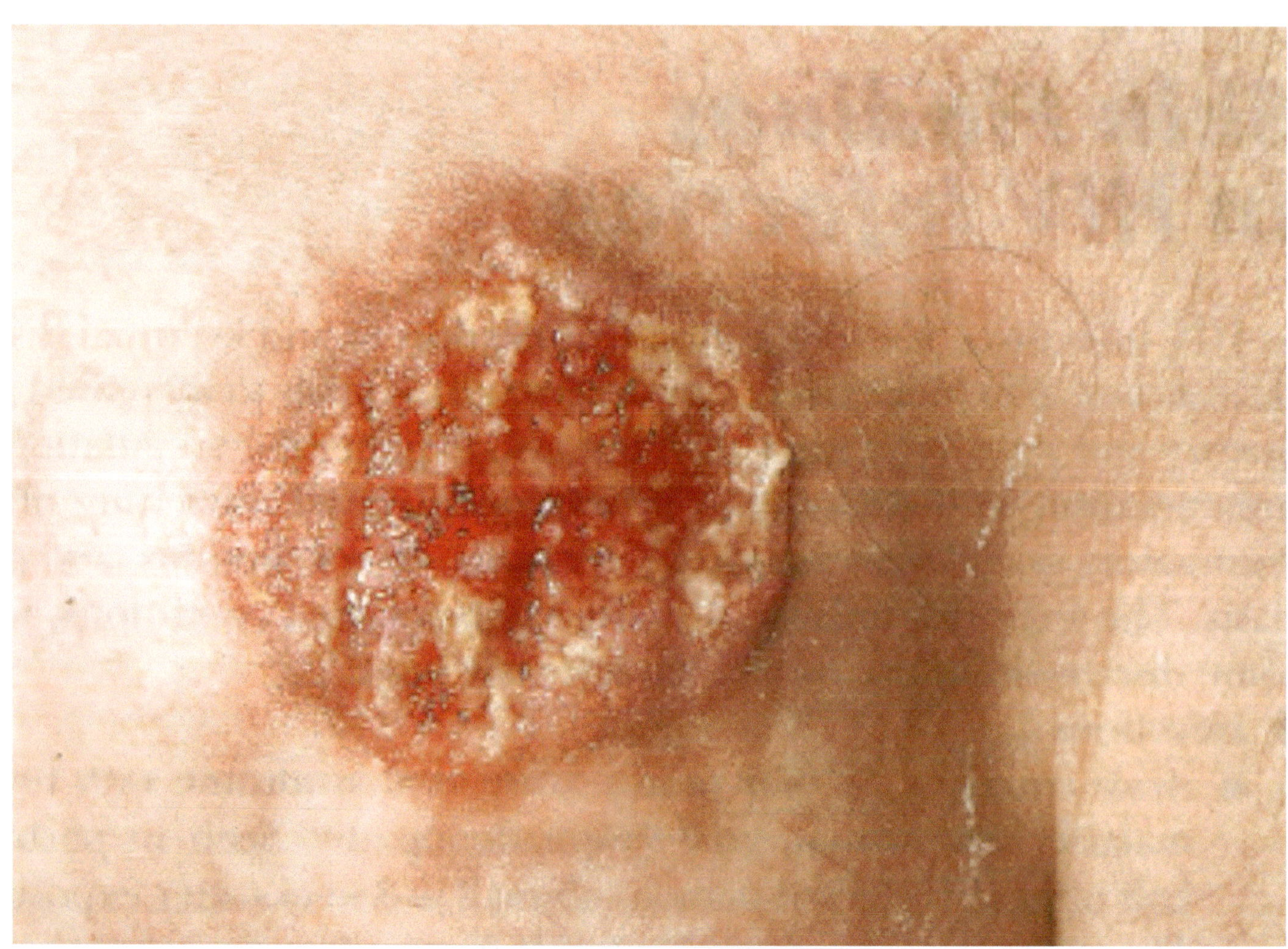

Chronic herpes simplex ulcer, present for 3 months on the left buttock near the intergluteal fold.

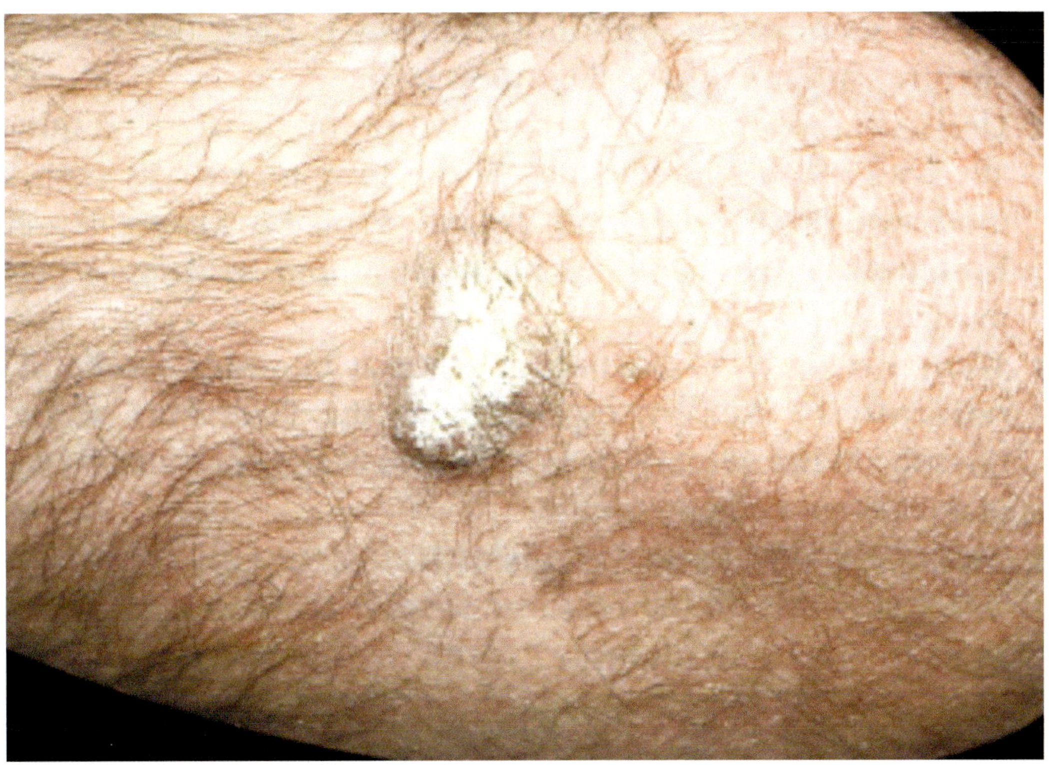

Chronic zoster forming hyperkeratotic papules.

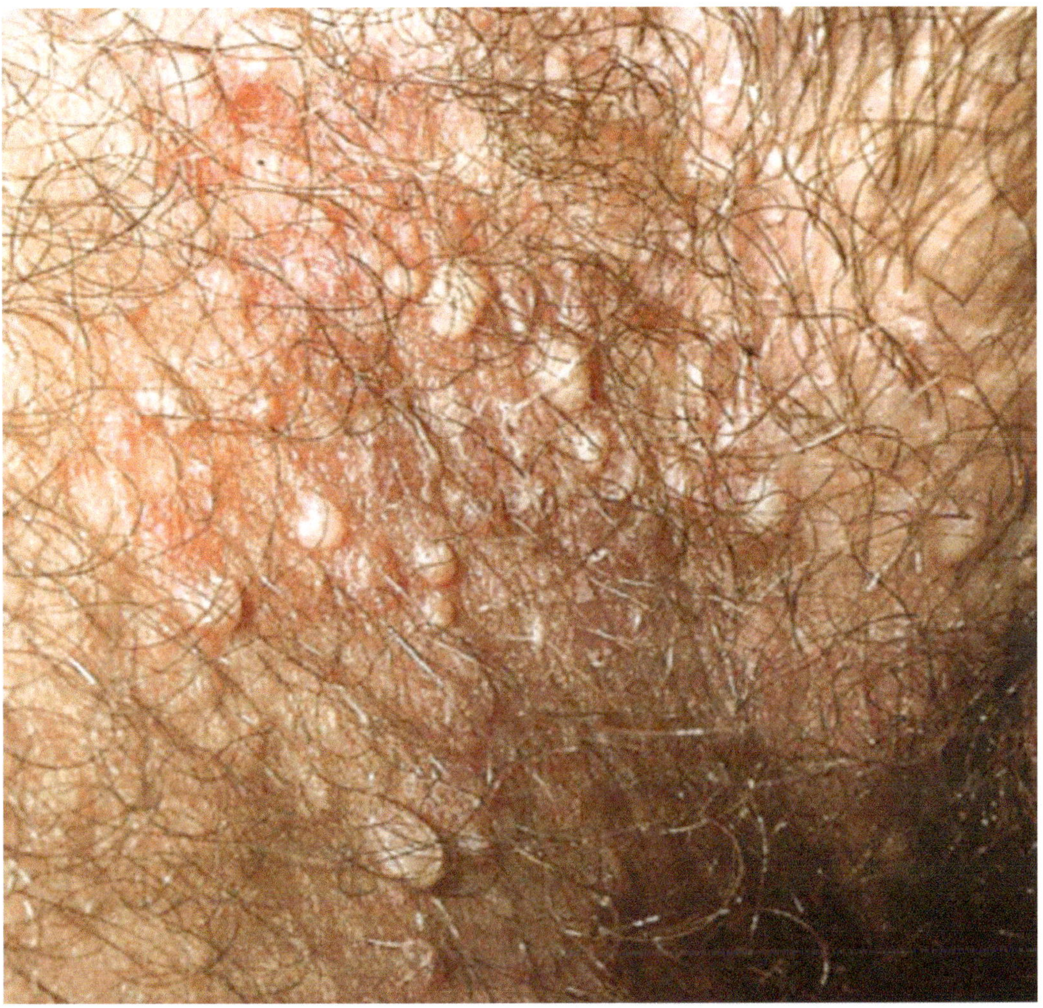

Bullous (staphylococcal) impetigo in the groin fold in a previously undiagnosed HIV-positive patient.

- *Deep fungal infections*
  - *Cryptococcosis.* Internal infections (usually manifested with neurologic signs) may be accompanied by skin lesions. They may be ulcers, abscesses, or nodules, but a common presentation is molluscum-like 2- to 6-mm papules with tiny necrotic centers. Biopsy is required for diagnosis.
  - *Histoplasmosis.* Nonspecific papules, nodules, or ulcers may be seen in patients with pulmonary disease. Biopsy confirms diagnosis
- *Bacterial infections. Staphylococcus aureus* is by far the most common skin organism. May manifest as impetigo (*See* page 159), folliculitis, or abscesses. Staphylococcal scalded skin syndrome and toxic shock syndrome have been rarely reported. Culture necessary to confirm diagnosis and sensitivities.
- *Syphilis.* *See* page 143.
- *Mycobacterial infections*
  - *Mycobacterium avium-intracellulare (MAI).* This is common in patients with acquired immunodeficiency syndrome (AIDS) but only occasionally has skin lesions, such as necrotic papules.

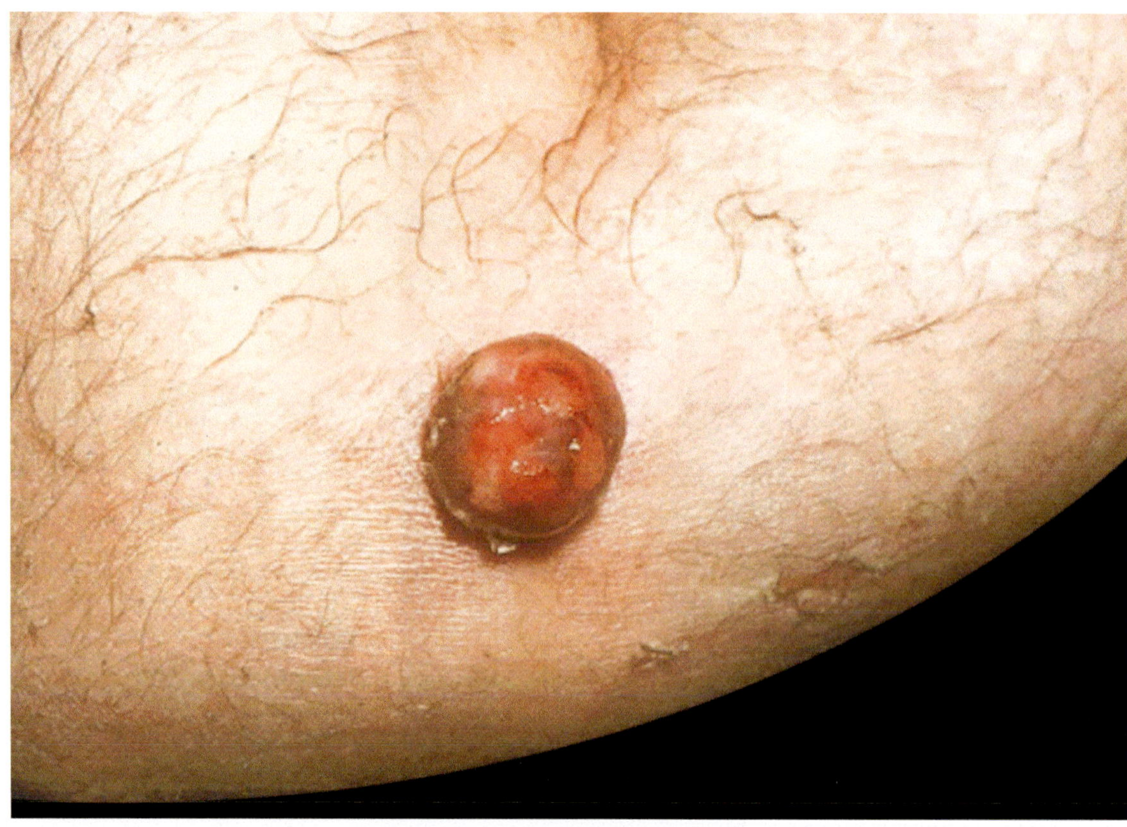

Angry red nodule of bacillary angiomatosis.

  - *Tuberculosis.* This is becoming more common in AIDS and may have granulomatous plaques (lupus vulgaris) or ulcers on the skin. Biopsy, acid-fast stain, and culture confirm the diagnosis.
- *Bacillary angiomatosis.* Caused by *Bartonella henselae* and *Barton ellaquintana,* these skin lesions resemble those of Kaposi's sarcoma (red to purple papules and nodules). Biopsy and Warthin-Starry stain confirm the diagnosis. Responds to erythromycin family of drugs.

■ Tumors

- *Kaposi's sarcoma.* This is a vascular proliferation caused by human herpesvirus 8. There are various subtypes, including one which is AIDS-associated. Most commonly located on the head, neck, and upper torso but may occur anywhere. Oral involvement common. Early is dusky blue macule, which then progresses to a plaque or nodule. May form ovals along skin tension lines, like pityriasis rosea (*See* page 125). Occasionally stabilizes and even regresses. The first-line treatment is the initiation or continuation of antiretroviral therapy. Treatment modalities for specific lesions consist of intralesional chemotherapeutic agents (vinblastine and vincristine), liquid nitrogen cryotherapy, excision, and radiation therapy. Systemic chemotherapy may be considered if there is systemic involvement.

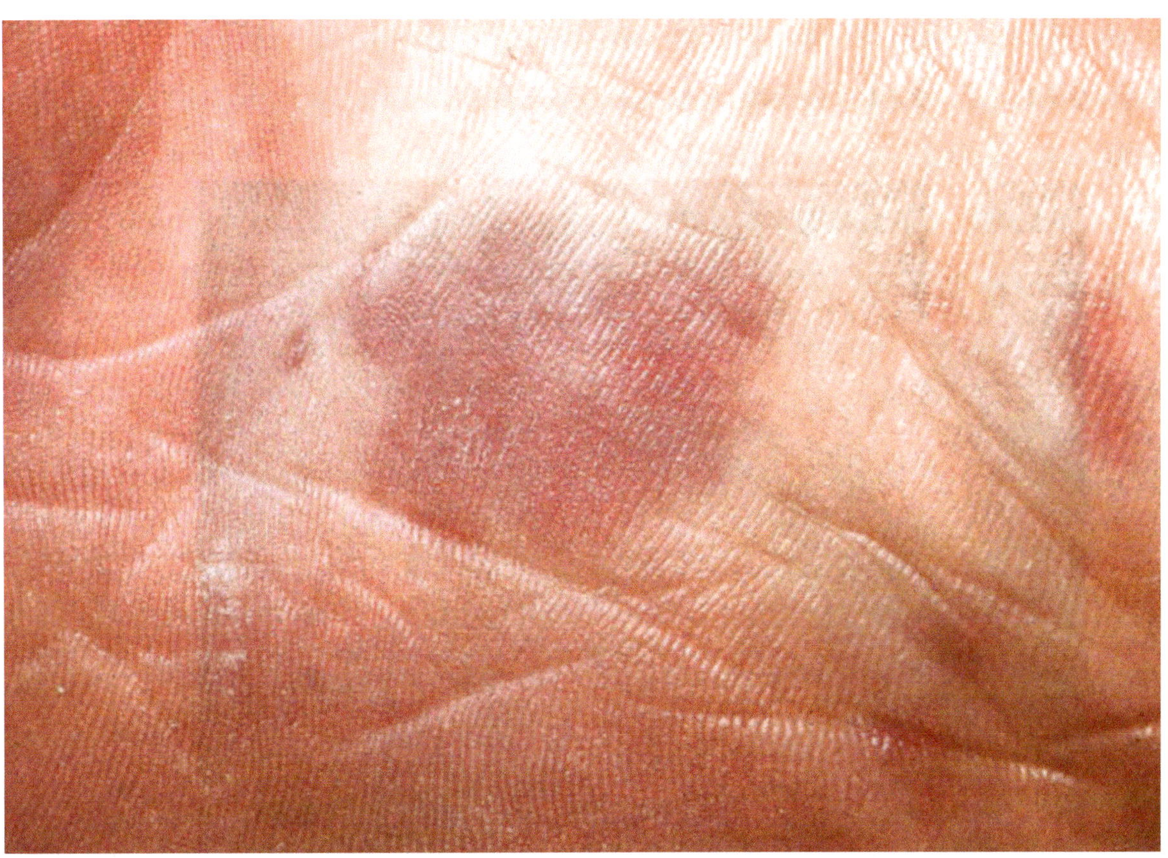

Very early Kaposi's sarcoma on the palm, presenting as a light purple macule.

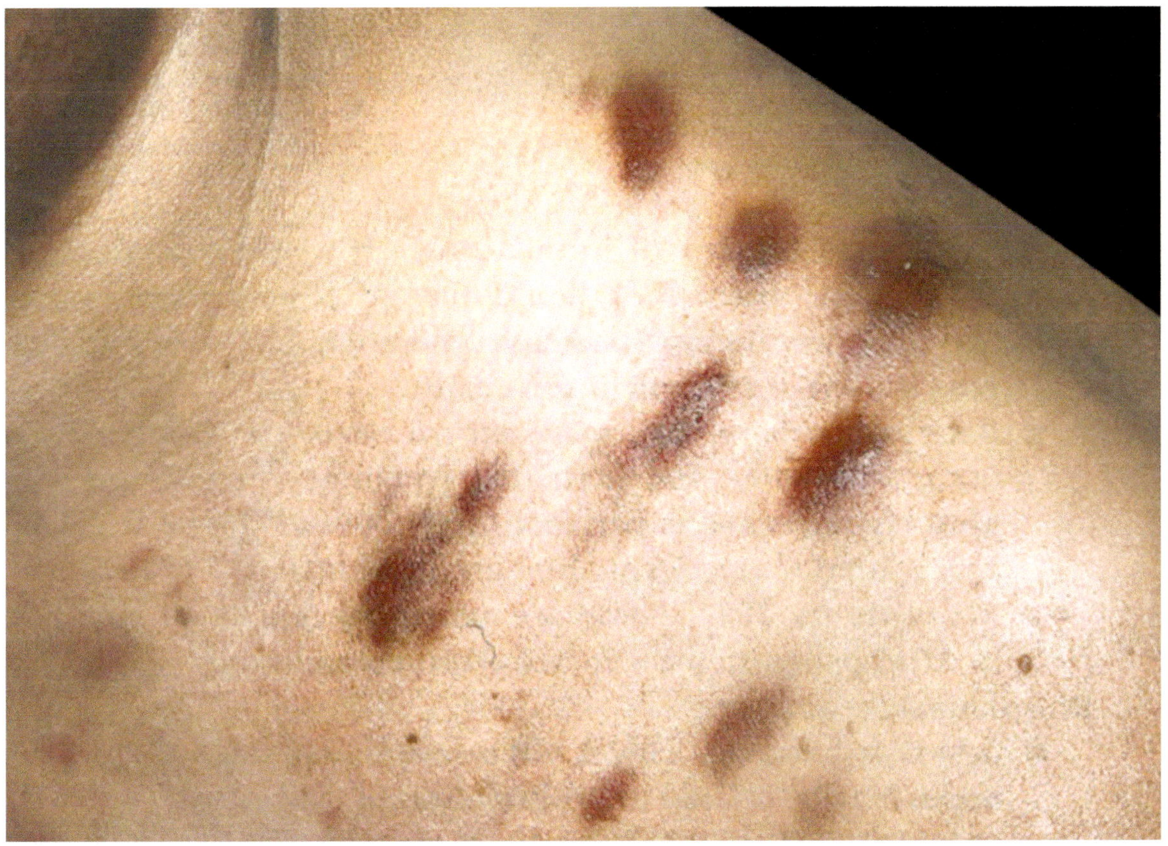

Late nodules of Kaposi's sarcoma, beginning to darken to a mahogany brown color.

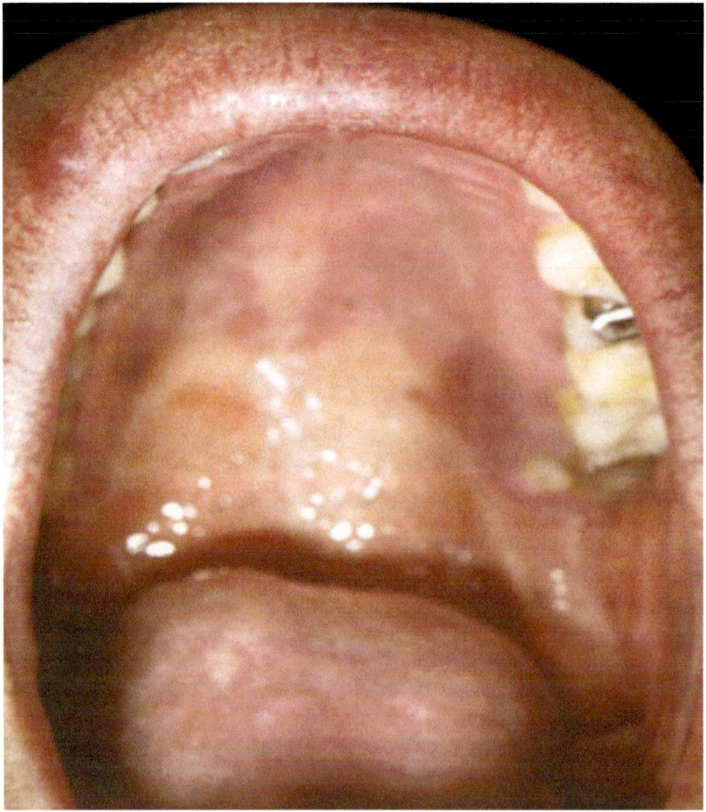

Kaposi's sarcoma of the palate.

- *Basal cell carcinoma and squamous cell carcinoma* (*See* page 213). These occur with somewhat increased frequency in HIV infection. Most characteristic is perianal squamous cell carcinoma, probably related to oncogenic human papillomavirus strains.
- *Melanoma* (*See* page 220). The incidence of melanoma is increased in AIDS patients.

▪ Inflammatory disease

- *Seborrheic dermatitis.* This is often severe and refractory to treatment. May be related to proliferation of the normal skin organism *Malassezia ovalis* but has been seen to occur severely in the face of systemic antiyeast medication, which kills this organism. May occur very early in the course of the disease.

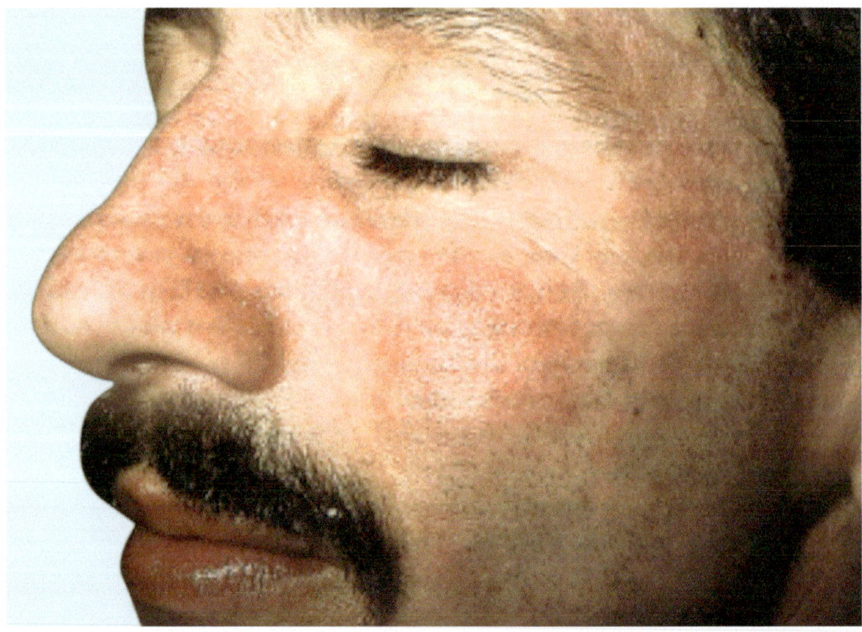

Extensive, recalcitrant seborrheic dermatitis in HIV. The CD4 count was above 400.

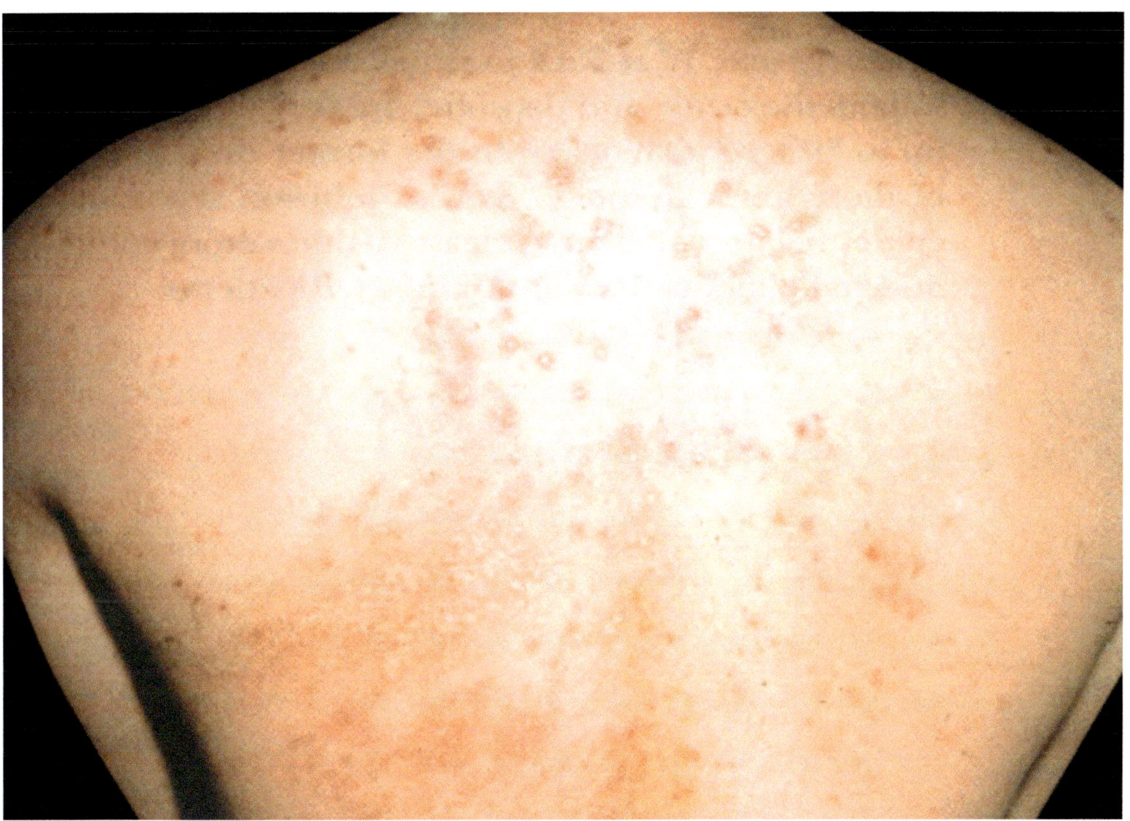

Intensely itchy follicular papules and pustules of eosinophilic folliculitis.

- *Psoriasis* (*See* page 117). Often flares as AIDS worsens and may present for the first time as CD4 count falls. May be severe and resistant to therapy. Reactive arthritis (which has psoriasis-like skin lesions) is also seen with increased frequency. Narrow-band UVB phototherapy, a mainstay for psoriasis, is safe in AIDS patients. Methotrexate and cyclosporine are relatively contraindicated.
- *Xerotic eczema and ichthyosis.* These are frequent findings in HIV.
- *Eosinophilic folliculitis.* This may be seen with moderate drop of the CD4 count. Presents as an itchy, follicular, red papular eruption, typically of the shoulders and the upper torso. Itching may be so severe as to be debilitating. Biopsies are characteristic and fail to show organisms. The most reliable therapy is narrow-band UVB ultraviolet light phototherapy, but symptoms may be controlled with topical corticosteroids, antihistamines, or oral itraconazole (200 mg bid). Itraconazole is thought to work as an anti-inflammatory, not as an antibiotic, in this setting. Other treatment options are oral isotretinoin, an acne drug shown to have immunomodulatory effects, or with metronidazole 250 mg tid for 3 weeks.
- *Drug eruptions.* Reactions to drugs, especially to trimethoprim/sulfamethoxazole and dapsone, are very common, occurring in up to 80% of patients given the former drug and 30–50% of those given dapsone. Stevens–Johnson syndrome and toxic epidermal necrolysis are 100 times more common in HIV-infected patients than in noninfected patients.

CHAPTER 6

Tumors, Lumps, and Marks

Moles (Melanocytic Nevi)

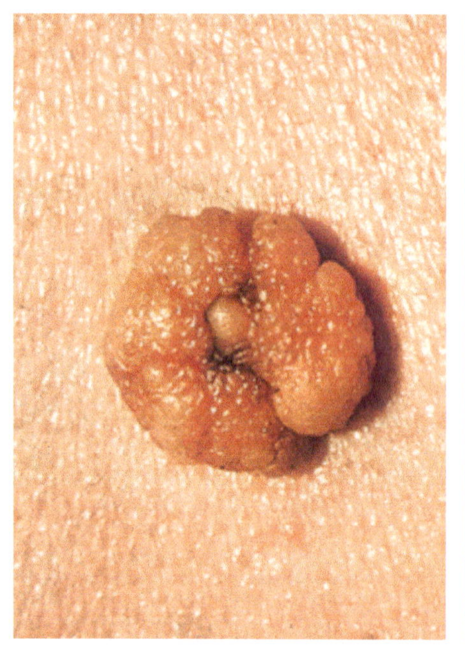

Cauliflower-like hyperplasia of dermal mole.

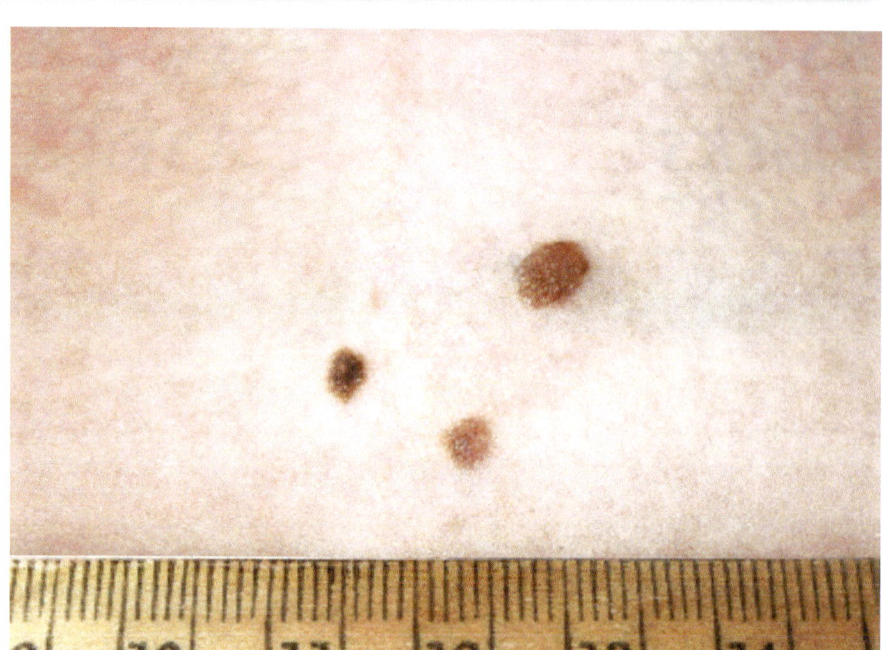

Typical flat "junctional" moles.

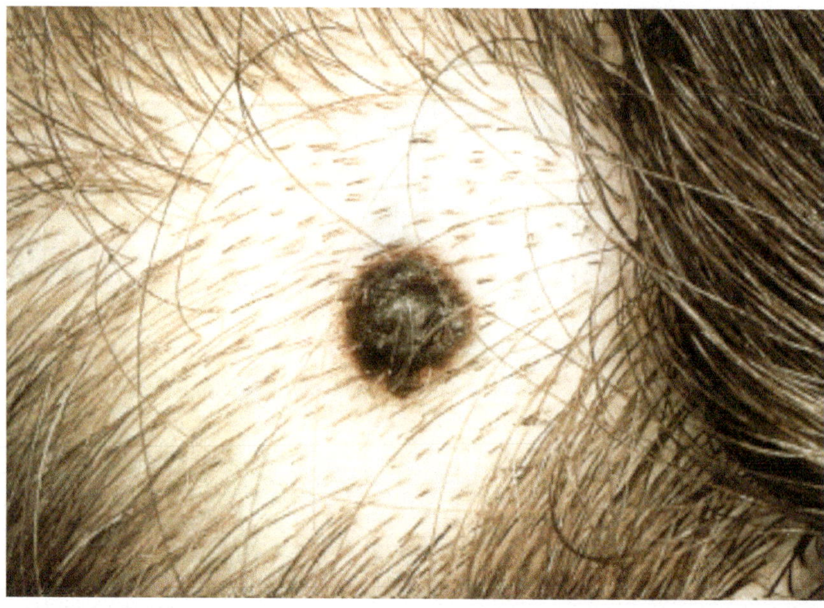

Dermal nevus in scalp.

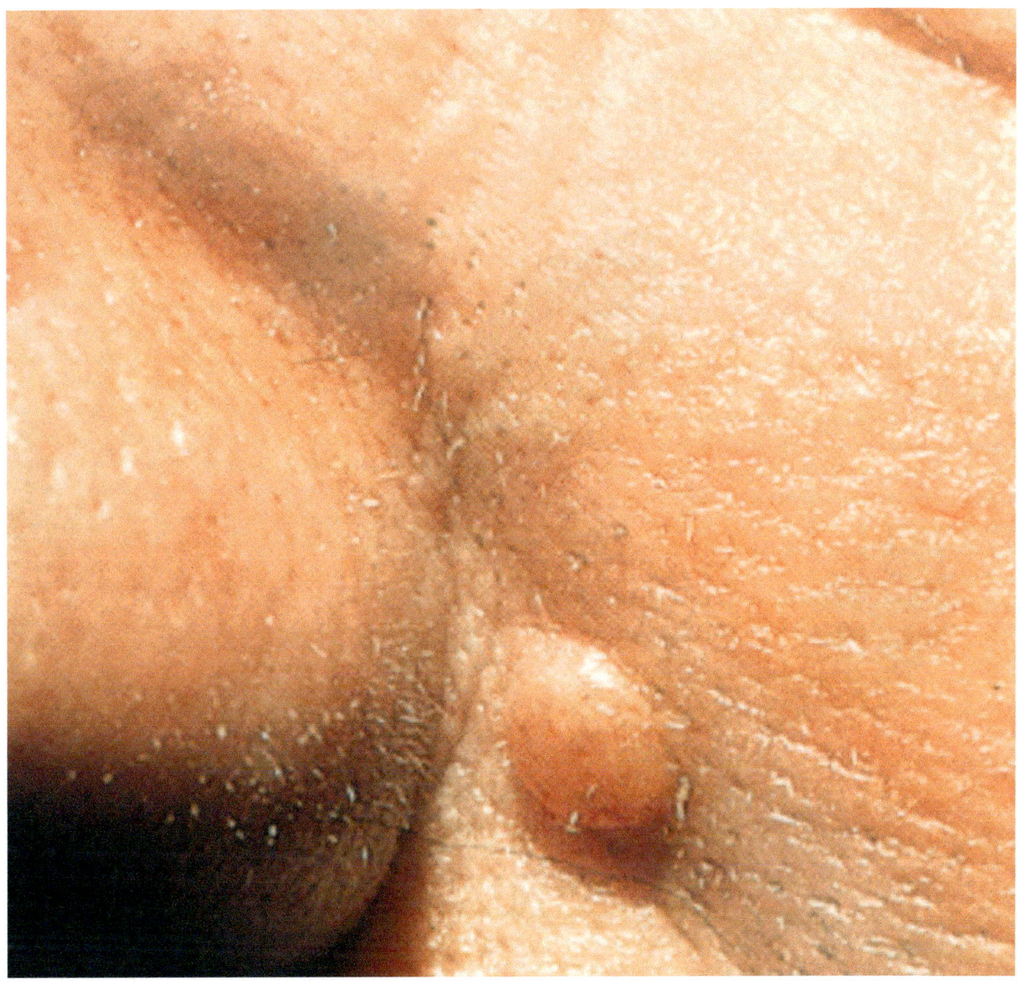

Nonpigmented dermal mole.

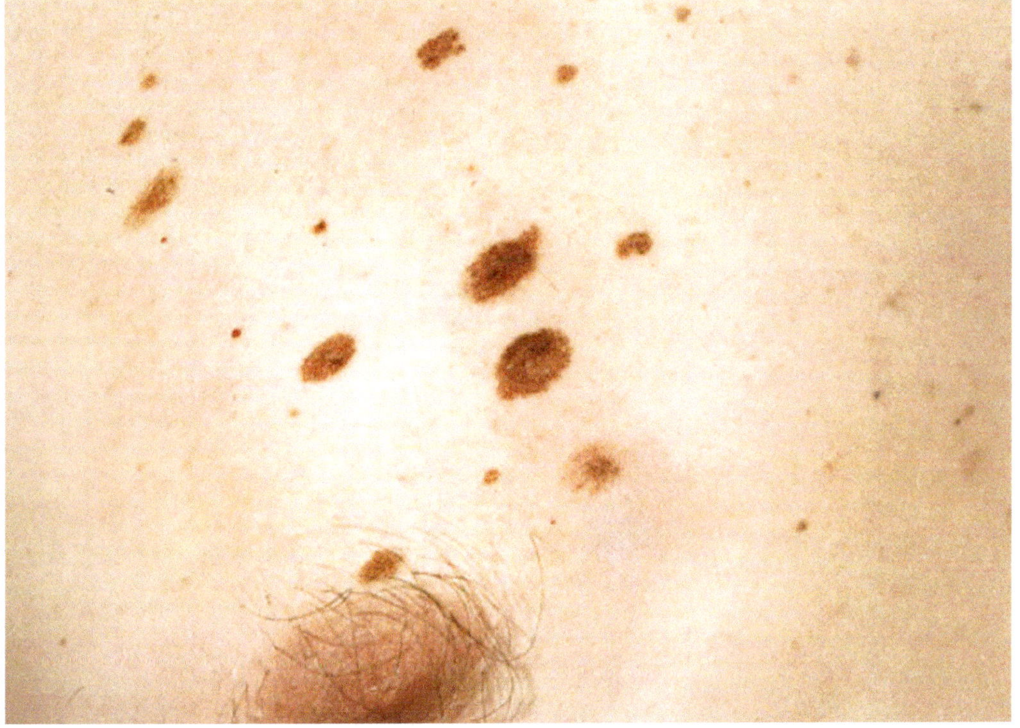

Many large, bizarre dysplastic nevi in person who has family members with similar lesions and melanomas.

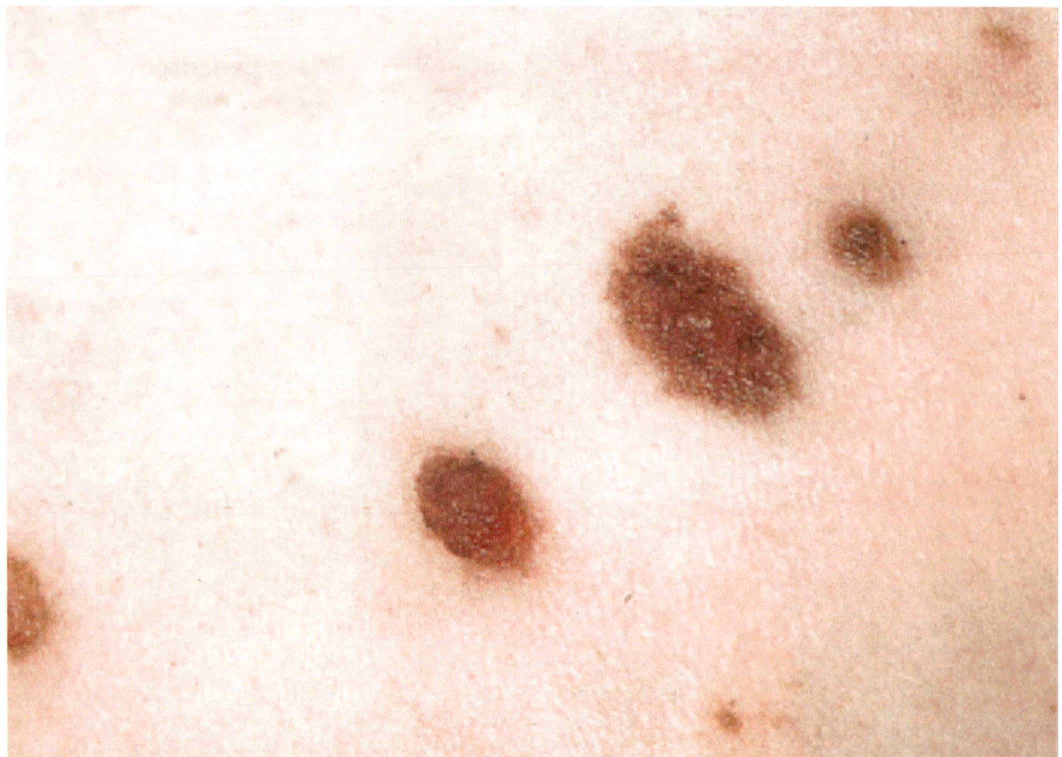

Close-up of some of many large, dysplastic nevi in familial setting. Close monitoring is indicated.

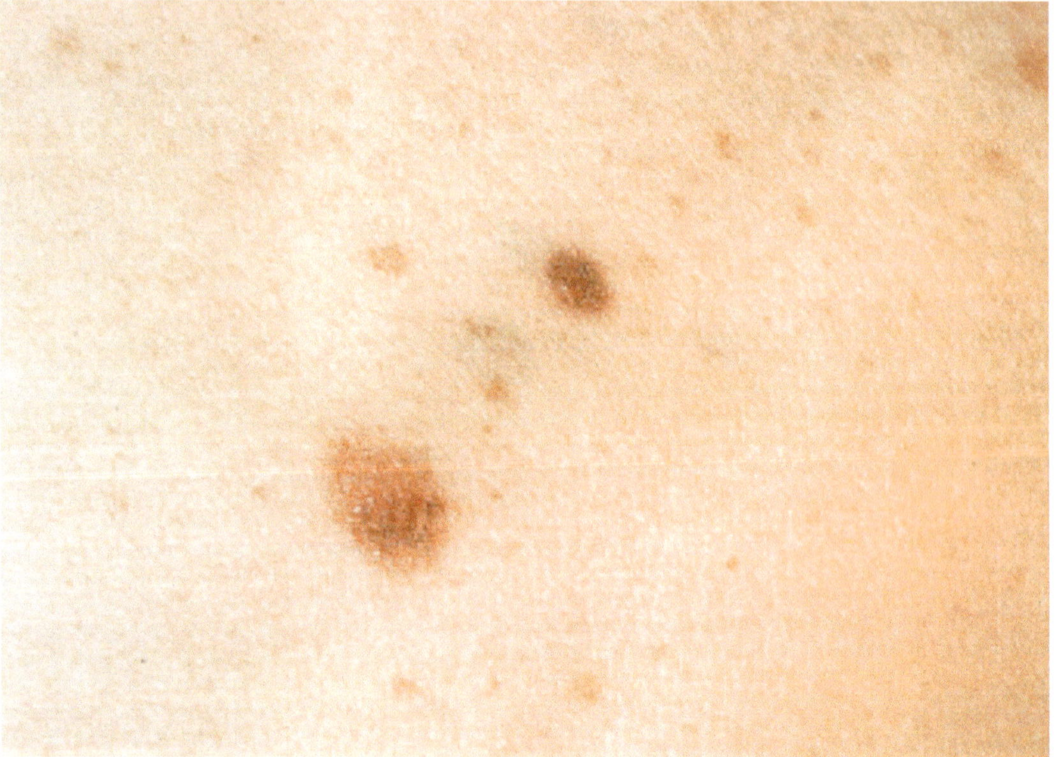

One small dysplastic nevus in a person who otherwise has only typical nevi. Significance is questionable.

CLINICAL

- These lesions contain a proliferation of pigment cells in the epidermis, dermis, or both.
    - The average white adult has about 35 moles, whereas dark-skinned people have few, if any.
- Moles are flat to elevated, flesh-colored to dark-brown macules and papules located randomly over the entire skin surface.

- Onset and course
  - Moles are occasionally present at birth.
  - They usually start appearing between 1 and 4 years of age and increase in number into adulthood.
- The surface may be flat, smooth, or cerebriform, but never keratotic. Moles in fold and friction areas may become pedunculated.
- They may contain a *few* coarse hairs.

- Clinical variants
  - "Giant hairy nevi," or large, hairy, congenital nevi
    - These are pigmented plaques >1 cm, which are present and bearing hair at birth.
    - The pigment may be variegated.
    - With age, such nevi often become irregularly papular and hypertrophic.
    - The rate of malignant transformation (to melanoma) is high (1–10%) for a large lesion. The rate is less for small lesions, but the risk is still greater than for noncongenital moles.
    - A large congenital nevus over the nape of the neck may be associated with leptomeningeal melanocyte proliferation, which may block the spinal fluid canals and cause hydrocephalus.
  - Halo nevi
    - These usually occur in young adulthood; depigmentation develops around one or several moles. The mole may then fade and disappear, leaving a white macular area, which then may repigment normally.
    - The process may be arrested at any stage.
    - Halo nevi seldom have pathologic significance. Halos occasionally develop around nevi when the body is fighting a metastatic melanoma.
  - "Blue nevi"
    - These are dark gray-blue or blue-black dermal papules with a smooth surface.
    - Onset is usually young adulthood.
    - These moles represent pigment cell proliferation deep in the dermis.
    - There is no malignancy potential, but blue nevi are often mistaken for melanoma.
  - Atypical or dysplastic nevi
    - Compared with ordinary nevi, these are often larger, with an irregular border and perhaps with irregular pigmentation. The most striking ones have a "fried egg" appearance with a brown papule in the center and a large (up to 2 cm), tan halo.
    - About 5–20% of adult whites have at least one small dysplastic nevus seen clinically and on biopsy.
    - Individuals with atypical or dysplastic nevi probably have a rate of conversion to melanoma that is slightly higher than those with ordinary nevi.
    - Presence of several dysplastic nevi indicates an increased chance of melanoma developing somewhere on the individual's skin. Familial multiple dysplastic nevi have a high rate (up to 50%) of melanoma, but families with this condition are rare.
- Relationship of moles to melanoma
  - Only 30% of melanomas arise in moles; the remainder arise in normal skin.

Clinical signs for melanoma rather than a mole:
- Rapid growth
- Variegated instead of homogeneous pigment (speckles of different color)
- Diffusion of pigment from papule into surrounding skin (resembles spread of ink on blotting paper)
- Inflammation of surrounding skin
- Bleeding, oozing, and crusting of surface

TREATMENT

- Indications for removal of moles
  - The changes just listed or the conviction of the patient that the mole has suddenly changed
  - A large congenital hairy nevus, when removal is feasible

- Surgical removal
  - Excision
    - This is necessary for diagnosis if melanoma is suspected.
    - The preferred method is to allow the linear scar to fall into natural skinfolds.
  - Surgical shave of a papular mole
    - After local anesthesia, shave the mole flat with a scalpel or snip scissors. Stop the bleeding with styptic (*See* page 244) or light electrodesiccation.
    - Do not shave if melanoma is suspected.
    - It is possible to achieve a good cosmetic result on the trunk and flat planes of the face with this technique.
    - Shaving may leave residual dermal cells that can grow back or produce pigment. Partial removal does ***not*** induce melanoma.
- Nonsurgical methods such as cryotherapy or chemical cautery should not be used to treat melanocytic lesions.
- Counseling (*See* Patient Guides, page 255)
  - White individuals should examine their skin at least twice a year.
  - New benign nevi may develop in middle age, and old flat ones may slowly become elevated.
  - Advise medical examination if there is:
    - Sudden appearance of rapidly growing pigmented lesion with unusual appearance
    - Rapid change in old mole, especially if one section is developing differently (e.g., darker, shiny, and oozing)
    - Pigmented lesion that becomes inflamed or is fragile.

Dermatosis Papulosa

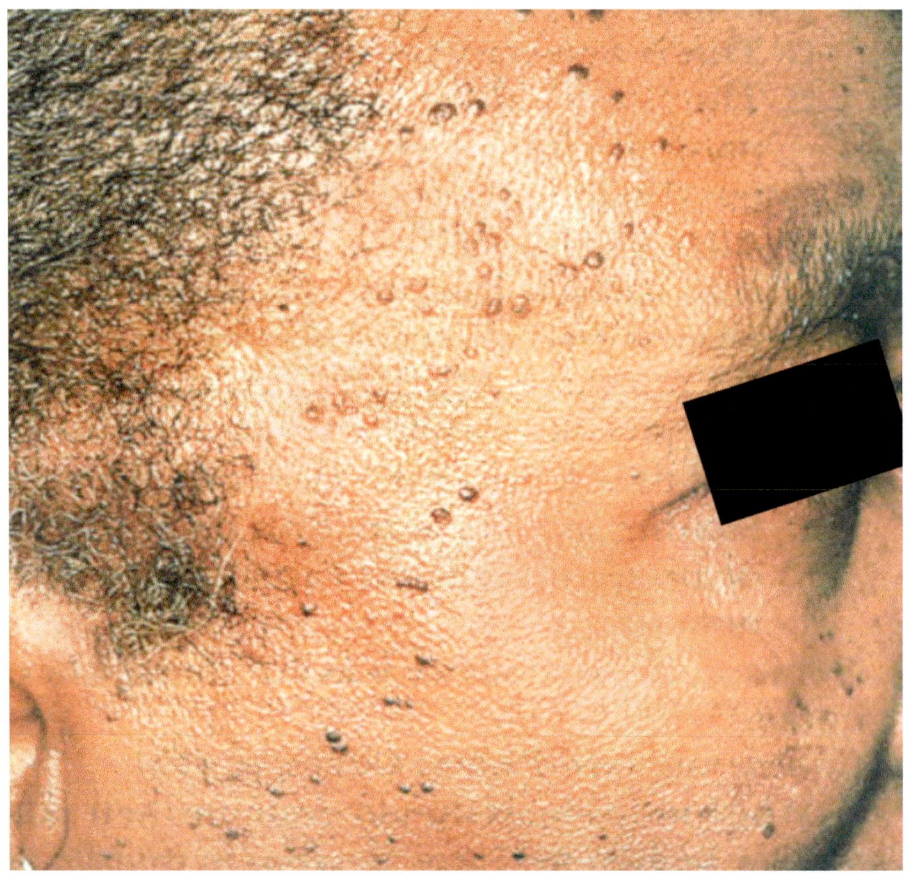

Typical soft, fleshy, pigmented papules of dermatosis papulosa on the cheeks.

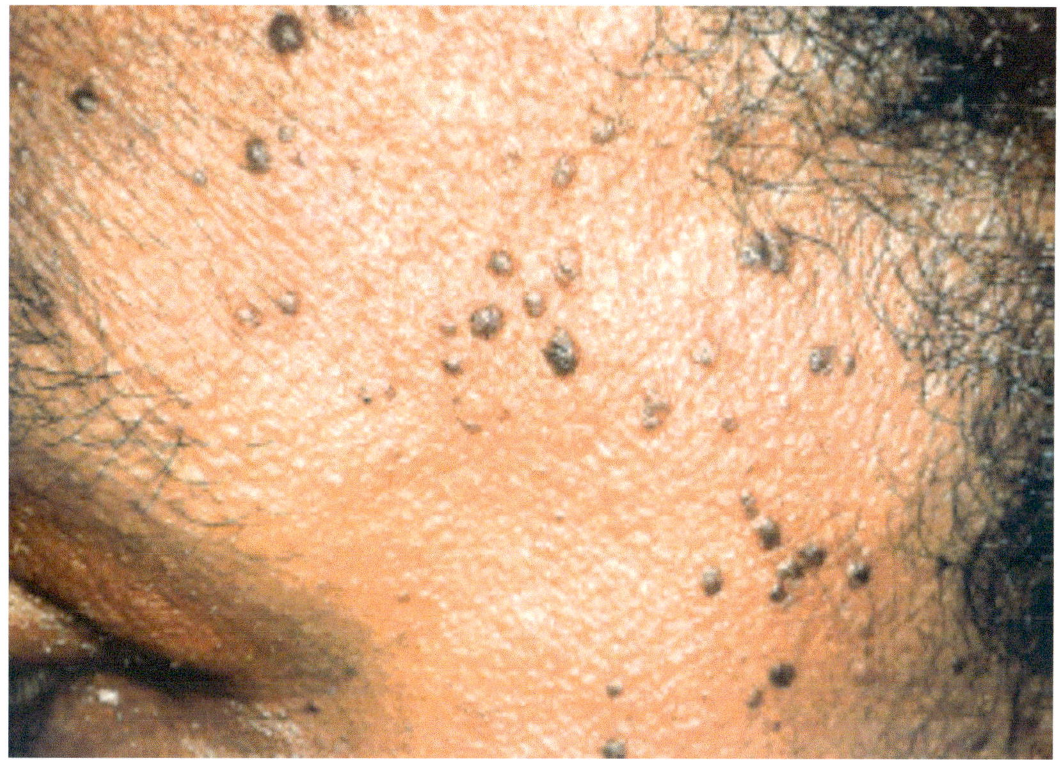

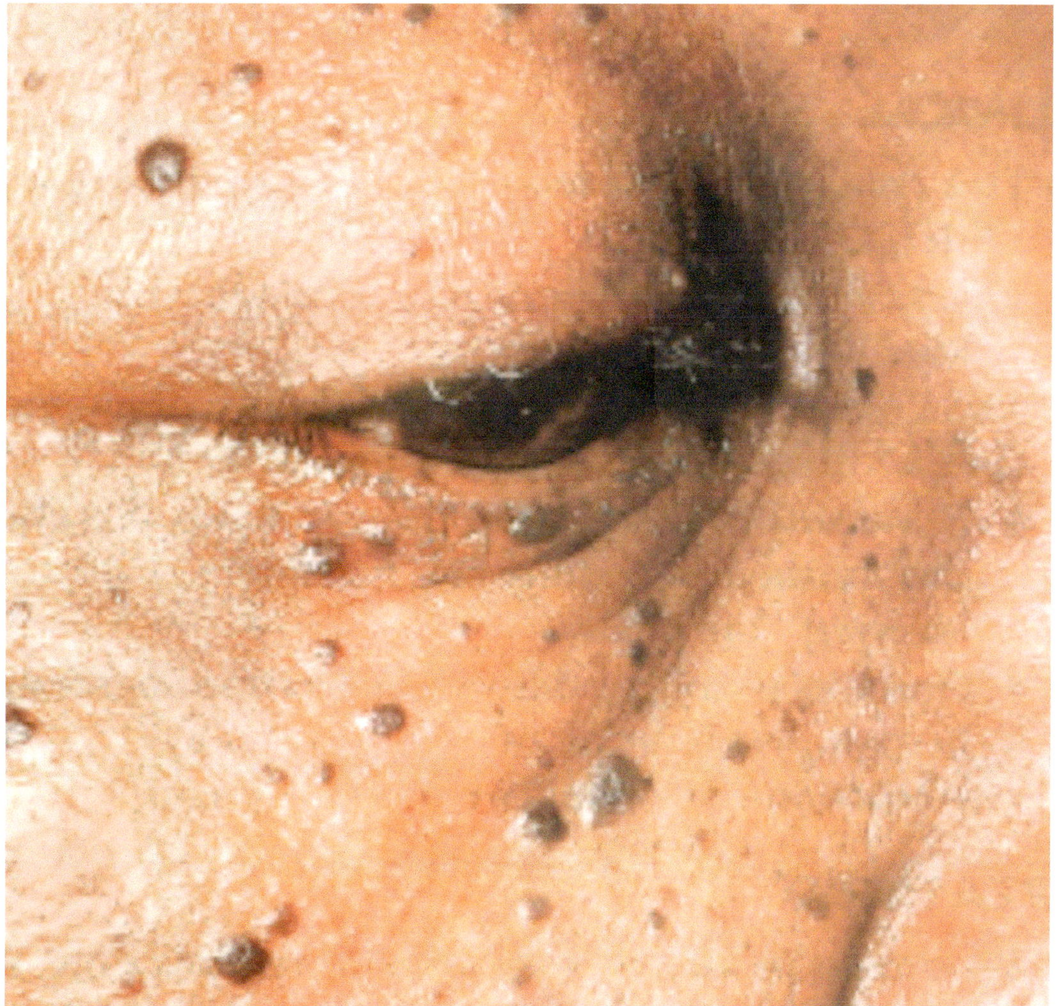

Lesions may occur on eyelids and may become filiform or verrucous, as here, lateral to the eye.

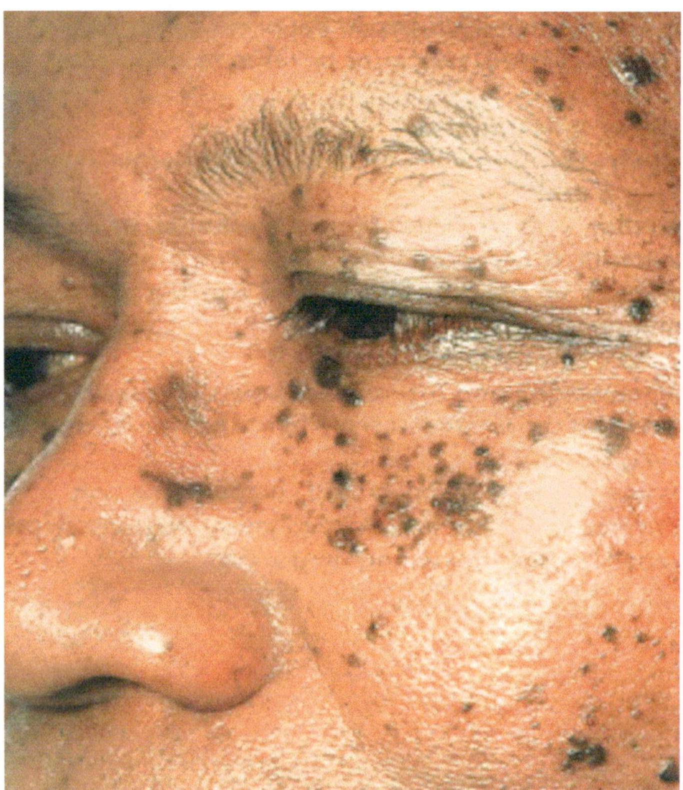

Clear area on left cheekbone is area in which lesions were shaved off 1 month before photograph was taken.

CLINICAL

- This condition, to at least a mild degree, occurs in up to 40% of dark-skinned adults.
  - Less common in Asians
  - Rare in whites
- The condition consists of soft, fleshy, and pigmented papules in a "mask" distribution around the eyes.
  - Occasionally the papules appear down the cheeks to the neck and on the forehead to the hairline.
- A "delayed" birthmark
  - Onset in young adulthood, the extent increasing with age
  - Benign proliferation of epidermal cells
- The condition does not become malignant.

TREATMENT

- Treatment should be done cautiously, to avoid scarring and hyperpigmentation.
  - Light electrocautery or electrodesiccation
    - This procedure is quick, simple, and effective for small lesions.
    - For tiny lesions, local anesthesia is not necessary if a very low current is used in brief pulses.
    - Scarring and pigment changes do not occur if only the lesion itself is lightly charred; care must be taken to stop at the skin surface.
  - Scalpel-shave or scissor-snip
    - If the papules are planed flat to the skin, little dermal damage or scarring is caused.
    - Stop bleeding with pressure or a mild cauterant, if necessary.
    - Electrocautery increases the chance of scarring and hyperpigmentation.
  - Liquid nitrogen cryotherapy
    - Hyperpigmentation and hypopigmentation are possible.
    - Lesions recur if the treatment is too light and scar if the treatment is too heavy.
  - Mild trichloroacetic acid or other acid chemodestruction
    - Experience and skill are necessary to get to the right depth and to avoid excessive pain and destruction.

Seborrheic Keratoses

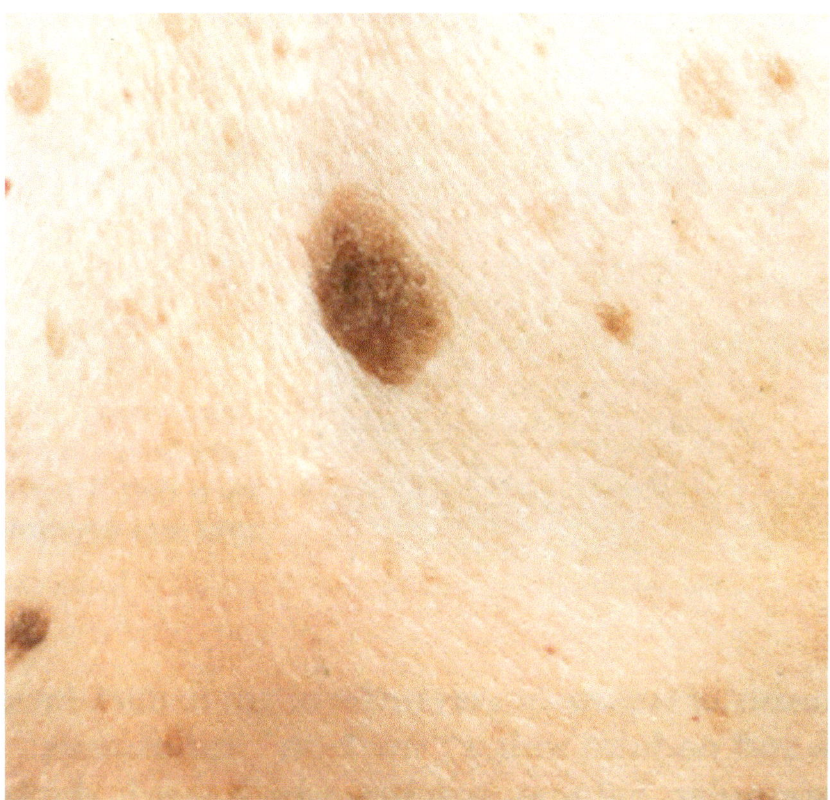

Typical "stuck-on" appearance of seborrheic keratoses on the back.

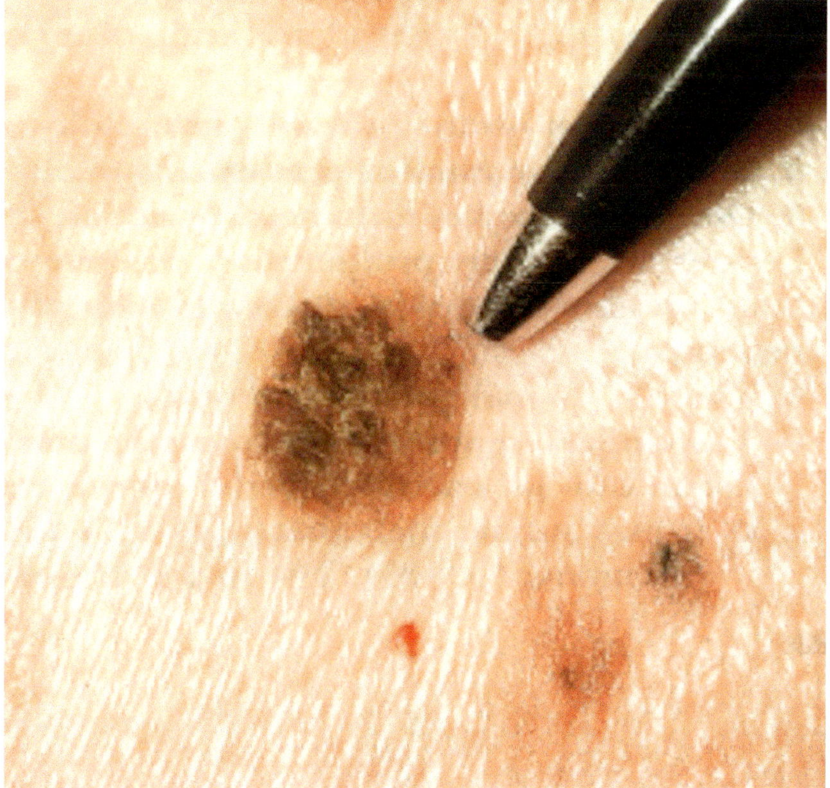

Early lesions are flat and faint-colored. Older lesion is dark and keratotic.

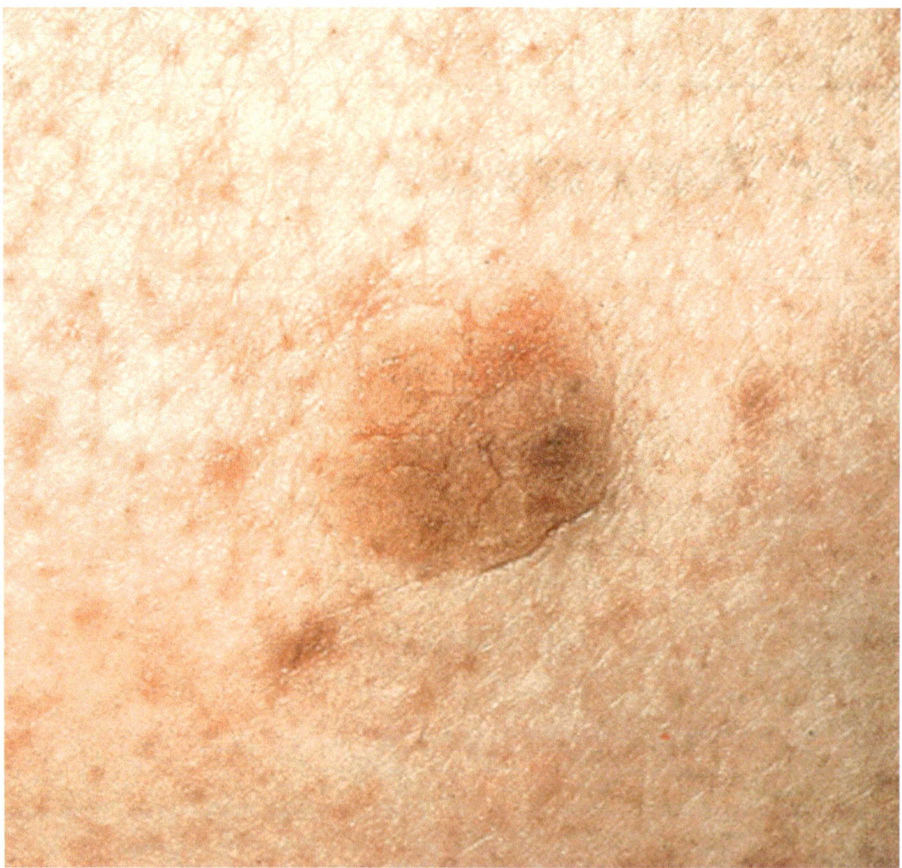

Seborrheic keratosis covered by a belt is softer and less keratotic.

CLINICAL

- This condition consists of rugose or cerebriform tan to dark-brown verrucous plaques and nodules with a "stuck-on" appearance.
  - It may start as granular, light-tan patches, which slowly thicken and darken.
  - The hyperkeratotic cap may repeatedly peel off and a new one accumulate.
  - It is found most commonly on the trunk, but the scalp, face, and extremities may be involved.
  - Lesions on the forehead and scalp often remain flat and slightly granular.
- This condition occurs primarily in middle-aged to older whites.
  - There is some familial predisposition.
  - Occurrence seems enhanced by actinic damage.
- Lesions are benign proliferation of epidermal cells and keratin piled up above the skin surface (which gives the "stuck-on" appearance).
  - There is no malignancy potential.
  - The clinical significance is cosmetic; nevertheless, possible confusion with potentially harmful lesions exists.
    - It may mimic melanoma (*See* page 220) or pigmented basal cell carcinoma (*See* page 213). The major distinguishing feature is that seborrheic keratosis is nearly always surmounted by a keratin cap that can be loosened with a fingernail, and the other growths are fleshy and not keratotic.

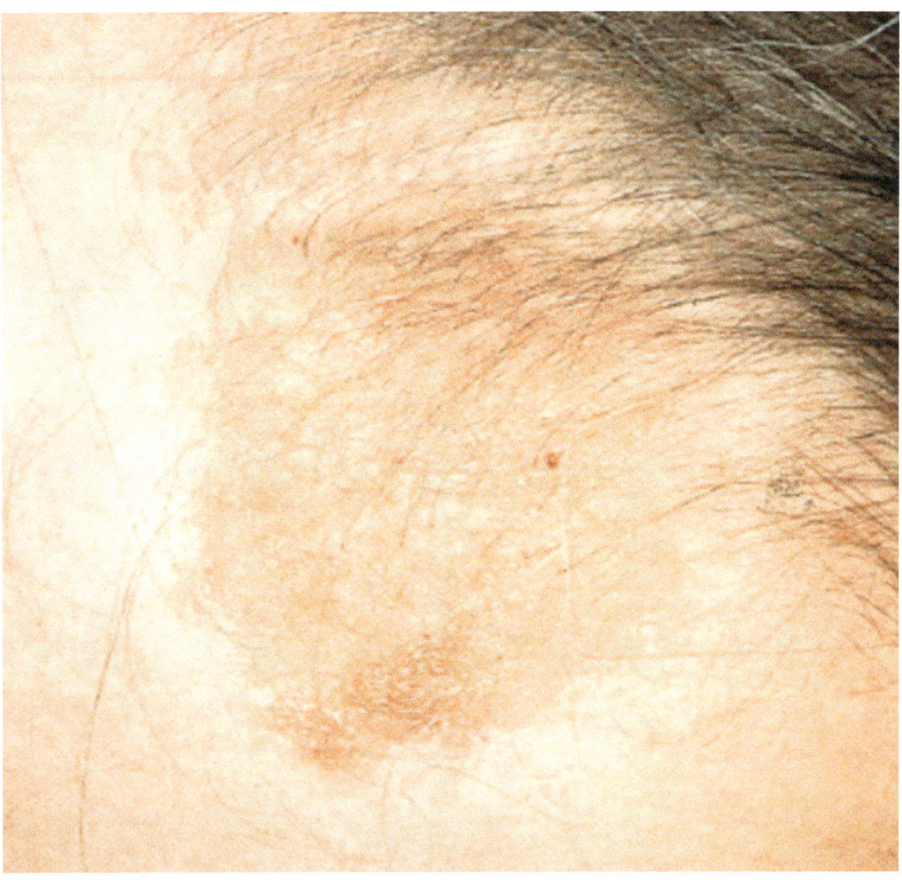

Large, flat seborrheic keratoses occur commonly on the face and balding scalp.

TREATMENT

- Treatment is cosmetic only, unless ruling out a suspicious lesion.
- Because these are growths of epidermis that protrude above the skin surface, destruction of the growth down to the dermal surface will heal by re-epithelialization without scarring. Avoid dermal injury with risk of scar formation. Do not excise.
    - Liquid nitrogen cryotherapy
        - A light application from 15 to 30 seconds is usually curative.
        - Check in 1 month for residua, which can be treated again.
    - Light curettage after ethyl chloride or anesthesia.
        - The spray freeze imparts stiffness to the skin, which facilitates curettage.
        - Spray anesthesia lasts for only 15–20 seconds, so quick, firm strokes of the curette are necessary. Curette only to the white, glistening surface of the dermis.
        - Stop bleeding with pressure or chemical styptic (*See* page 244). Do not stop bleeding with electrocautery, as this increases the likelihood of scarring.

Dermatofibroma (Histiocytoma)

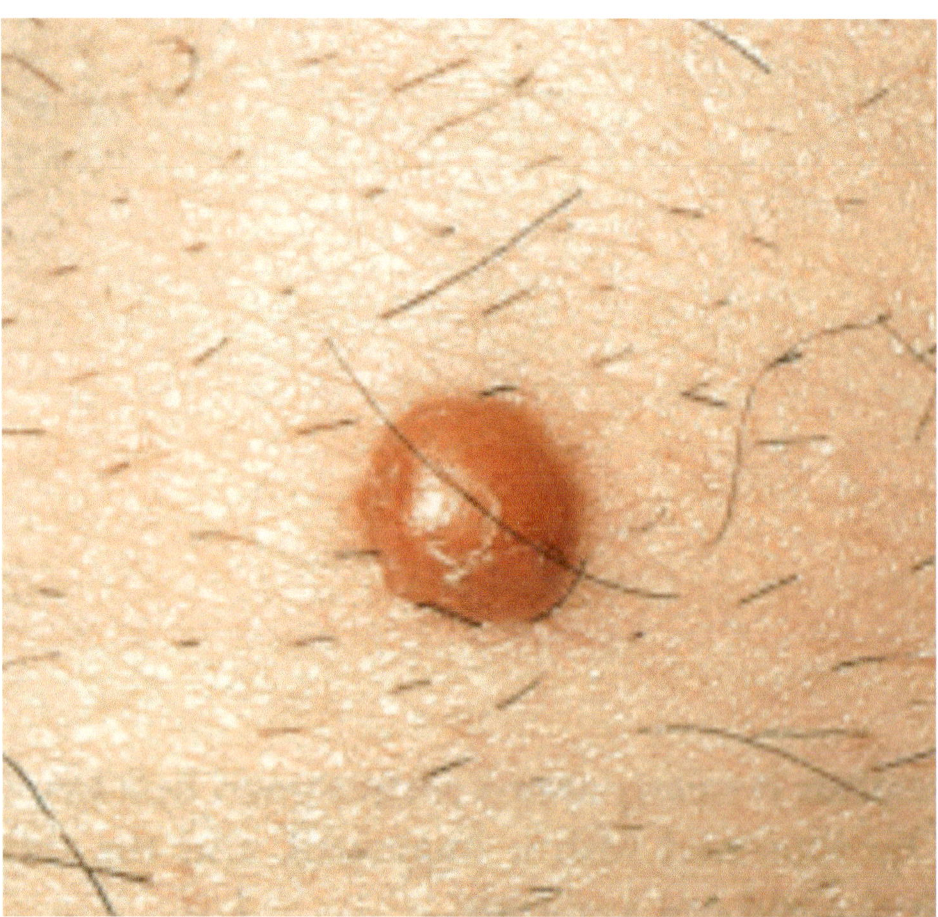

This dermatofibroma is orange because histiocytes within it contain phagocytized lipid.

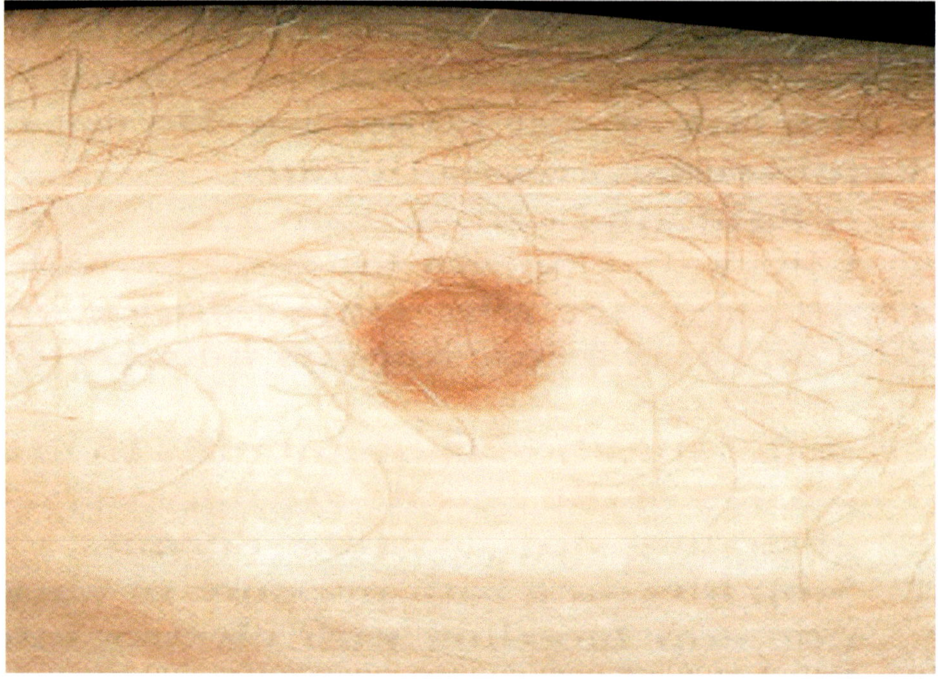

The brown color here is from melanin and hemosiderin.

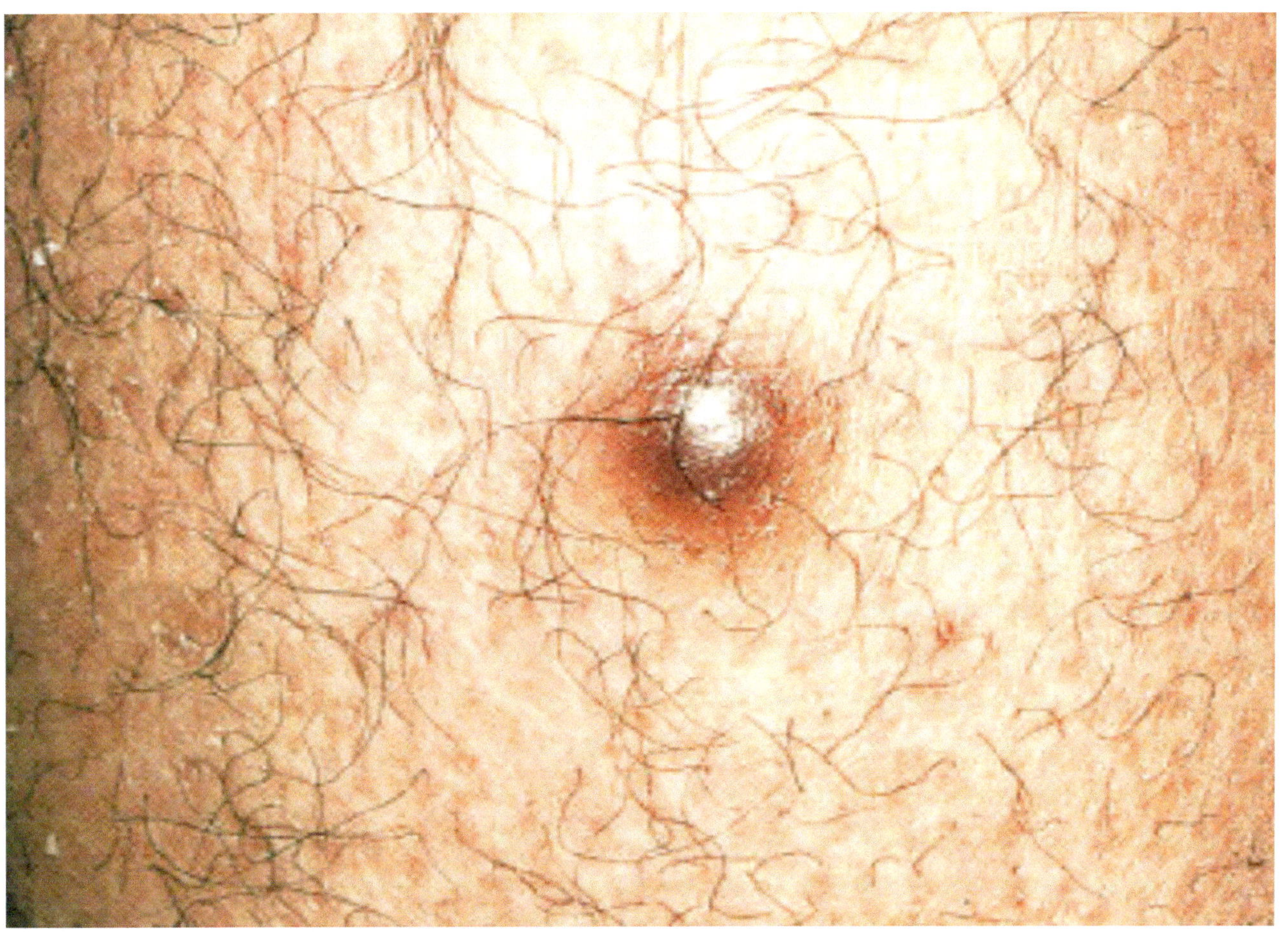

Numerous capillaries in this lesion impart a blue color.

CLINICAL

- This condition consists of firm, buttonlike, intradermal papules or nodules.
  - Up to 1 cm
  - Orange tan to dark brown
  - Smooth or rough and granular surface
  - Typically, when the surrounding skin is gently squeezed, the lesion puckers down and away from the surface.
- The papules usually appear on the extremities of young adults and remain throughout life.
- They are a benign growth of fibroblasts, histiocytes, or both, in a dense collagen stroma.
  - The color depends on the presence of phagocytized lipid, hemosiderin, or both.
  - Fibrosis connects with fiber bundles in subcutaneous fat, which accounts for dimpling behavior when squeezed.
  - There is no malignancy potential.

TREATMENT

- Assure the patient that the condition is benign and that no treatment is necessary.
- Excision is definitive but leaves scarring.
  - Location on a leg or arm often tips cosmetic consideration in favor of no treatment, because surgical scars on those sites are often wide and unsightly.
- Cryotherapy is occasionally used by experienced physicians, but it must be deep and it runs the risk of delayed healing and unsightly scar formation.

Skin Tags (Acrochordons)

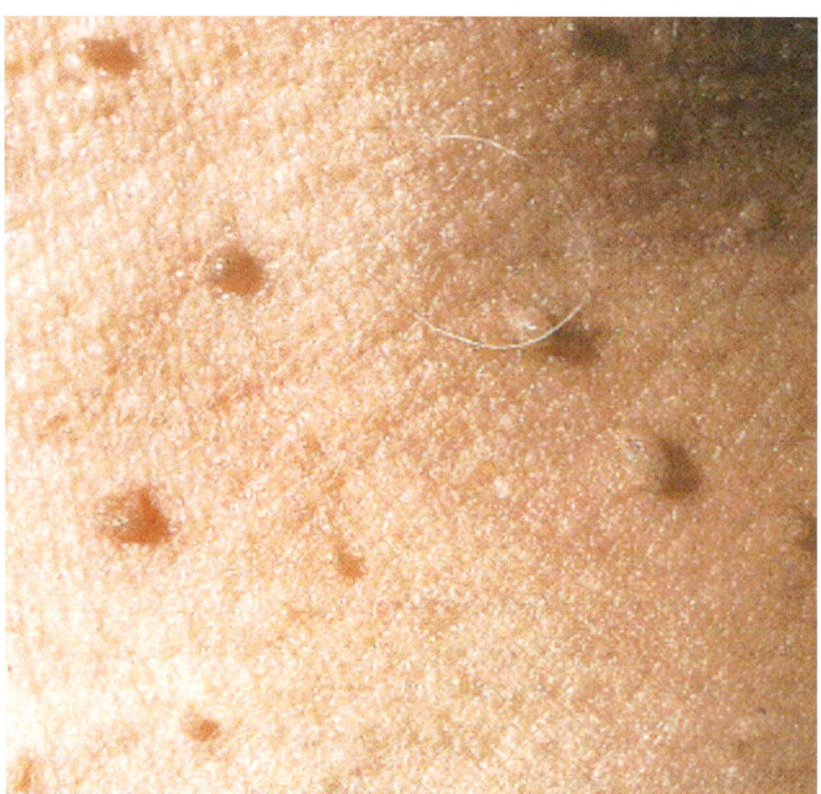

Skin tags often are multiple and on fold areas, as are these on the neck.

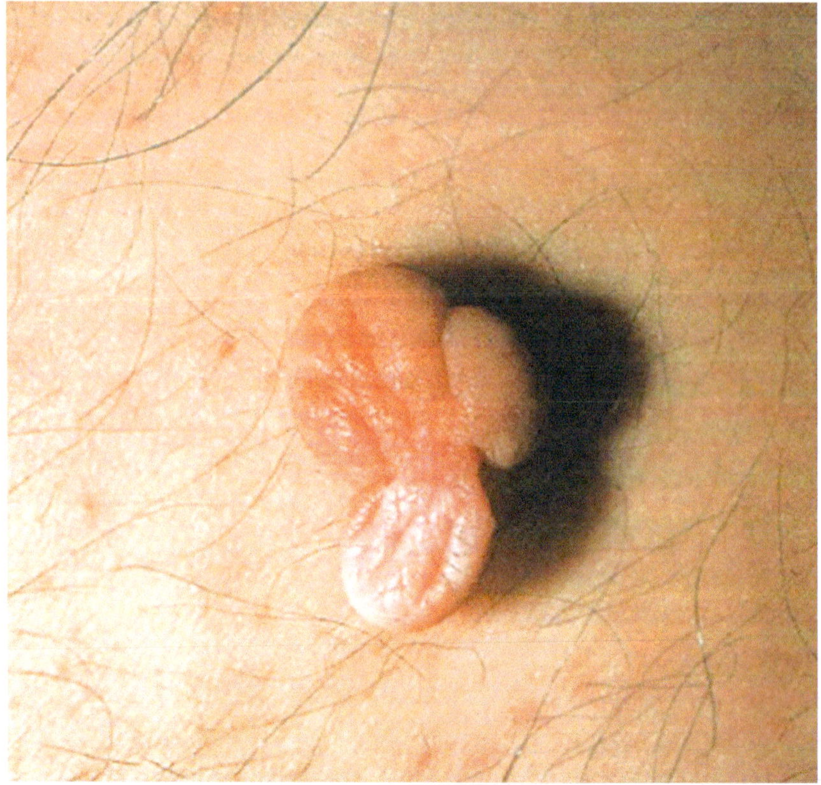

Skin tags can become quite large and pedunculated.

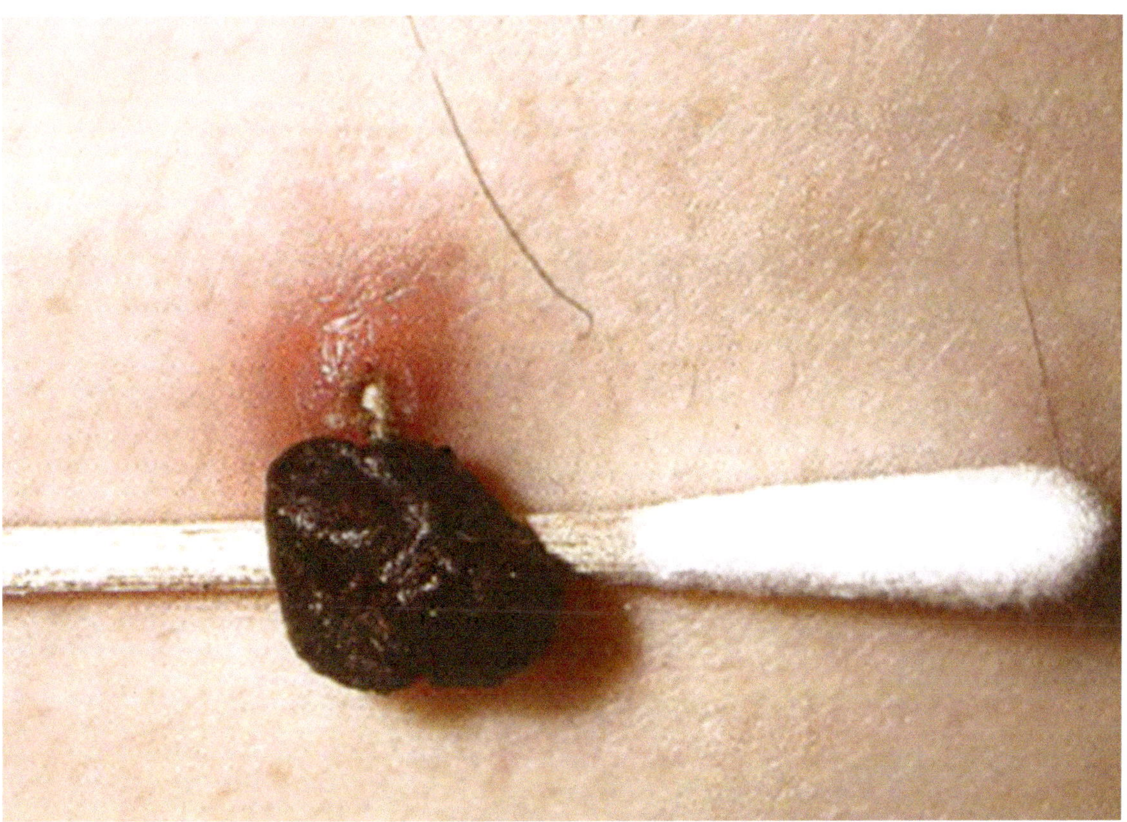

Pedunculated tags may twist on their stalks and infarct spontaneously.

CLINICAL

- This condition typically consists of small (1- to 3-mm), fleshy, filiform or pedunculated papules.
    - They are often hyperpigmented.
    - They are occasionally hyperkeratotic.
    - They are occasionally large (5–30 mm).
    - They are located on:
        - Friction areas (neck, axillae, and groin)
        - Eyelids
- They occur in:
    - Adults
    - Individuals in whom there is a familial tendency
    - Obese individuals
- They have no medical significance, but occasionally twisting of the stalk causes infarct and inflammation.

TREATMENT

- Tiny lesions can be lightly cauterized without anesthesia.
- Small lesions can be snipped quickly without anesthesia.
    - Grasp the fold of skin between thumb and index finger to position tag on its apex. This allows the tag to be snipped without inadvertently cutting or pinching surrounding skin.
    - A quick snip is practically painless; a slow, pinching snip is painful.
    - Stop bleeding with pressure or a dab of styptic (aluminum chloride 30%) (*See* page 244). Bleeding is often delayed for up to 15–30 seconds by arteriolar spasm, so check all sites before the patient dresses.
- Larger lesions require local anesthesia and electrocautery to control arterial bleeding.

Pyogenic Granuloma

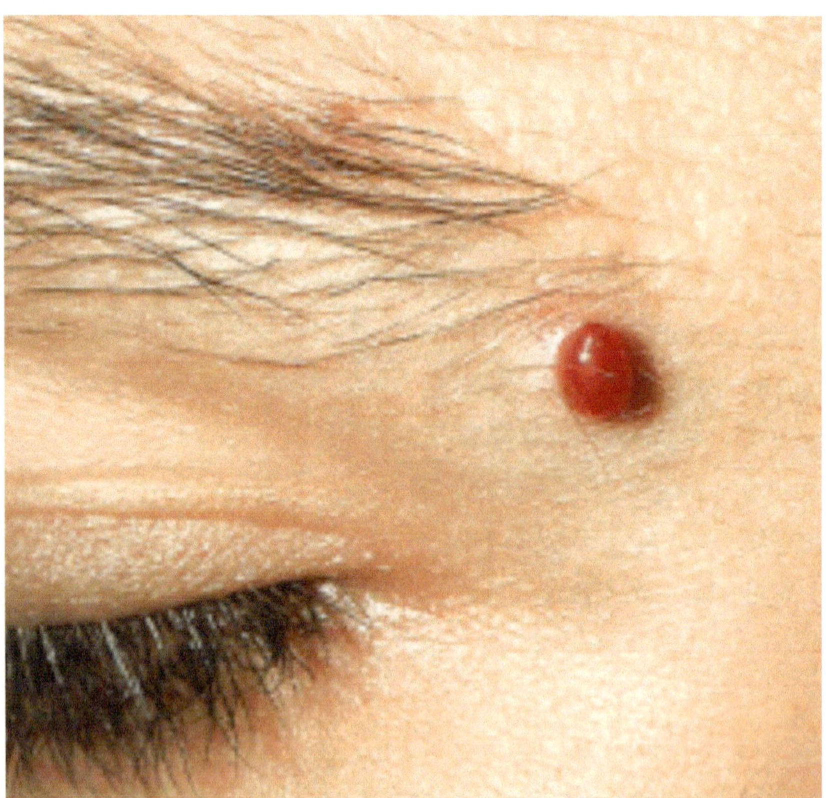

Early (2 weeks), bright red pyogenic granuloma.

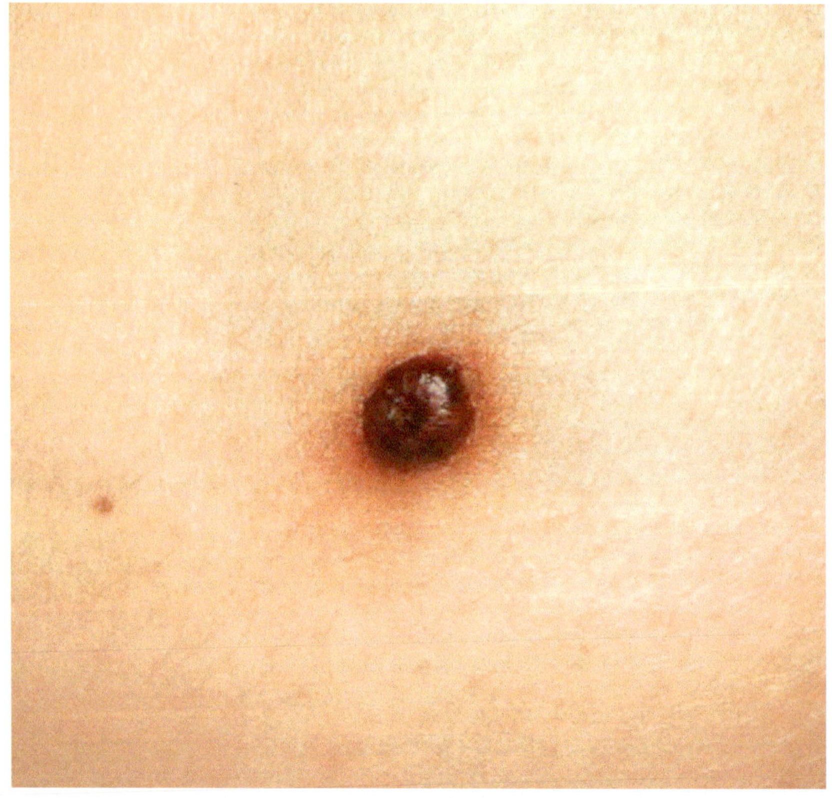

After several weeks, fibrosis begins to replace the vessels.

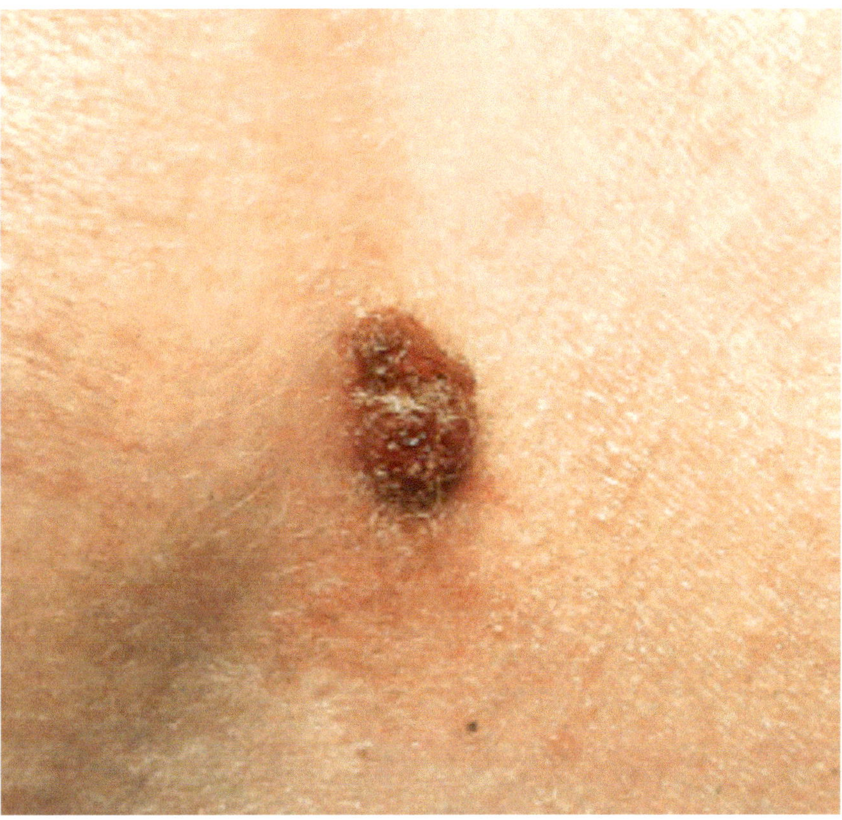

Fibrosis is nearly complete.

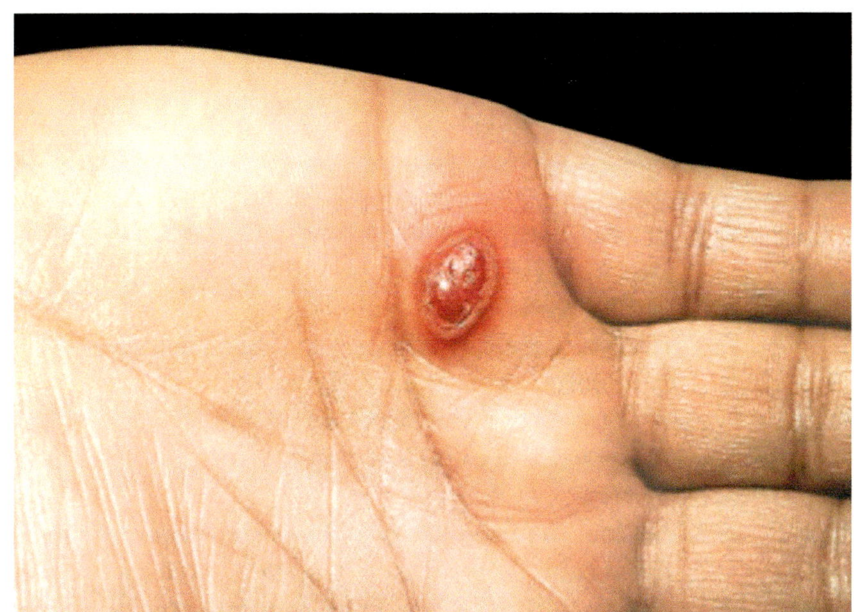

A keratotic collar may be evident, especially on thick-skin areas.

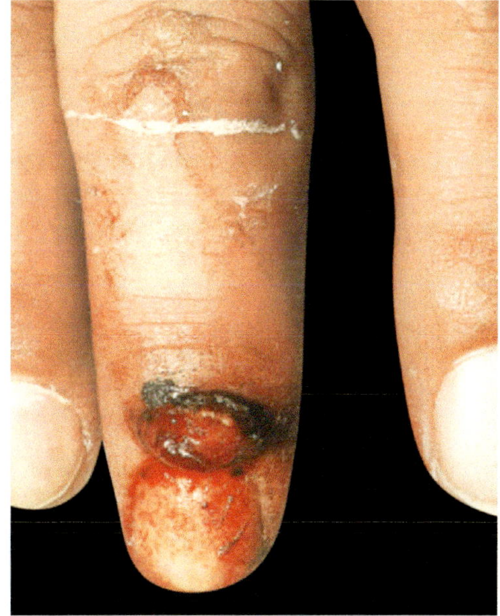

Trauma may cause bleeding. This lesion could easily be mistaken for a melanoma.

CLINICAL

- This condition consists of the sudden appearance and rapid evolution of:
  - Bright cherry-red, glistening papules, with fine keratin collar
    - Somewhat friable, fragile, and bleed easily
  - After a few weeks of growth, the papules become dull red and the surface becomes rougher.
  - After several weeks or months, the papules may involute completely or become flesh-colored and fibrotic.

- The condition occurs most commonly in young adults and during pregnancy.
  - It may arise spontaneously or at the site of minor skin injury.
    - It may occur a few weeks after tattoo or vaccination.
  - During pregnancy the condition may occur on the gums as "epulides."
- The condition is a growth of granulation tissue (proud flesh), consisting of immature capillaries and collagen.
  - The name is a misnomer. It is neither pyogenic nor a granuloma.

TREATMENT

- Treatment is usually advised because:
  - Involution is rarely complete if the condition is untreated.
  - If the condition is not treated early, the papules may grow larger.
  - Biopsy specimen rules out nonpigmented melanoma (*See* page 220).
- The type of treatment depends on the size and location of the papules.
  - If the papule is small, scoop-shave (scoop deeply in dermis with a number 15 scalpel blade) or snip with a curved, small scissors.
    Electrodesiccate or cauterize base.
    - This procedure leaves a small, flat, and round scar.
    - The lesion may recur in 5–10% of cases if destruction is not complete; treat again.
  - If papules are large (up to 1 cm) or in a wrinkle line of the face, excision with suture closure has a low recurrence rate and gives a good cosmetic result.

Cysts

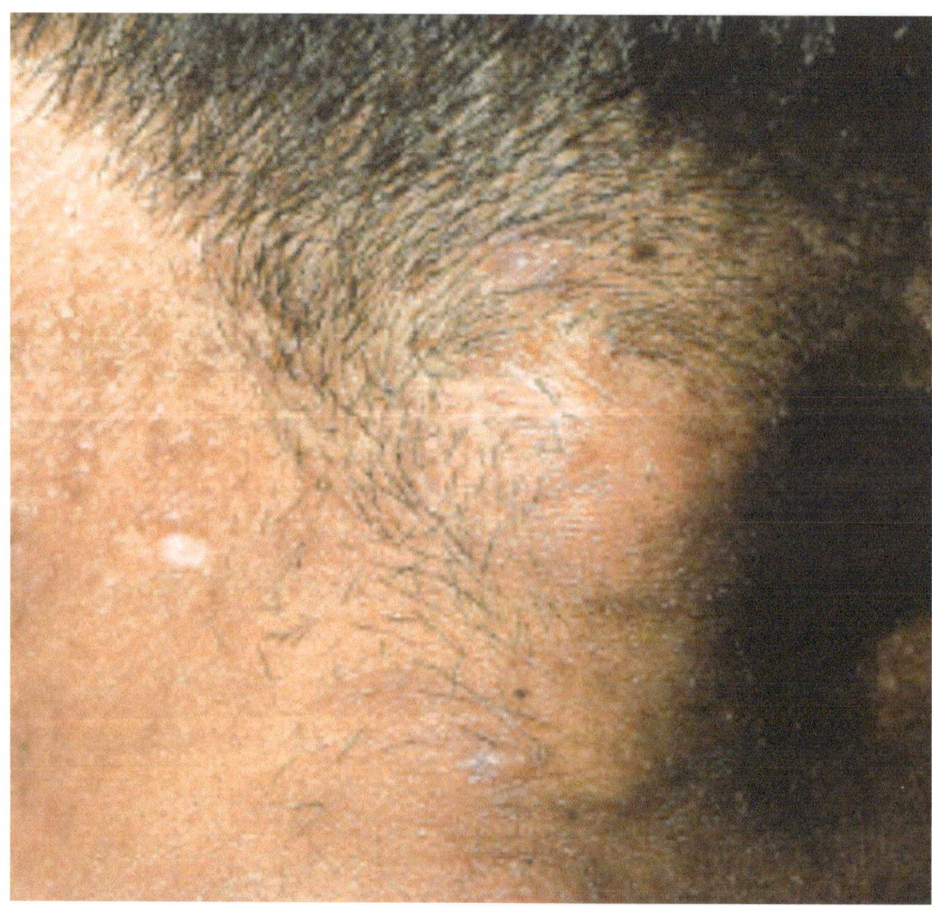

Inflamed and swollen epidermoid cyst at nape of neck.

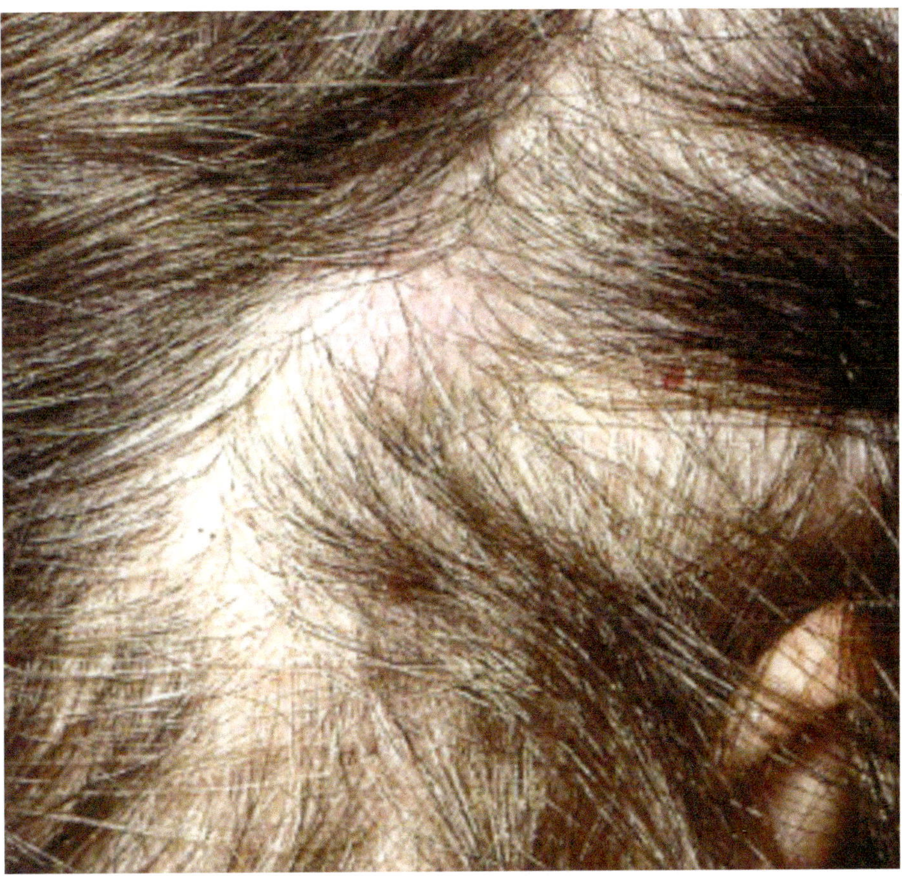

Pilar cyst of scalp. These cysts are more obvious on palpation than on inspection.

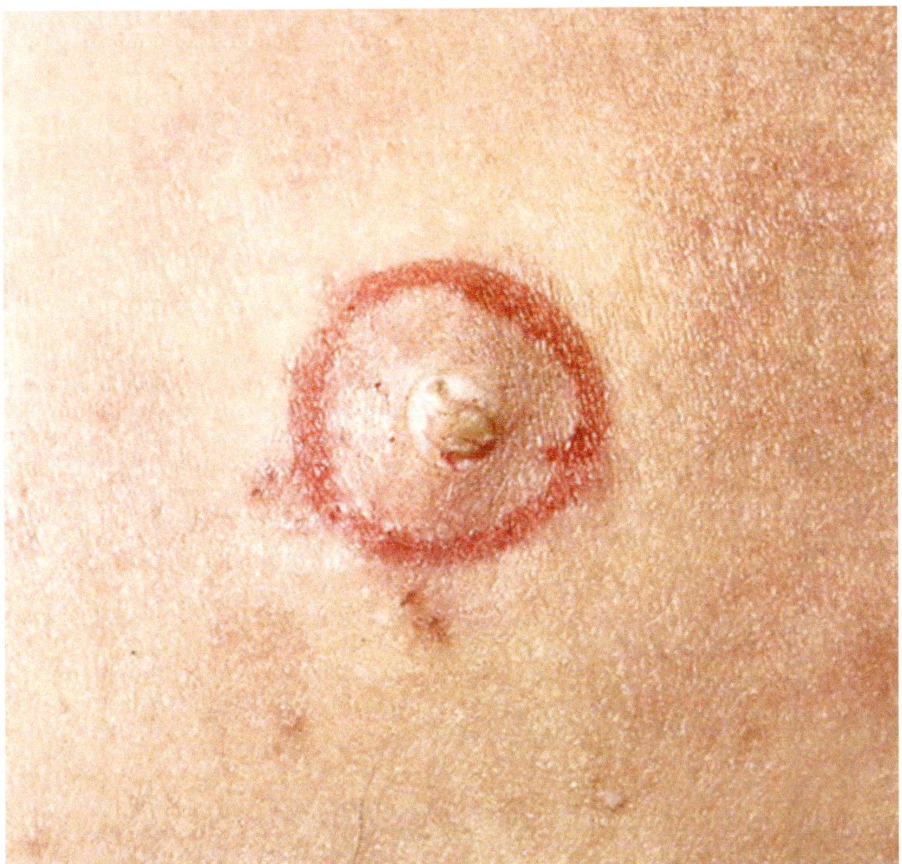

Epidermoid cyst (extent outlined in red) anesthetized and incised by a 3-mm punch.

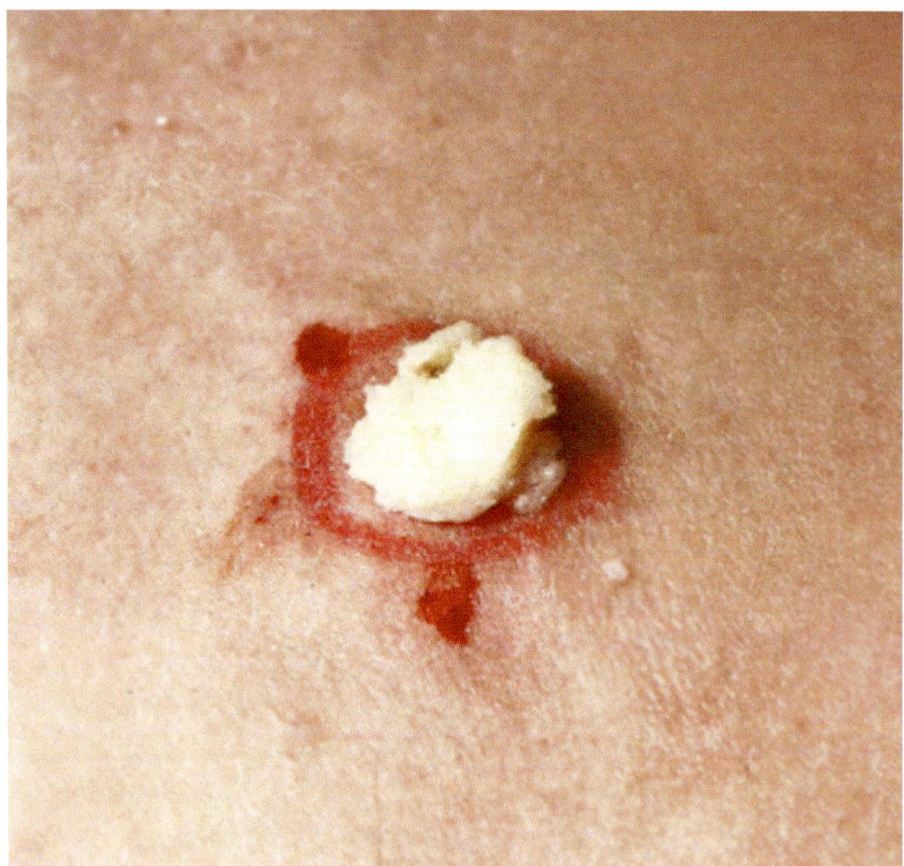

Cyst contents forcibly expressed.

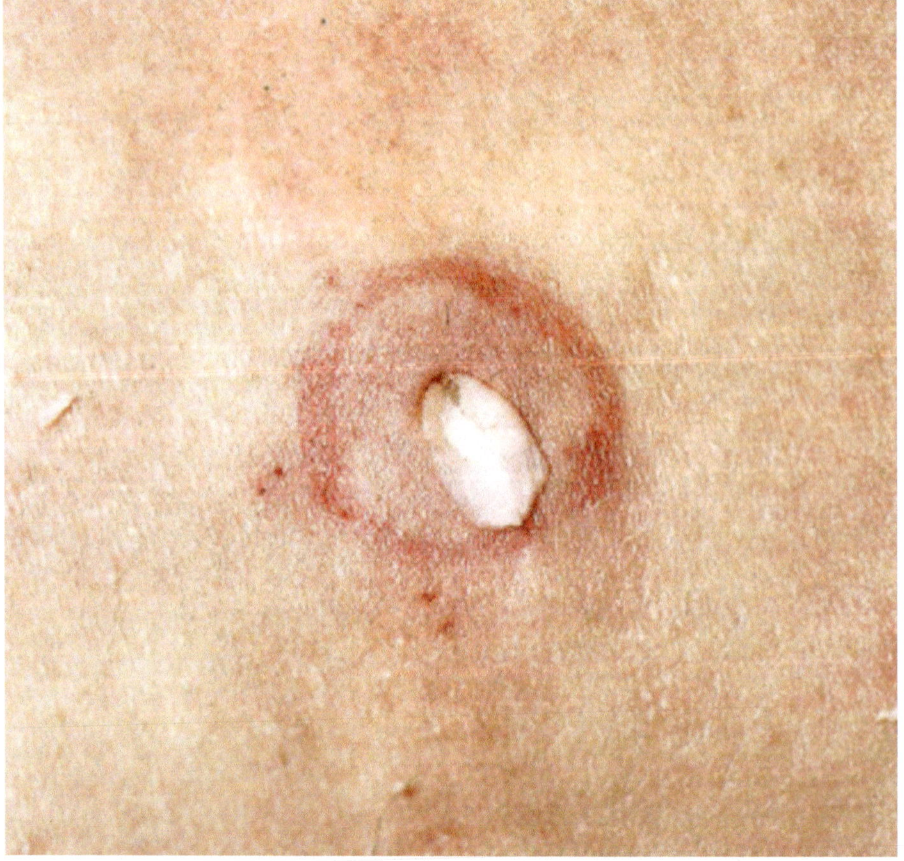

Wiping away debris reveals filmy cyst wall protruding from incision.

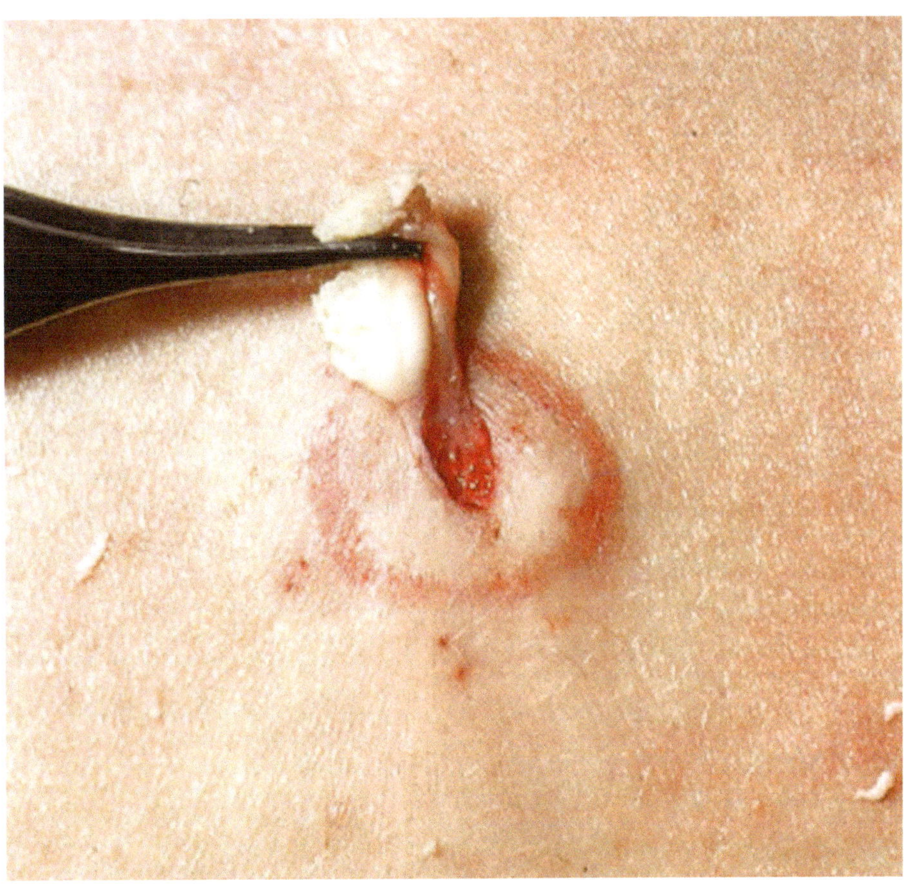

Entire wall is gently teased out, usually using fine, curved scissors.

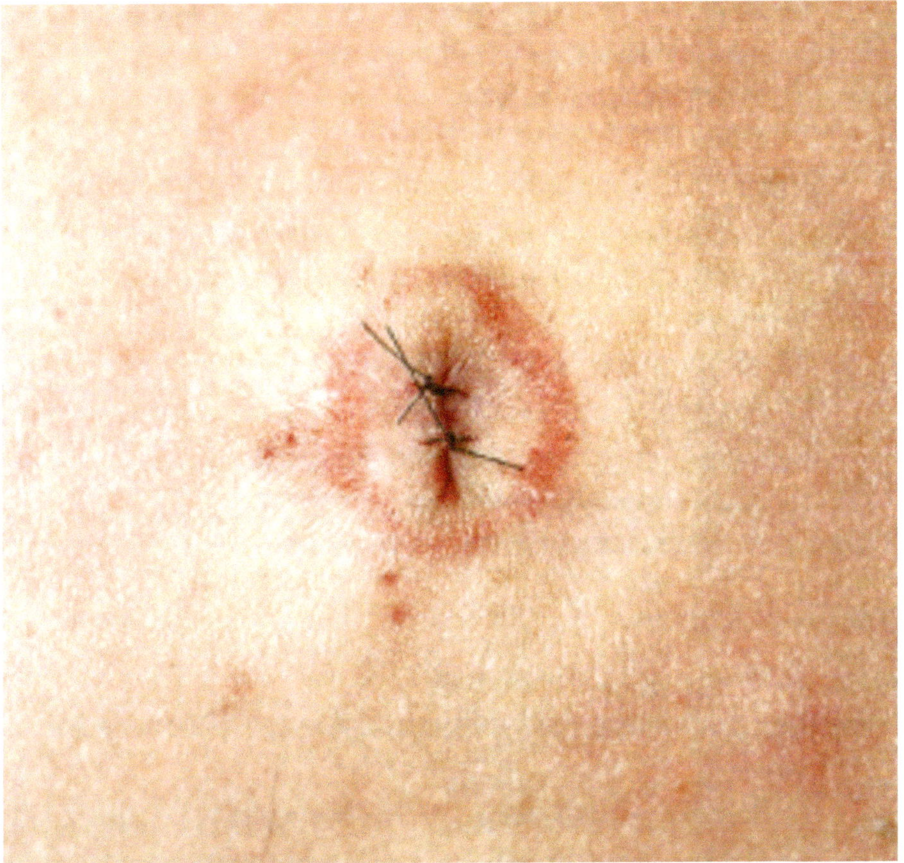

Closure results in a scar much smaller than the cyst itself.

CLINICAL

- An **epidermoid** cyst is a sac-like growth of the upper portion of a follicle. The wall is like epidermis; the contents are immature keratin and cellular debris.
  - It is a soft, hemispherical, subcutaneous nodule usually surmounted by a comedo or dilated pore.
  - It is usually located on the face, neck, and upper trunk.
    - More common in males and in individuals with large oil glands and acne
  - It occasionally drains cheesy material or the patient expresses such matter through a dilated pore.
    - The foul odor is rancid lipid and cellular debris—*not* infection.
    - The lesion will refill after emptying because the intact cyst wall continues to shed keratin.
  - Occasionally the cyst will be red, tender, and swollen.
    - This represents rupture of the cyst wall with leakage of the contents into the dermis, provoking an intense inflammatory response like a large pimple.
    - It is *not* infected but is often misdiagnosed as such. Incision and drainage reveal a soupy, smelly debris that looks like purulence but is only keratin and cellular debris mixed with tissue fluid and inflammatory cells.
- A **pilar** cyst is a sac-like growth of the middle portion of a follicle.
  The wall is like the follicle; contents are hair-cuticle-like material.
  - A hard, hemispherical, subcutaneous nodule without an overlying pore
  - Most frequently located on scalp
    - May be familial
    - Often multiple and/or in clusters
    - May develop overlying alopecia
  - Does not drain or become inflamed

TREATMENT

- Inflamed epidermoid cyst
  - Do not incise and drain unless the thinned roof is ready to rupture
    - Incision is likely to leave an enlarged pore or sinus.
    - The contents will re-form because the cyst wall is still present.
  - Is difficult to excise when inflamed because the wall is fragile, hard to differentiate from surrounding tissue, and heals poorly when sutured
  - Requires intralesional or perilesional corticosteroid injection (*See* page 240) (e.g., triamcinolone acetonide 5–10 mg/mL, 0.1–0.4 mL)
    - Pain and tenderness improve in 12 hours and resolve in 2–4 days.
  - May be excised 3–6 weeks later when it is not inflamed
- Noninflamed epidermoid cyst
  - *Excision. See* farther on, under pilar cyst.
  - If the cyst is not inflamed or scarred from a previous inflammation, make a 3- to 4-mm incision into the cyst or, better still, a 3- to 4-mm circular punch. Express the contents firmly and the cyst wall will rise to the opening. Grasp gently with forceps and tease out the cyst wall, using fine, curved scissors to dissect it from surrounding tissue. This maneuver is similar to turning the finger of a glove inside out from within. An absorbable subcutaneous suture may be required to close dead space. Close the skin opening. If cyst has been inflamed in the past, scar tissue may prevent teasing out of the cyst wall.
- Pilar cyst
  - *Excision.* The wall is thick and the contents are hard. Incise over (not into) the cyst and it will often pop above the skin surface. Snip the few fibrous threads attaching it to the dermis and remove the cyst. If the cyst is in a hair-bearing scalp, the wound can be closed with absorbable suture. This will leave stitchmark scars, but they will be hidden by hair, and the patient need not return for suture removal.
  - An **epidermoid** cyst can be excised in similar fashion, but the skin over it is thin and the cyst wall is thin and fragile. Care is needed in gently freeing the cyst from the surrounding tissue to avoid rupture.

Warts (Verrucae)

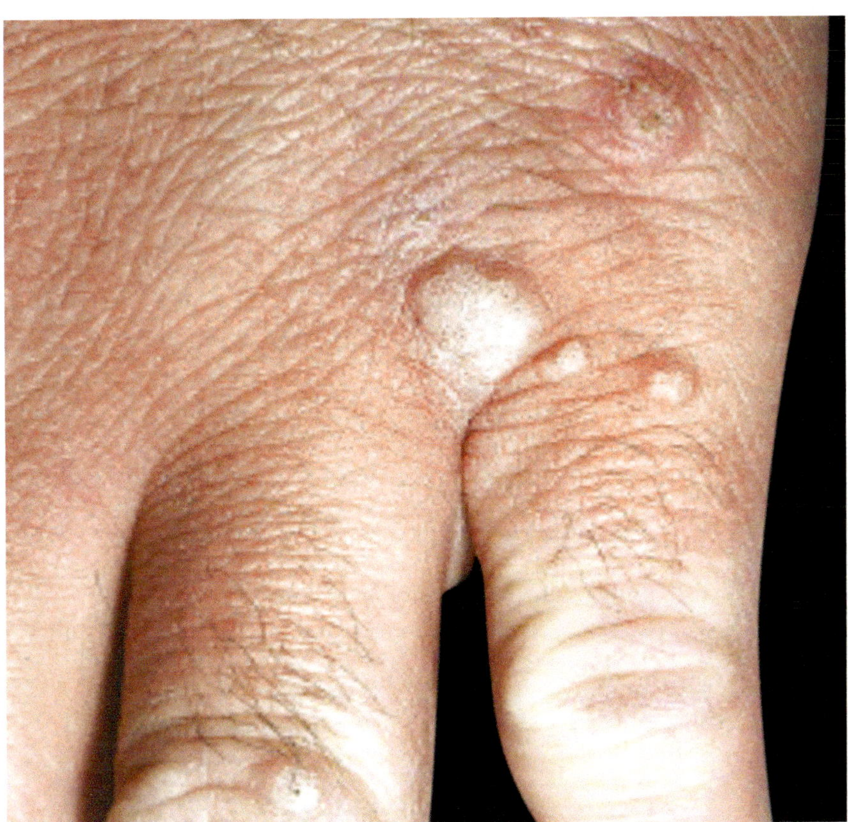

Common warts in a common location.

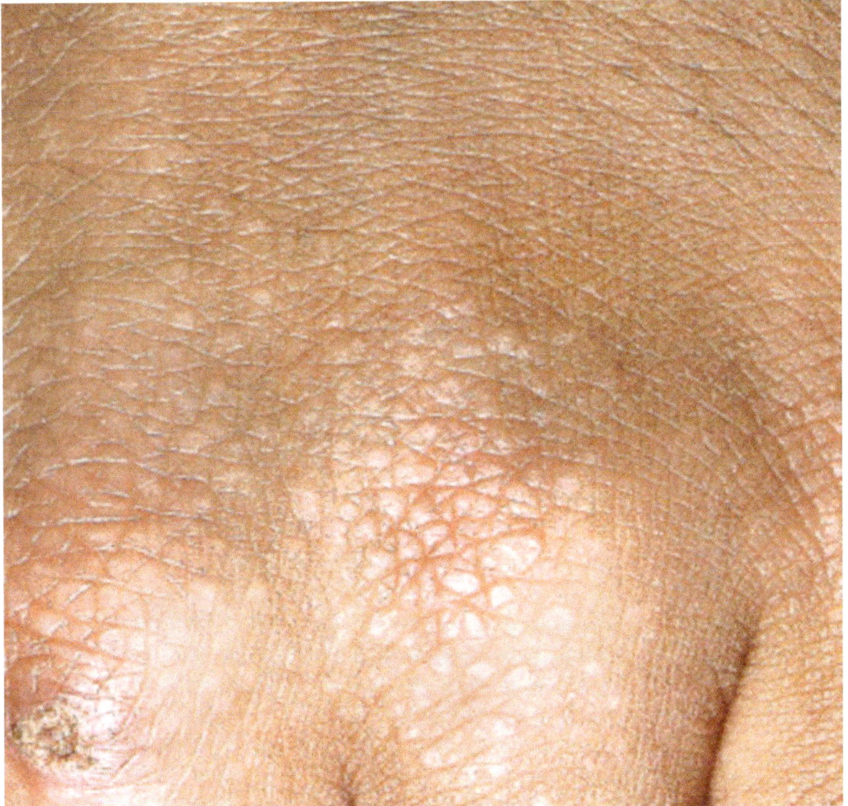

Plane or flat warts often occur as many lesions closely packed.

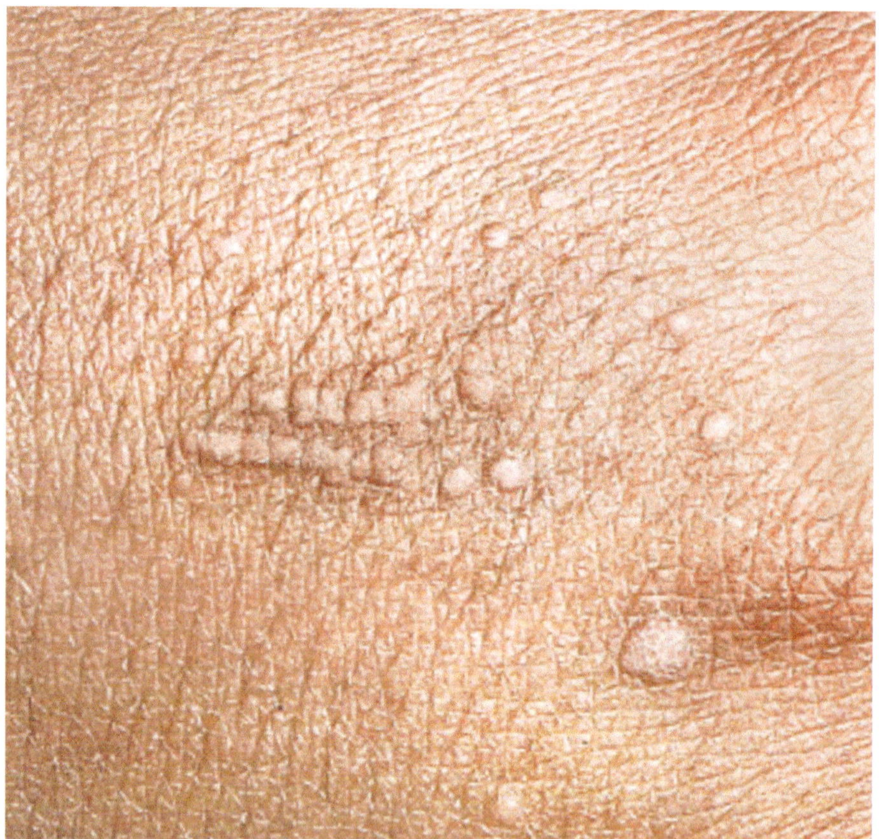

The wart virus can be seeded from one source in sites of trauma.

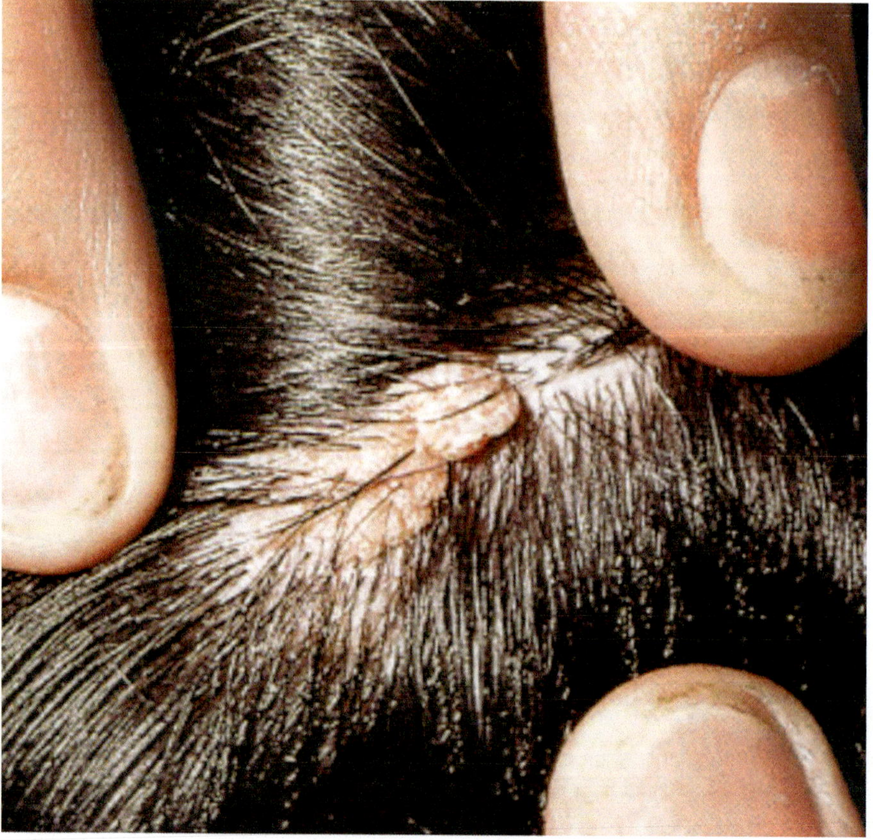

Exuberant wart growth in scalp.

CLINICAL

- Warty keratotic papules and plaques are most common in children on the hands and arms.
  - Sometimes occur in groups or in areas of trauma (e.g., scratches or cuts)
  - Usually asymptomatic but may crack and bleed
- They are caused by the human papillomavirus implanted in the skin.
  - Incubation period: 2 to 4 months or longer
  - Seed into areas of broken skin
  - Disappear spontaneously when immunity develops. Except for plantar (*See* page 94) and periungual (*See* page 91) warts, the duration is approximately 6 to 24 months in children, but in adults they may last for many years.

TREATMENT

- General (*See* Patient Guides, page 255)
  - If asymptomatic, warts require no treatment unless for cosmetic reasons (except for genital warts, which may be oncogenic).
  - Discourage picking of warts or shaving the area, which may cause spread of lesions.
    - Young children will often not hold still because of pain. Do not treat.
    - Do not see patient again for 3 weeks, as inflammation and scab mask site. Re-examine the patient in 3–4 weeks and treat any tiny residual warts again.
    - Warts may recur at the site of treatment for up to 6 months. Warn patient of this possibility.
  - Light electrodesiccation and curettage
    - Requires local anesthesia
    - Insert treatment electrode into the wart and apply the current until wart tissue whitens, swells, and softens (usually 5–10 seconds). Lightly curette.
    - Skillful use leaves little, if any, scarring and is effective. Excessive electrodesiccation causes scarring.
  - See also facial warts (*See* page 42), genital warts (*See* page 57), periungual warts (*See* page 91), and plantar warts (*See* page 94).

Actinic Damage and Sun Protection

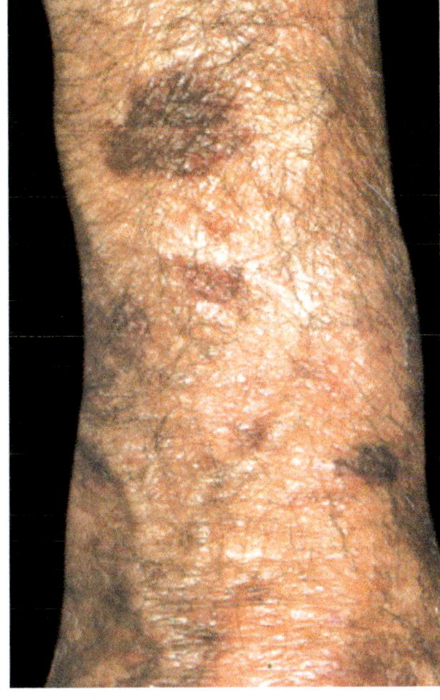

Marked dermal atrophy, loss of normal elasticity of skin. Marked purpura secondary to minor trauma to damaged vessels.

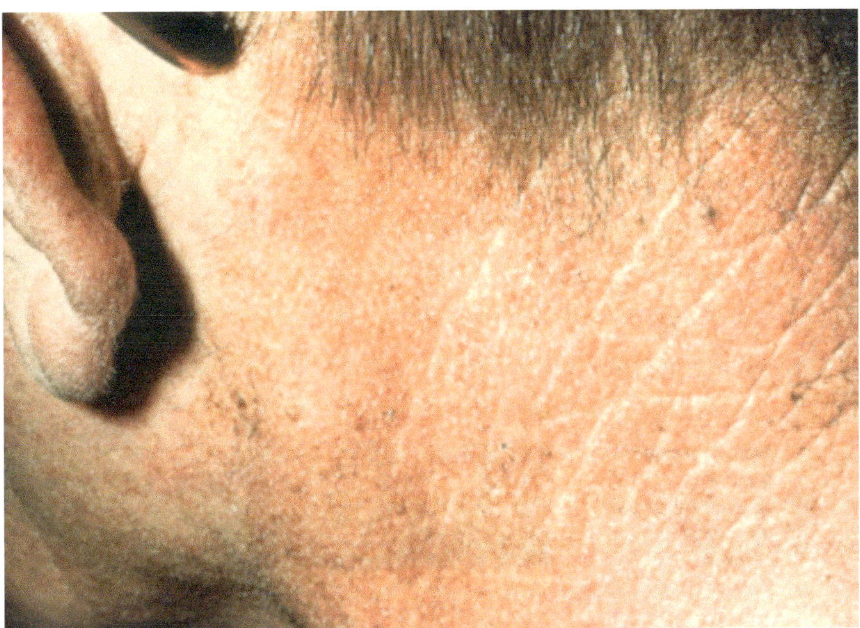

Hyperpigmentation, leathery thickening, and wrinkling from chronic sun exposure.

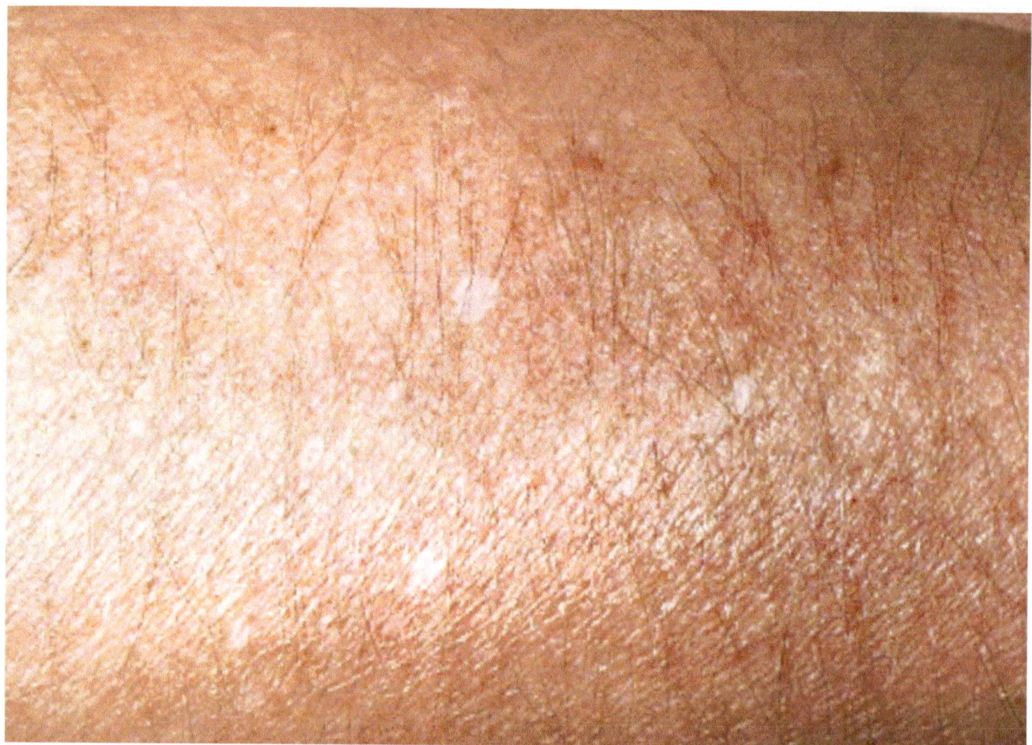

Idiopathic guttate hypomelanosis: small, polygonal hypopigmented macules, probably from actinic damage to melanocytes.

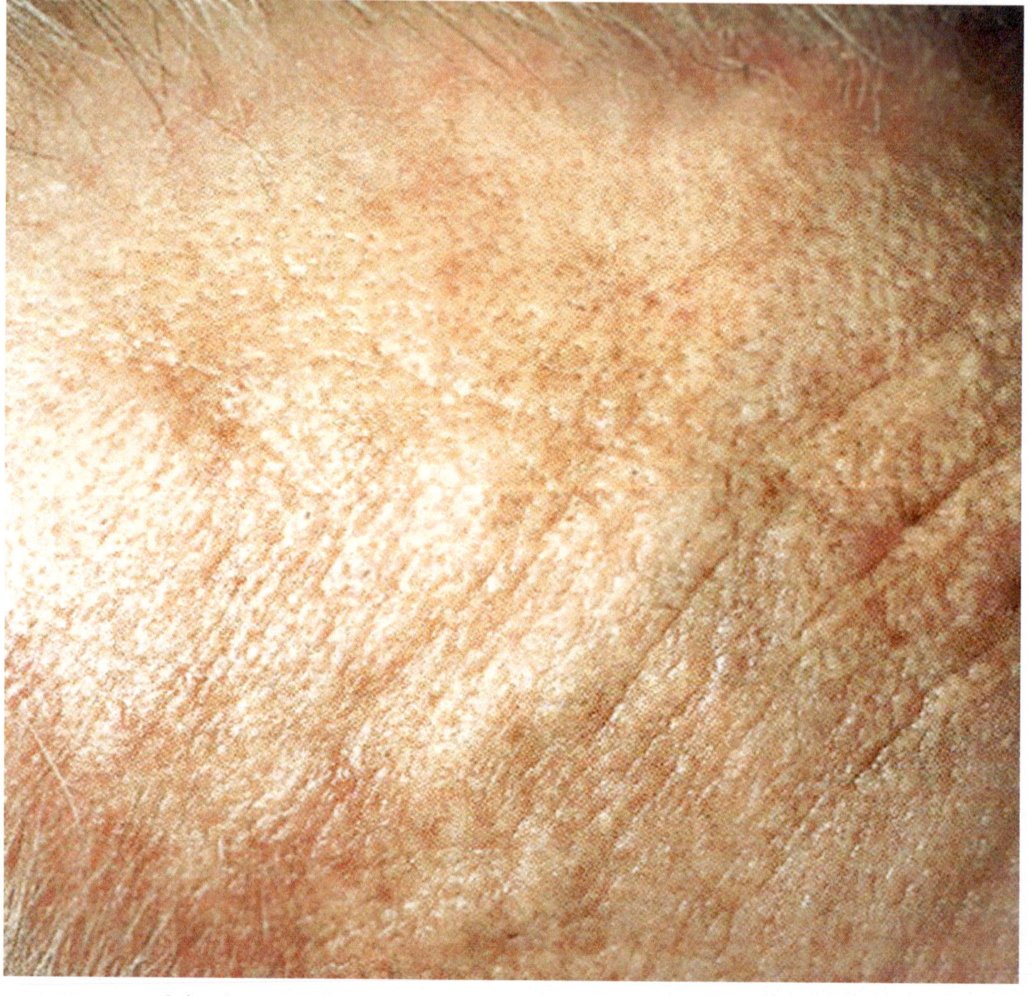

Solar elastosis: Yellow, dermal plaque is degenerated sundamaged collagen.

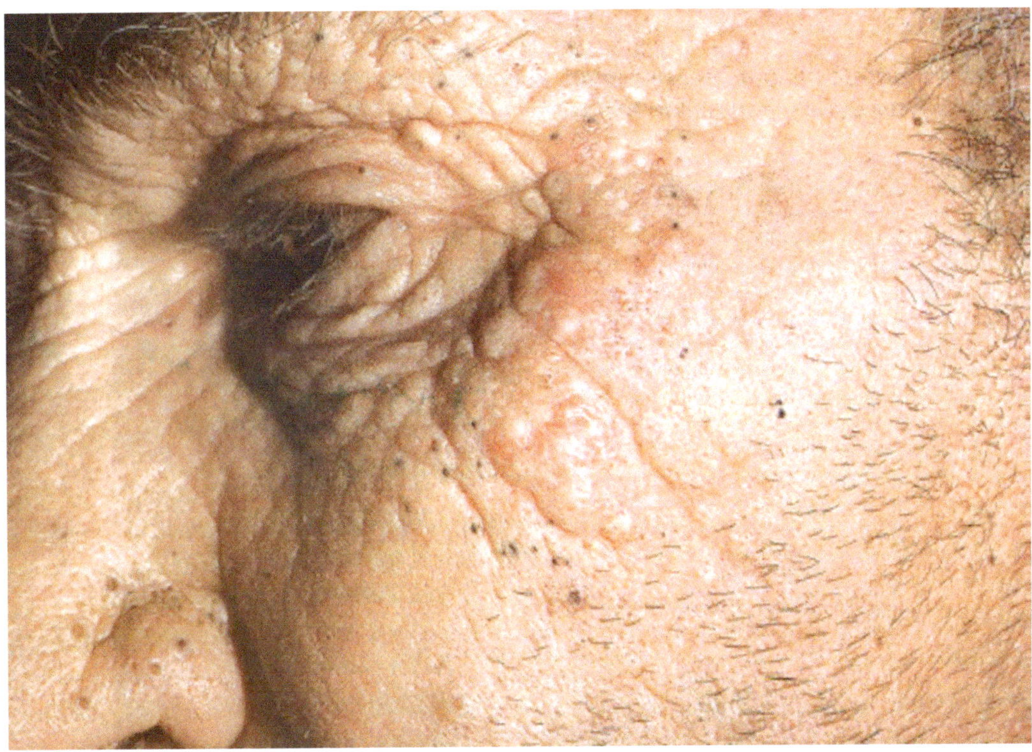

Solar comedones and wrinkling.

CLINICAL

In actinic damage, penetrating ultraviolet rays damage the epidermal cells, melanocytes, dermal collagen, blood vessels, and even the pilosebaceous structures. Clinical manifestations are:

- Epidermal
  - Dryness and scaling
  - Epidermal atrophy
  - Actinic keratoses (*See* page 207)
  - Carcinomas (*See* page 213)
- Melanocytes
  - Freckling, diffuse punctate pigmentation
  - Lentigo (*See* page 206)
  - Lentigo maligna and, possibly, melanoma (*See* page 220)
  - Hypopigmented spots (idiopathic guttate hypomelanosis)
- Dermal
  - Wrinkling
  - Solar elastosis (yellow plaques of collagen degeneration at the temples)
  - Dermal atrophy (thinning of the skin)
- Blood vessels
  - Telangiectasia (*See* page 205)
  - Hemorrhage and easy bruising, especially on the dorsa of the hands and arms
- Pilosebaceous
  - Milia
  - Solar comedones, or blackheads

TREATMENT

- Solar damage of the skin is cumulative during a lifetime, so intelligent precautions should be taken during childhood and practiced routinely thereafter. Skin changes will occur late in life, even if the skin is then protected, if excessive sun exposure has occurred during childhood and young adulthood. Continued sun exposure worsens the changes.

- Protection
  - Minimize sun exposure.
    - Avoid the sun from 10 AM to 2 PM, the time that 60% of the day's ultraviolet light reaches the earth.
  - Wear protective hats and clothing.
  - Use sunscreens. They are ranked for sun protection factor (SPF), usually from 5 to 50, denoting a multiple of the regular length of sun exposure before overt sunburn occurs. So, if burning usually occurs after 30 minutes of exposure to the noonday sun, then an SPF 5 preparation will safely allow 2.5 hours of such exposure. Sunscreens with SPF higher than 50 offer very little more protection than one with 50, so their use is not necessary. Sunscreens should be applied 30 minutes before sun exposure, to allow skin binding, and should be reapplied after swimming or vigorous sweating. Sunscreens marked "water resistant" are required to state whether the sunscreen remains effective for 40 minutes or 80 minutes when swimming or sweating. Allergy and photoallergy to sunscreens occasionally occur.
  - Special factors enhancing sun damage
    - Burning occurs more quickly in a humid environment than in a dry one and in turbulent rather than in still air.
    - Ultraviolet penetration is enhanced by the presence of oil or grease on the skin, as in "sun tan oil."
    - Reflection from water, sand, and snow is intense, so protection by a beach umbrella may be inadequate.
    - Ultraviolet penetration through wet white cloth is substantial, so wearing a T-shirt while swimming is only minimally protective. Clothing specifically designed to block ultraviolet rays is available.
    - Ultraviolet intensity increases greatly with altitude because of less filtration by the thinner air. At higher altitudes particular caution must be used, even by individuals who rarely burn.
  - *See* Patient Guides (page 253)
- Treatments covered elsewhere
  - Actinic keratoses (*See* page 207)
  - Carcinomas (*See* page 213)
  - Lentigines (*See* page 206)
  - Lentigo maligna and melanoma (*See* page 220)
  - Telangiectasia (*See* page 205)
  - Milia and solar comedones: *See* page 33 for treatment of comedonal acne. Topical use of retinoids and comedo removal in the office are effective. Aged, dry skin is easily irritated by retinoids, so begin with alternate-day applications.
- Topical retinoids (*See* acne treatment, page 30)
  - May slowly reverse freckles and fine wrinkles caused by the sun (but not due to age) and may slowly improve or resolve actinic keratoses but often only after a brisk inflammatory response for weeks or months.
  - Start with the lowest concentration and build up as tolerated
  - Increased sun sensitivity (faster sunburning) is noted by many patients, so sunscreens must be worn regularly. This sensitivity lasts at least 2 weeks after discontinuing retinoids, so it cannot be stopped just before a sunny vacation to avoid increased burning.
  - The improvements in pigment, wrinkles, and keratoses likely slowly reverse when the retinoid is stopped, so its use is probably lifelong, although perhaps at a diminished frequency (2 nights a week) after the first year.

> Cataracts and retinal damage can result from accumulated ultraviolet exposure. Older plastic sunglasses, even with dark lenses, often did not filter out ultraviolet rays. In the United States, most sunglasses now filter all or some ultraviolet light, but the consumer should look for a tag stating "complete" or "maximal" protection. Ultraviolet-filtering pigment can be added to prescription lenses on request.

Telangiectasia and Spider Angiomata

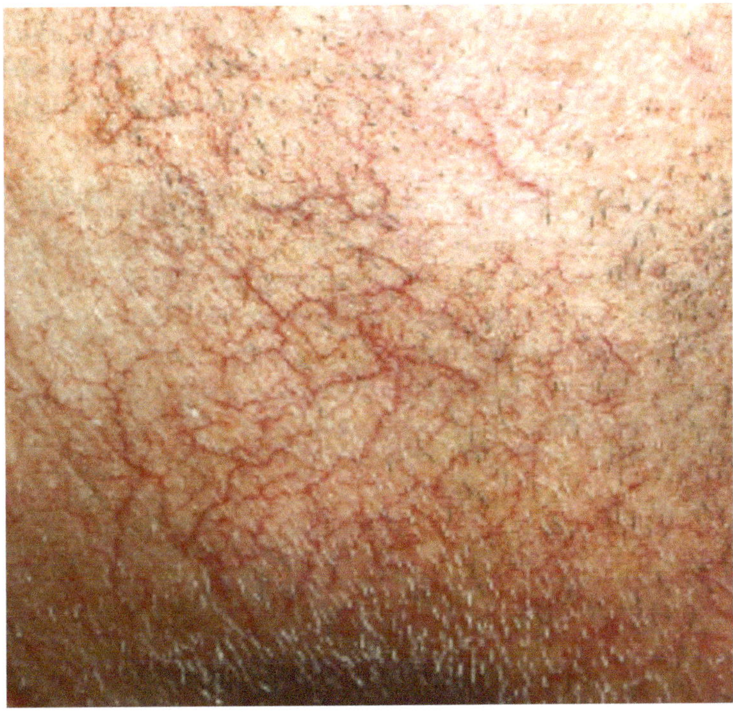

Profuse telangiectasia from chronic sun exposure.

CLINICAL

- Telangiectasia is a series of visible, dilated capillaries, usually on the nose and cheeks of fair-skinned individuals.
  - It is a form of chronic sun damage.
  - Check for keratoses and carcinomas.
- Spider angiomata are red dots with dilated capillaries radiating from the center (like legs radiating from a spider's body). They represent dilated arterioles with surrounding engorged capillaries.
  - They occur in healthy young adults on the face (especially just below the lower eyelid) and the backs of the hands.
  - They occur more frequently and in greater numbers with pregnancy, estrogen therapy, and chronic liver disease.

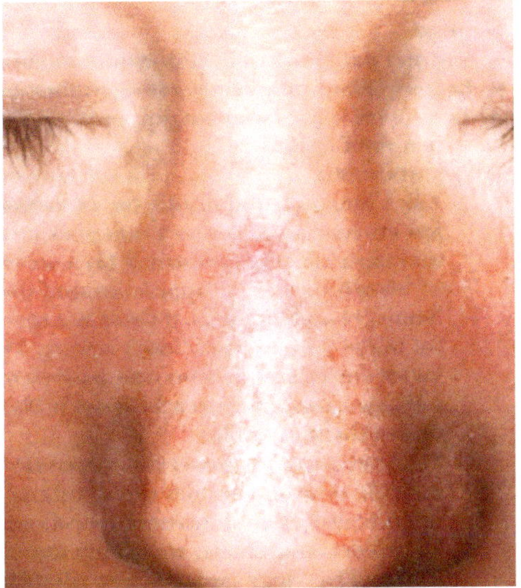
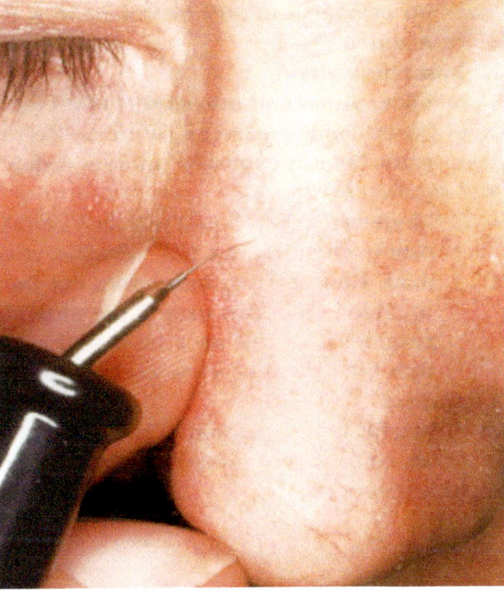

Spider angioma, treated by light electrodesiccation.

TREATMENT

- General
  - Instruct patients in sun protection and avoidance (*See* page 253).
  - Inquire about pregnancy, estrogen therapy, and alcoholism.
  - Treatment is for cosmetic purposes.
- Destruction of lesions
  - Electrocautery
    - Use a fine epilating needle on a treatment probe set at a very low current. Insert up to 1 mm of electrode tip into the vessel and tap activating foot switch for a second or two. A tiny zone of blanching should appear around the tip. If a large (2- to 3-mm) blanch appears, if there is a spark, or if it is very painful to the patient, use a lower setting. The proper dial setting varies considerably from one patient to the next. Local anesthesia cannot be given because it blanches the vessels and makes them invisible.
    - For telangiectasia, insert the electrode as far "upstream" as possible or at the branch of the tributaries. Treatment there often blanches all downstream outflow.
    - For spider angiomata, treat only the central "body" of the spider. The "legs" will collapse on their own.

  Note: Relapse or appearance of new vessels is common; follow-up examination and treatment in a few weeks are recommended.
  - Laser destruction
    - Older argon and other lasers often left scars.
    - Pulsed dye laser is painless, effective, and does not leave scars, but may leave a bruise for a few days.
- Cosmetics
  - A helpful hint to patient: The addition of a small amount of green color to the cosmetic greatly enhances its effectiveness in hiding redness.

Solar Lentigo

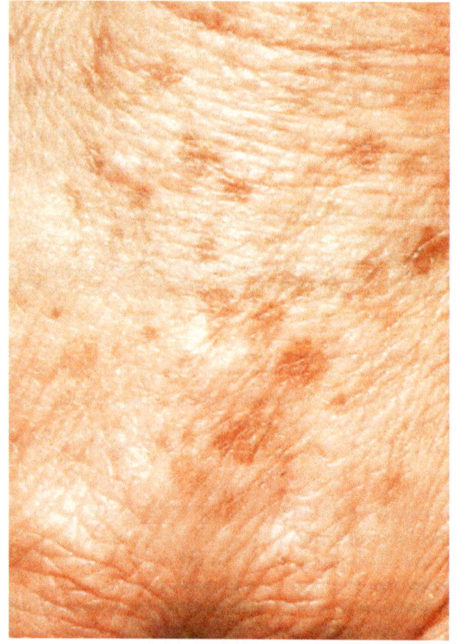

Typical early lentigines.

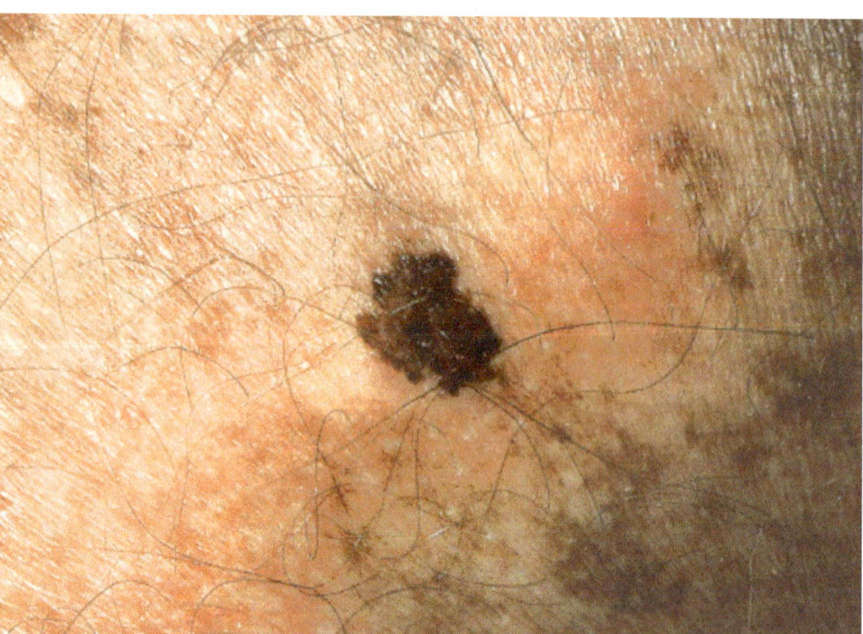

Dark lentigo and mottled hyperpigmentation in very sun-damaged skin.

CLINICAL

- Solar lentigo consists of flat, homogeneous, 2- to 30-mm tan or brown spots with well-defined borders.
  - They occur on sun-exposed skin of middle-aged to elderly adults.
    - Face, especially forehead and temples

  - Dorsa of forearms and hands
  - Less commonly, trunk and legs
- Occasionally, there is slight scale or rough surface.

- Lentigo is caused by sun damage and genetic predilection.
  - It results from increased activity and slightly increased number of melanocytes in the epidermis.
  - There is no malignancy potential.

TREATMENT

- General
  - The appearance of lentigines indicates ultraviolet damage to the skin. Examine sun-exposed areas for solar-induced tumors. Discuss sun protection with the patient.
  - Removal of lentigines is for cosmetic purposes only.
- Epidermal peeling
  - Inducing epidermal peeling removes the abnormal melanocytes. New epidermis, which regenerates from surrounding skin and follicles, bears normal melanocytes. Incomplete peeling results in mottled residual pigment, but the treatment can be repeated. Excessively strong attempts at peeling may injure the dermis and produce a permanent scar, so err on the side of inadequate peeling. Agents used are:
    - Light liquid nitrogen cryotherapy (5–15 seconds). Melanocytes are more sensitive to cold than are epidermal cells, so this method is preferred.
    - Light electrodesiccation, usually with a fine epilating needle on desiccating current; control is excellent, but it is easy to damage dermis with too much current.
- "Bleaching" agents
  - Hydroquinone may slowly (over months) decrease darkness of lentigines, but only slightly, and the color usually returns when its use is discontinued.
- Tretinoin may mildly to markedly lighten lentigines over a period of many months. *See* page 204 for details.

Actinic Keratoses

Note: Actinic keratoses are also called "solar keratoses." These and seborrheic keratoses (*See* page 185) have been called "senile keratoses," but that term is inaccurate and pejorative.

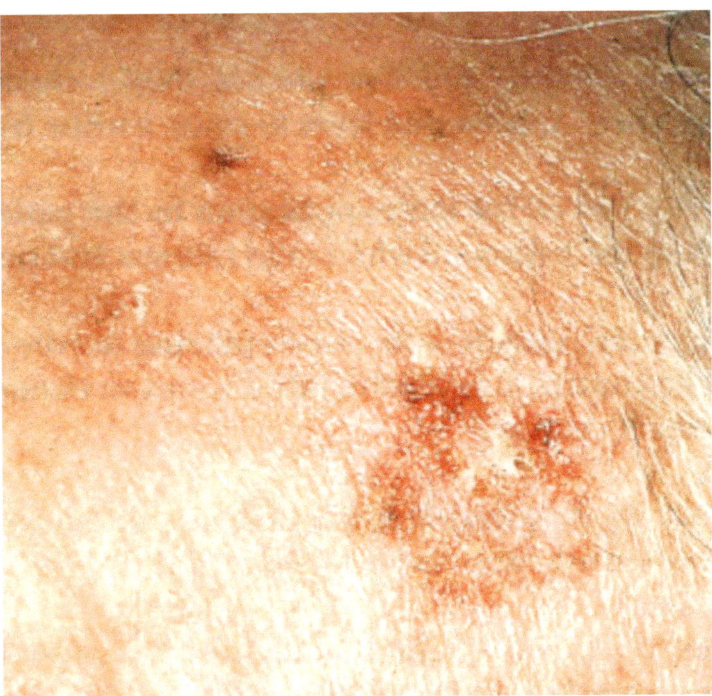

Slightly eroded, scaly actinic keratosis. Higher on the forehead, additional granular keratoses could be easily palpated.

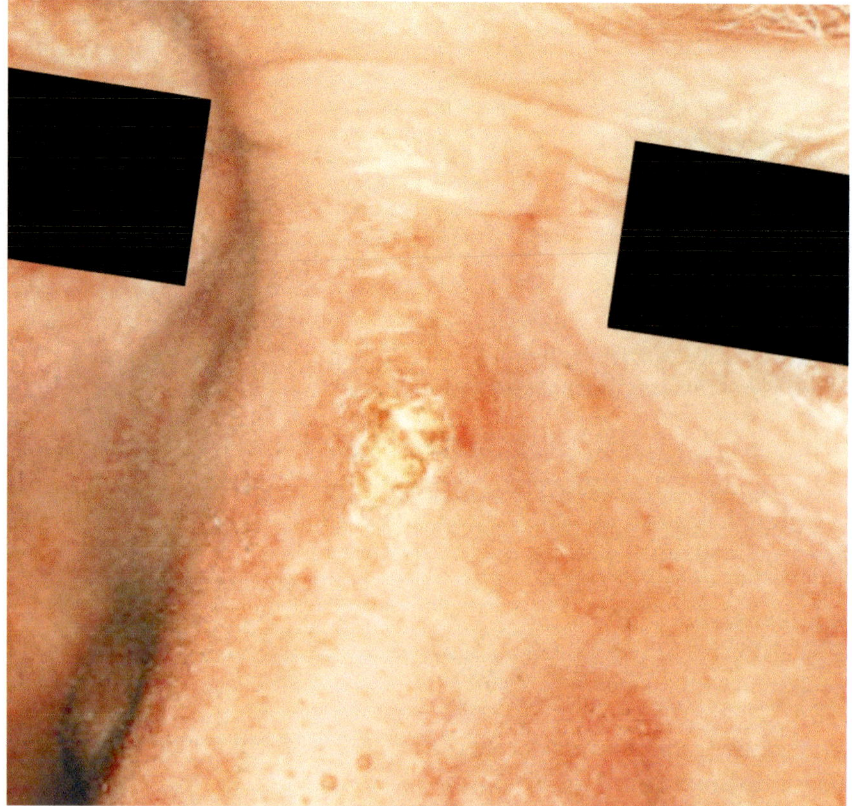

Very keratotic solar keratosis. Note also telangiectasia and dilated pores.

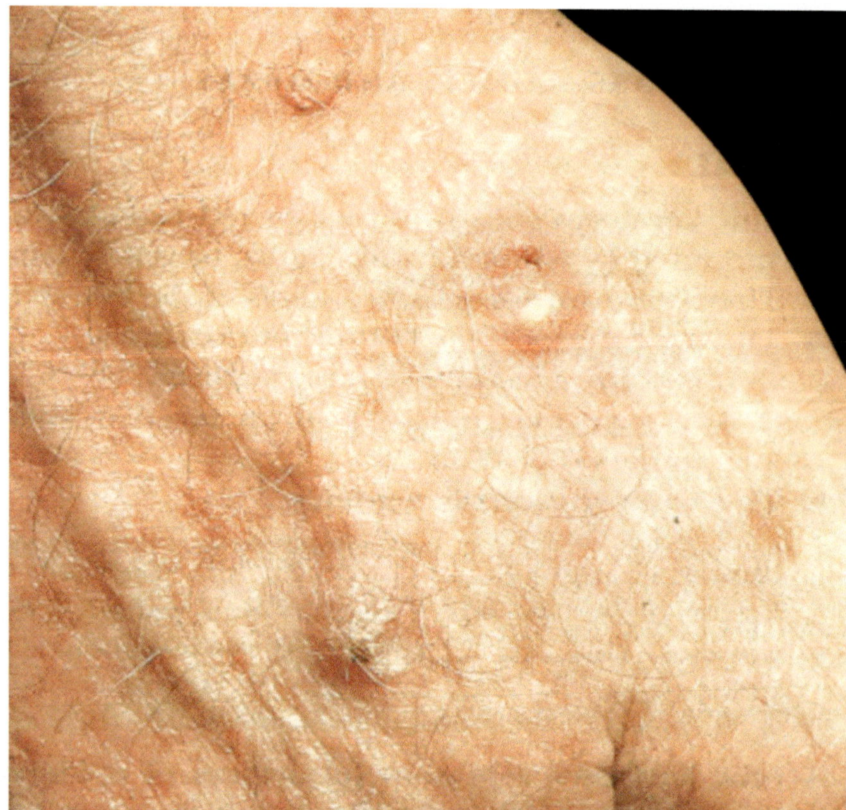

Fleshy actinic keratoses. Squamous cell carcinoma was considered, but biopsy showed that atypical cells were not invading through the basement membrane.

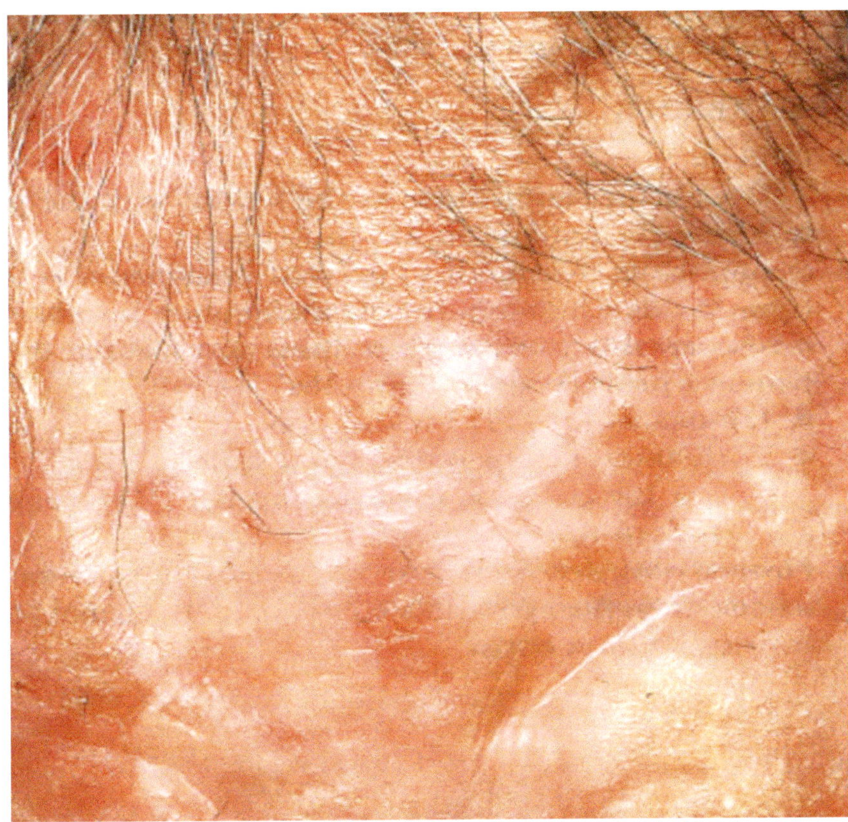

Almost confluent actinic keratoses in area of vitiligo (lower half of photograph), none in area of normal pigmentation.

CLINICAL

- Actinic keratoses consist of pink or red macules or fleshy papules surmounted by adherent white, gray, or yellow lamellar scale.
  - They occur on sun-exposed areas of the fair skinned.
  - The scale periodically falls off but re-forms.
    - It is painful to remove it prematurely.
    - The scale may not re-form on macular areas, leaving only roughened erosion.
  - They are occasionally tender.

Similar changes can occur on the lips, especially on the lower lip, as *actinic cheilitis.* This may be focal or diffuse. Scale is minimal (because of the moist environment), but the lips may fissure.

- Actinic keratoses represent focal areas of epidermal cell atypia, forming abnormal keratin. By definition, such keratoses do not extend through the epidermal basement membrane into the dermis, although fingerlike projections may protrude into the dermis. Actinic keratoses may become squamous cell carcinoma, but this is uncommon and late. Actinically induced squamous cell carcinoma (*See* page 213) metastasizes infrequently and late. Actinically-induced squamous cell carcinoma developing on the lip is more aggressive than that on the skin.
  - Examine all sun-exposed skin for the presence of other sun-induced changes (*See* page 201).

TREATMENT

- General
  - Discuss the significance of the lesions with the patient.
  - Advise the patient on sun protection.
- Symptomatic treatment to prevent malignancy is unnecessary because the development of true malignancy is unlikely and delayed; it is acceptable to treat for redness and scaling; then monitor the patient's progress every 6 months.
- Physical destruction may be the treatment of choice. Any method that destroys the epidermis is adequate. If dermal injury is avoided, scarring will not occur.
  - *Cryotherapy:* Liquid nitrogen application by cotton-tipped applicator is the preferred treatment, as it causes minimal dermal damage.

- Curettage is performed by a light, quick flick with a skin curette after local anesthesia. With experience, it is possible to avoid significant dermal injury.
    - Stop bleeding with pressure or styptic (*See* page 184).
    - Such treatment is difficult on soft areas, such as the central cheek, where the skin "skates away" from the pressure of the curette.
- Electrocautery and chemodestruction (phenol 88% or trichloroacetic acid 60%) are difficult to control and easily cause scarring.

- Topical chemotherapy destroys clinically undetectable incipient lesions as well as visible ones. The drug is applied to involved areas, as well as to areas suspected of bearing actinic keratoses.
    - 5-Fluorouracil (5-FU) (*See* page 244)
        - Traditional program is application twice daily. Inflammation usually develops in a few days; treatment is continued for 2–4 weeks until lesions are flat and nonkeratotic. There usually is marked redness, soreness, and even oozing in many of the keratoses.
        - "Pulse therapy" method is application once or twice weekly for 2–3 months. Inflammation is usually much milder than with the traditional program. Duration of benefit after treatment is known to be a few years with the traditional program but is not as well known for the pulse method. Treatment can be repeated months to years later if relapses or new lesions occur.
        - Absorption and response occur more reliably and promptly on the face than on the arms. Usual treatment course for traditional twice-daily treatment is 3 weeks on the face. Avoid the eyes, nasolabial folds, and mouth; material collects in the folds and is irritating.
        - Response is slow and possibly incomplete on the arms. Occlusion or the addition of tretinoin cream or gel may be necessary to obtain penetration and effect. Treatment twice daily may take 6–8 weeks to achieve benefit. Treat the thickest lesions by individual destruction.
    - To minimize irritation from 5-FU, a potent topical corticosteroid may be used. There is disagreement as to whether suppressing the inflammation diminishes effectiveness.
    - A course of treatment may need to be repeated every few years.
    - Imiquimod 5% cream is applied twice weekly for 16 weeks. Preparations containing 2.5% and 3.75% imiquimod are also available and are applied once daily for 2 weeks, followed by a 2-week pause and then a second cycle of 2 weeks.
    - Tirbanibulin cream is applied once daily for 5 consecutive nights, and then washed off after 8 hours.

Keratoacanthoma

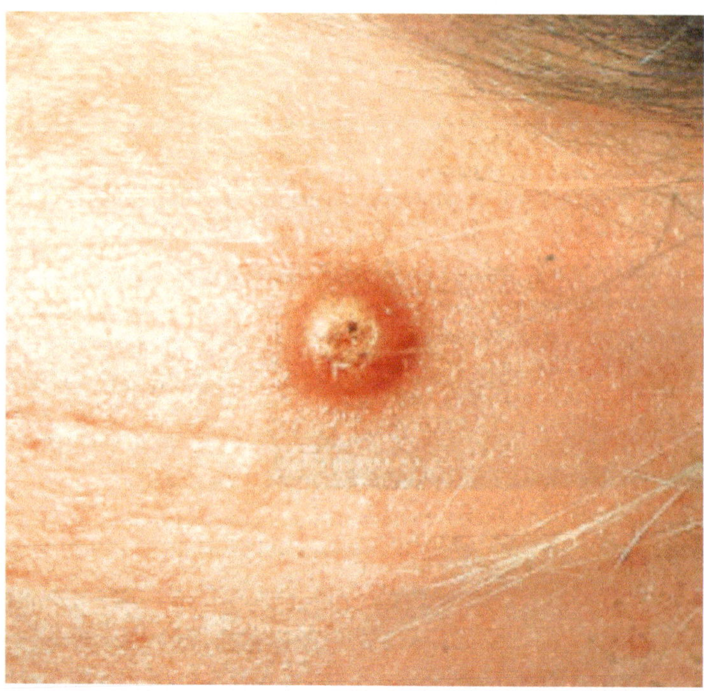

Early keratoacanthoma: a fleshy nodule just beginning to develop a keratotic core.

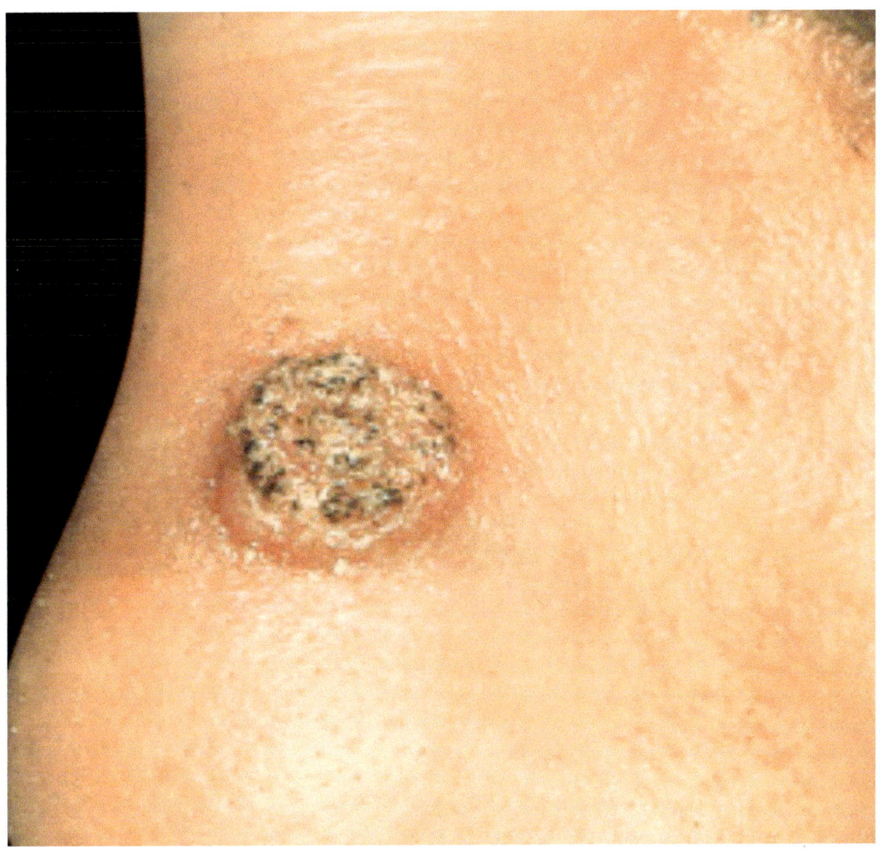

Keratotic core more developed in a later lesion (present 3–4 weeks).

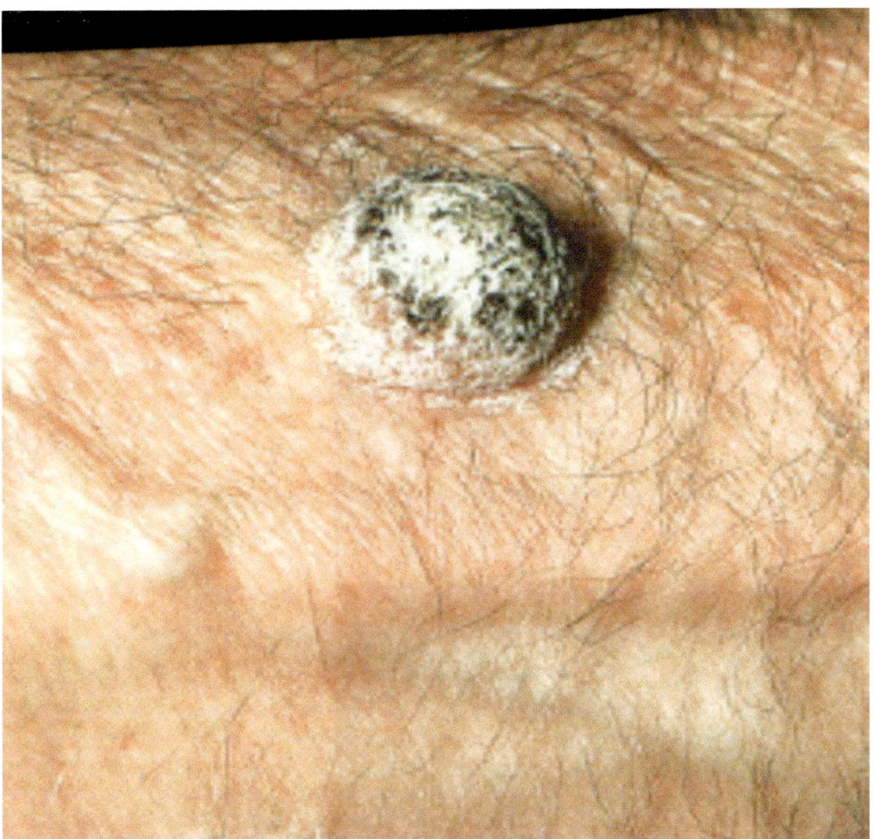

Keratotic cap in keratoacanthoma (present 4–6 weeks).

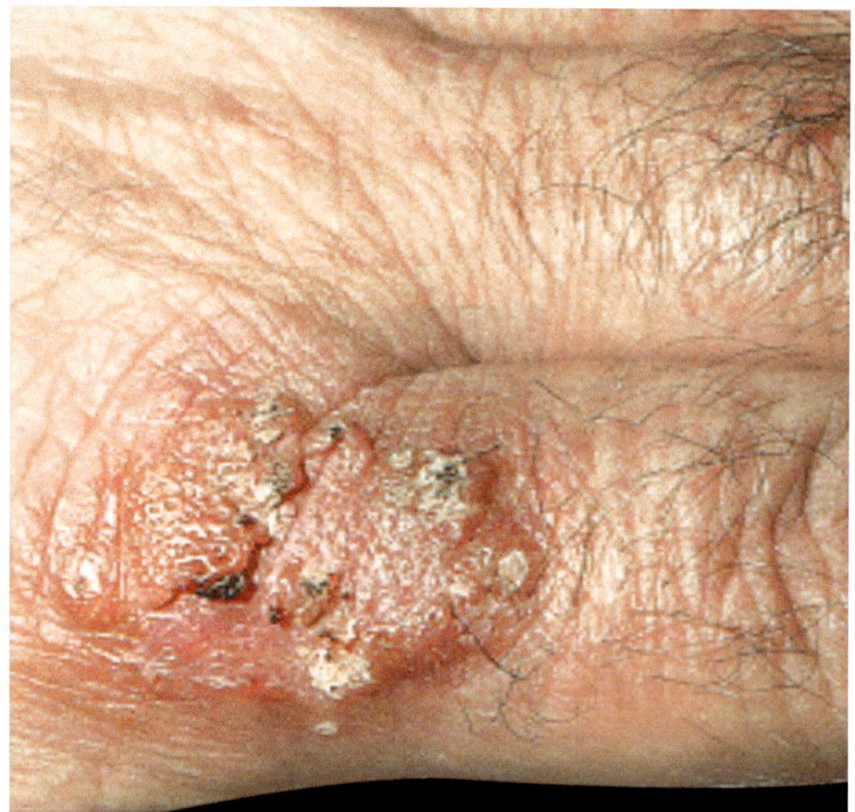

Keratoacanthoma almost completely involuted after 3 months.

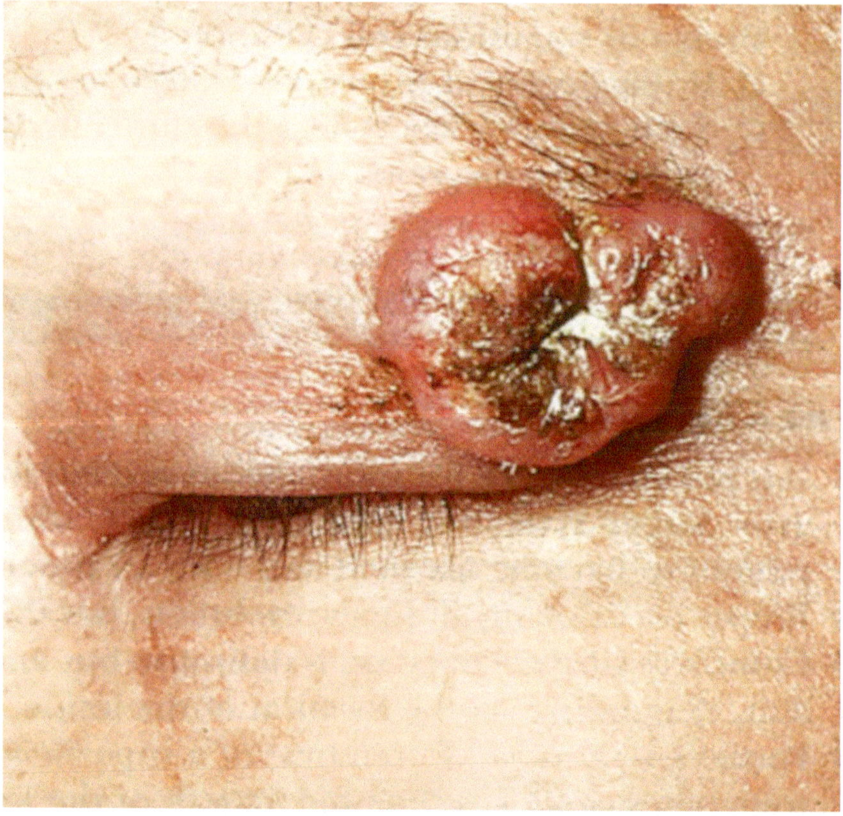

Keratoacanthoma recurrent only 1 month after presumably complete excision.

CLINICAL

- Keratoacanthoma consists of a fast-growing nodule on the sun-exposed skin of fair-skinned adults.
  - Starts as a slightly keratotic fleshy papule, rapidly develops a keratotic core and a fleshy rim; the core may then fall out, leaving a fleshy, umbilicated nodule. The condition usually resolves spontaneously in about 3–6 months, leaving an atrophic scar.
  - Usually reaches maximum size (about 1 cm) in 3–4 weeks. Occasionally grows to 3–4 cm and, rarely, to 10 cm or more.
  - Most common in sun-damaged skin
  - Occasionally multiple occurrences, sometimes with dozens of lesions
- Histopathologic examination of keratoacanthoma shows dysplastic growth of epidermal prickle cells.
  - Biopsy of a piece of the lesion is indistinguishable from squamous cell carcinoma.
  - It is necessary to have a section of the entire lesion or a biopsy specimen from border to border, showing the entire architecture, to confirm the pathologic diagnosis.
  - There have been some reports of conversion of keratoacanthoma to squamous cell carcinoma.
    - If this occurs, it is rare.
    - Such reports may reflect the difficulty in making the initial pathologic diagnosis.

Diagnosis of keratoacanthoma is clinical or a combination of history, clinical appearance, and pathologic findings.

TREATMENT

- It is possible to wait for spontaneous resolution, but the lesion may grow larger (resulting in a larger scar), which often causes the patient to become alarmed and want treatment.
- Biopsy occasionally induces resolution, but this is unpredictable.
- Complete surgical excision is definitive but may leave an unsightly scar, depending on the location of the lesion.
- Partial excision, shave removal of a superficial portion, or biopsy sometimes provokes renewed growth of the lesion to a larger size (3 to 4 cm).
  - This is especially true of lesions on the nose or central face.
  - Partial removal of these recurrent lesions usually provokes more growth.
- Intralesional injection therapy
  - This usually causes lesions to resolve in a few weeks. Treatment is usually initiated only after clinical diagnosis, making follow-up essential.
  - Infiltrate the fleshy portion of the lesion with 0.1–0.5 mL of solution at weekly intervals.
    - 5-FU 50 mg/mL (from vial for intravenous use)
  - The lesions should be smaller in 1 week and will regress completely in 3–4 weeks.

If there is no change, excise the lesion to rule out squamous cell carcinoma.

Basal Cell Carcinoma and Squamous Cell Carcinoma

Basal cell carcinoma (BCC) and squamous cell carcinoma (SCC) are discussed together here because of similarities in their biologic behavior and treatment.

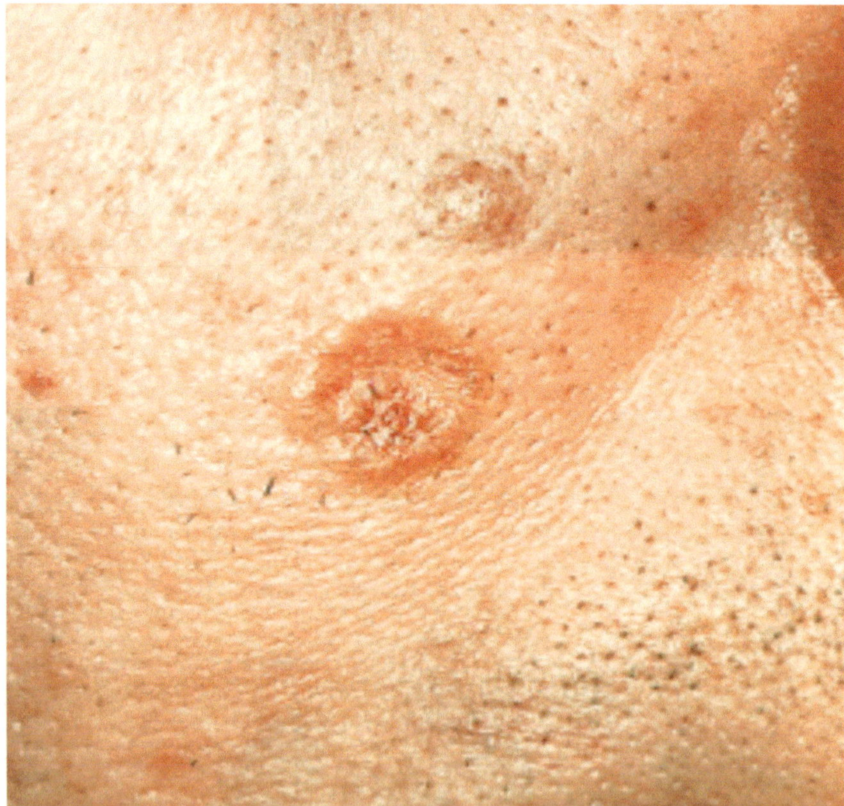

Classic basal cell carcinoma: pearly (translucent), flesh-colored papule with depressed center, rolled edge, and telangiectasia. Lesion above it is nonpigmented mole.

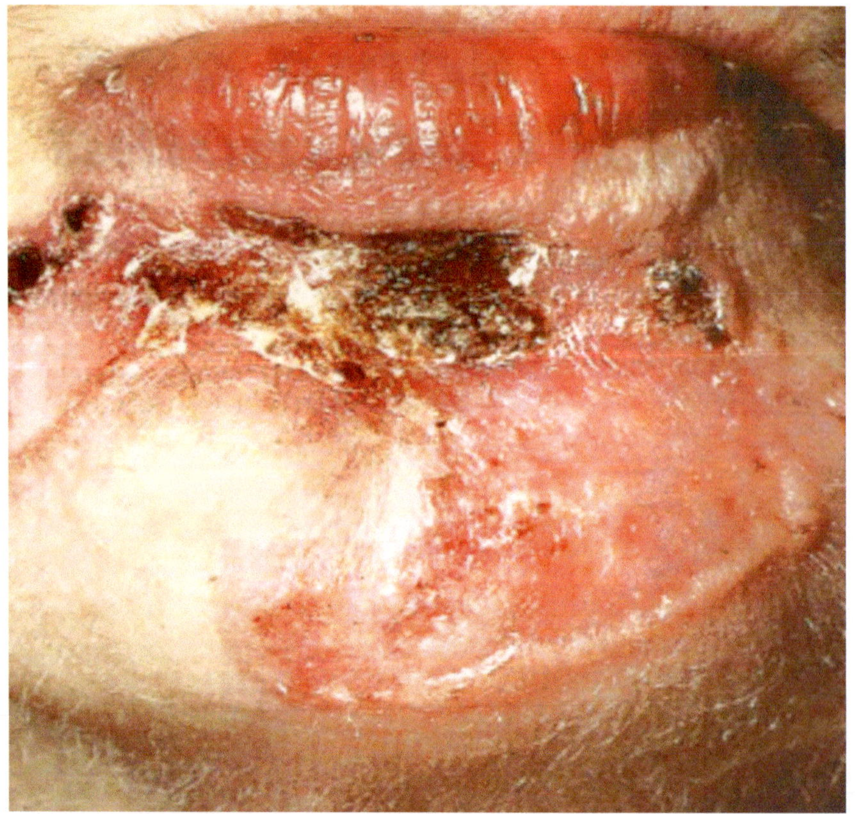

Neglected basal cell carcinoma has enlarged superficially for years. Note rolled border and scarred appearance.

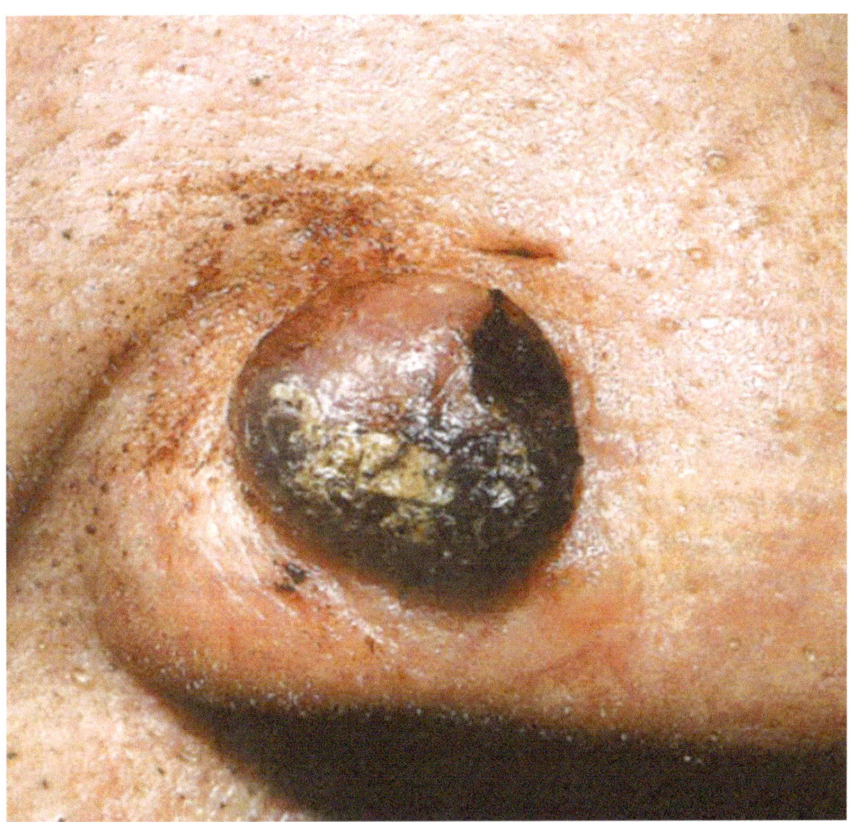

Cystic or nodular basal cell carcinoma.

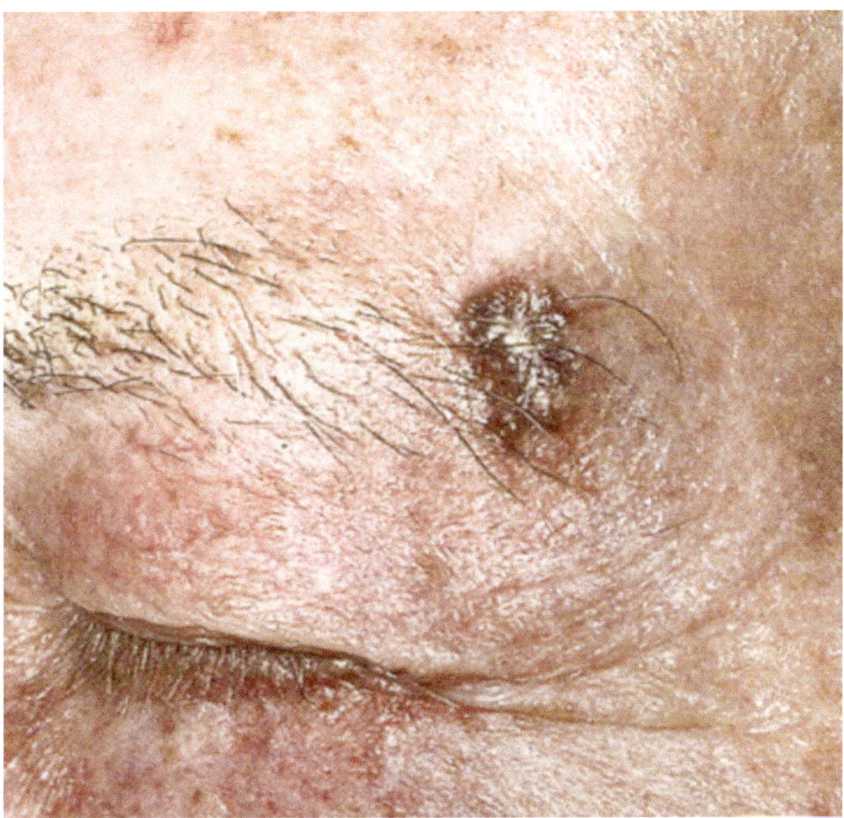

Pigmented basal cell carcinoma still displays pearly quality and depressed center. Note sundamaged skin.

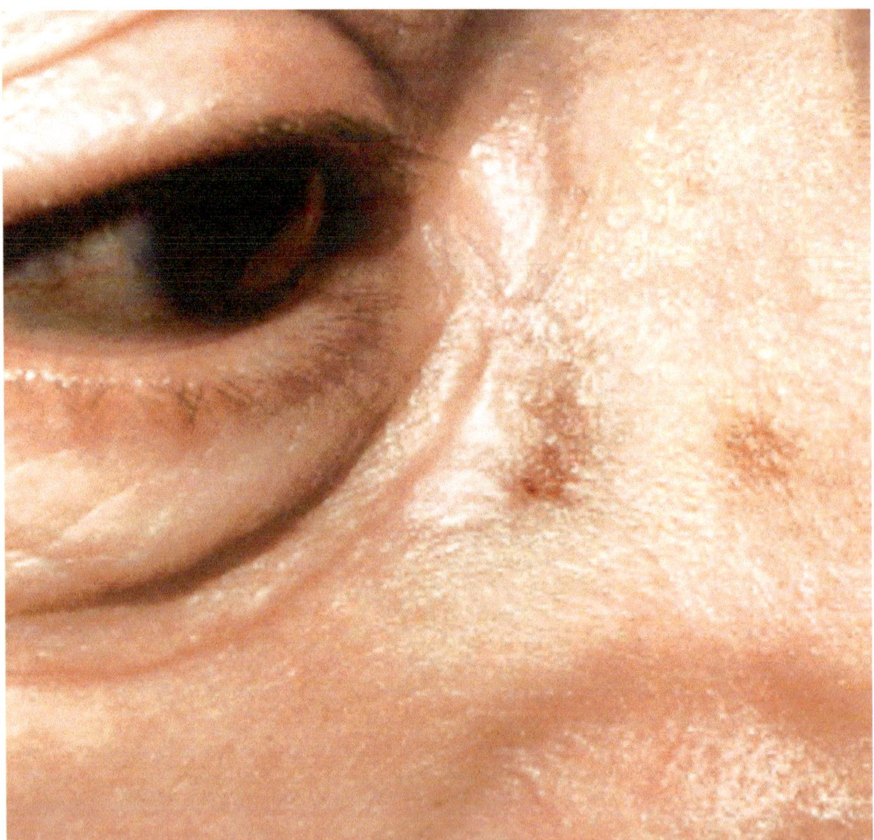

Subtle sclerosing or scarring basal cell carcinoma below indentation from glasses nosepad. Very firm on palpation.

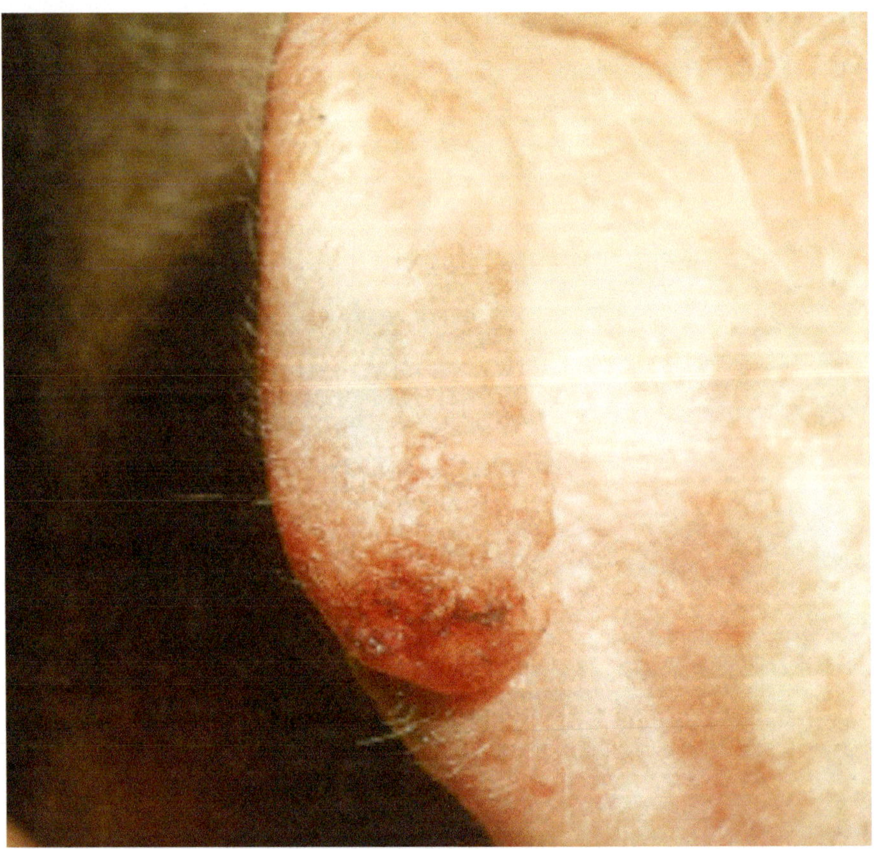

Early squamous cell carcinoma. Surface is fragile and bleeds easily.

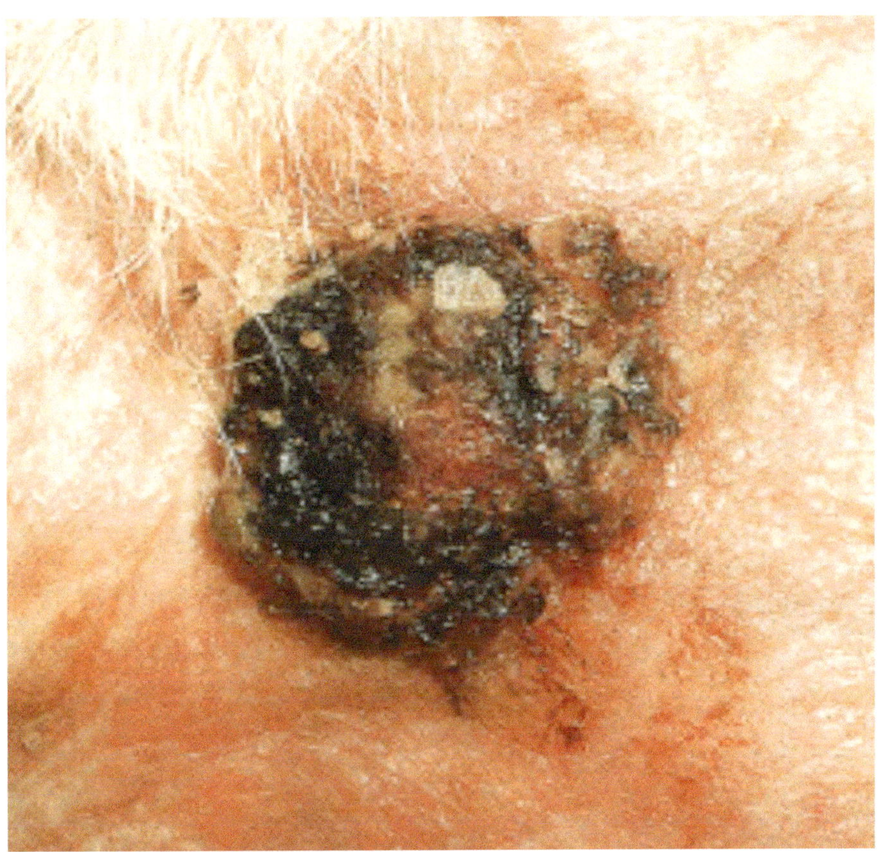

Neglected squamous cell carcinoma.

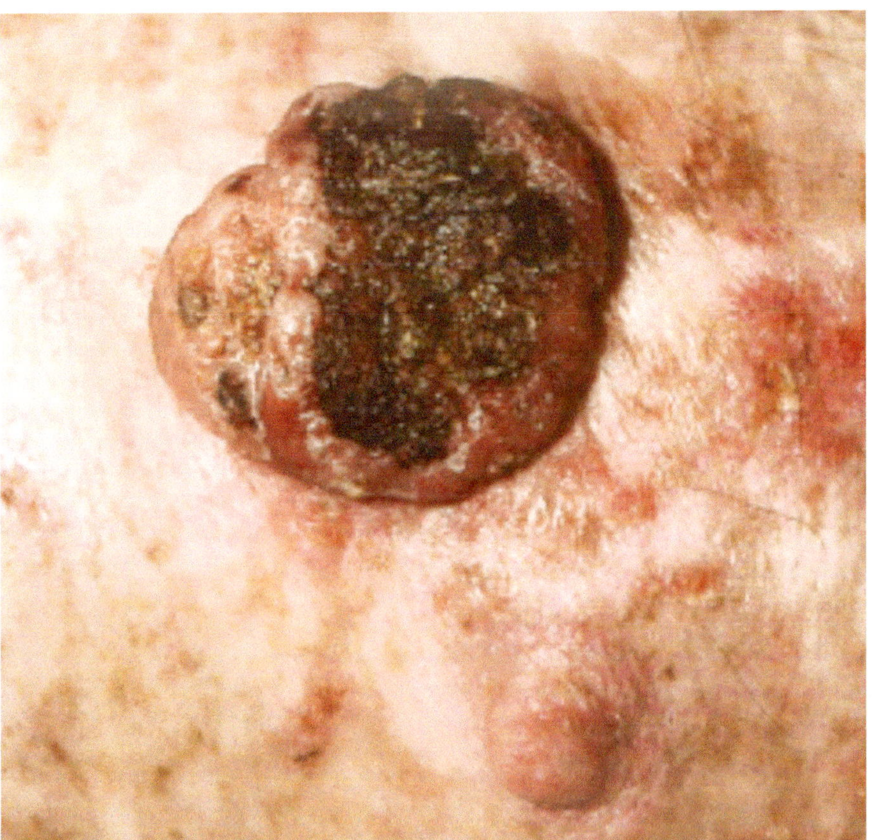

Huge squamous cell carcinoma (note nipple for size comparison) and severely sun-damaged skin. Eighty-year-old man had been a lifeguard for 40 years.

CLINICAL

- Both tumors
  - Are seen mainly on the sun-exposed skin of fair-complexioned people
    - Basal cell carcinoma is occasionally seen in dark-skinned people and on sunsheltered skin.
    - Squamous cell carcinoma and, to a lesser extent, BCC are occasionally seen at sites of chronic inflammation, such as osteomyelitis sinuses, old radiation burns, discoid lupus erythematosus, and hidradenitis suppurativa. In these locations SCC is more aggressive (20% metastasis) than when actinically induced.
  - Have a low rate of deep tissue invasion or metastasis (except at sites of chronic inflammation)
    - They are usually seen in growths neglected for years.
    - In BCC, metastasis rarely occurs to local nodes; in SCC, metastasis may be generalized.
    - The major clinical complication is local extension into complex structures such as the orbit, sinuses, or calvarium.

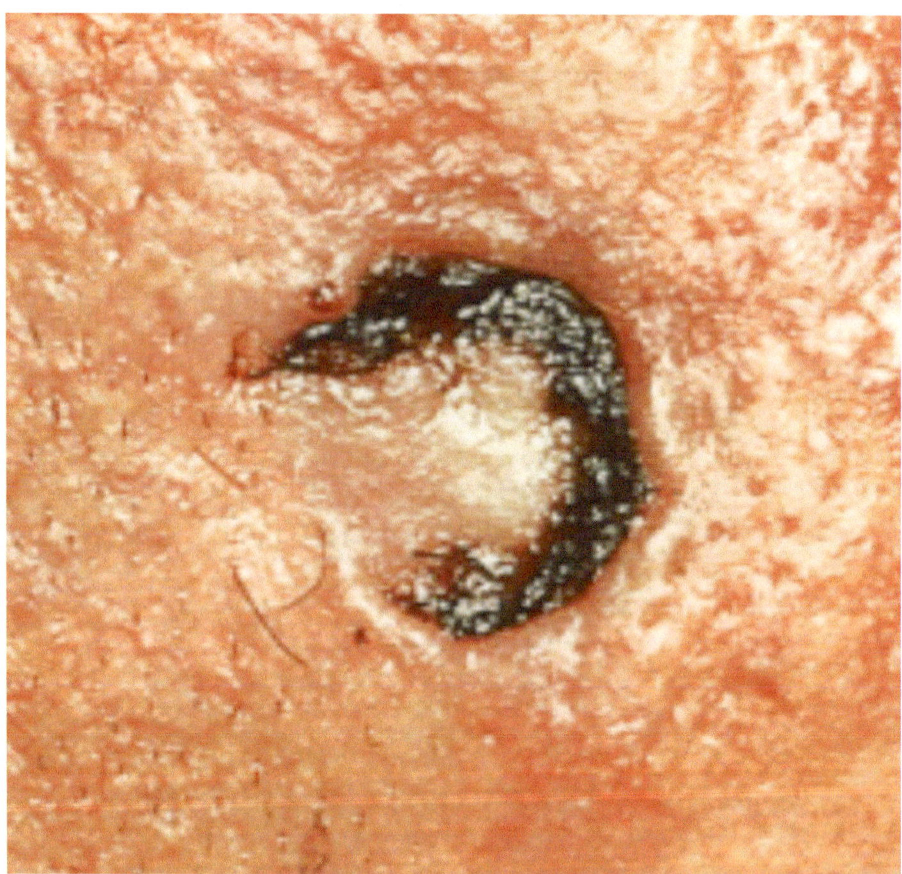

Infiltrating squamous cell carcinoma.

- Typically, *BCC* consists of a translucent (pearly) fleshy papule or nodule with an umbilicated or depressed center and a rolled border, often containing ectatic capillaries.
  - It is not keratin-producing, so the lesions are not scaly or hyperkeratotic, but occasionally there is mild oozing and crusting.
  - Clinical variants
    - Nodular or cystic: Tense and shiny
    - Superficial: Shiny, thin patch or plaque
    - Pigmented: Ranges from a few specks to completely black pigmentation. Translucent quality differentiates it from melanoma (*See* page 245).

- "Rodent ulcer": The central umbilication burrows in to form a pit. This often oozes. It is usually near the nose.
- Sclerosing, scarring, or morpheaform: Firm, fibrous reaction with subtle, tiny pearly papules at the border. This often extends more deeply and is more lateral than it appears on the surface.

- *SCC* consists of an opaque, pink, or skin-colored fleshy papule, nodule, or plaque that is usually scaly, keratotic, or eroded.
  - Hyperkeratosis may be verrucous, crumbly, or in the form of a cutaneous horn.
  - The tissue is fragile, so oozing and bleeding are common.

TREATMENT

- General
  - Examine all sun-exposed skin for evidence of solar damage (*See* page 201) and other tumors.
  - Discuss sun damage and sun protection with the patient (Patient Guides, *See* page 253).
  - If the lesion is small, it can be promptly treated by one of the methods to be discussed. If it is large or in a difficult site (eyelid, ear, or burrowing deep into the nose), perform a biopsy or refer the patient to a dermatologist or an appropriate surgeon.
- Destructive treatments all have a cure rate of >95% in uncomplicated cases. Each method has advantages and drawbacks. Site, tumor type, patient age, and cosmetic needs all help to determine the method that is right for the patient.
  - Surgical excision is generally the preferable treatment if the lesion is small, simple, and easily closable. Usually the procedure is quick and postoperative inconvenience is slight, cosmetic outcome is good, and, most importantly, the margins of the surgical specimen can be checked for adequacy of excision.
  - Curettage and electrodesiccation are excellent treatments for simple, superficial lesions, and even for those with a large diameter. An unsightly scab is present for weeks. Residual scarring is usually marked but may be slight on certain areas of the face. The adequacy of treatment is detected by the "feel" of the curettage in the hands of an experienced therapist. The surgical specimen is fragmented and useless for determining margins. Curettage and desiccation should be performed only by adequately trained individuals.
  - Cryotherapy consists of profound tissue freezing with liquid nitrogen spray or metal applicators. A generous margin is selected clinically to ensure adequate treatment. Post-therapy pain, swelling, tissue necrosis, and oozing may last for days to weeks. There is surprisingly little scarring. Cryotherapy spares cartilage, so it is useful for complex tumors on the nose and ear. It should be performed only by an experienced cryotherapist.
  - Chemotherapy, now FDA-approved, is usually supervised by specialists.
  - Radiation therapy is appropriate for complex tumors but is particularly harmful to cartilage. It requires 10–20 office visits and is followed by weeks of inflammation. The scar has a good early appearance but looks worse with the passage of years and may undergo malignant degeneration, generally restricting the use of this modality to patients over the age of 60 years.
- Treatment of recurrent and complex tumors
  - **Complex tumors** are treated by wide excision and complex closure, cryotherapy, or radiation therapy. All such cases should be referred to the appropriate therapist.
  - **Recurrent tumors** have a cure rate of only 50% when treated by curettage, cryotherapy, chemotherapy, or radiation therapy. Surgical excision with examination of specimen for margins is the best treatment. For difficult primary or recurrent tumors, the preferable treatment is often Mohs' chemosurgery, or microscopically controlled serial excisions. The tumor is mapped and excised and the margins are immediately checked on frozen sections. Areas abutting positive margins are immediately excised and checked, and this continues until all specimens are clear. The cure rate for primary and recurrent tumors is over 95%. It is advisable to send patients with complex recurrent tumors to the nearest center for obtaining this treatment.
- Follow-up examinations should be performed at 3, 6, and 12 months and yearly or semi-yearly thereafter. Look for tumor regrowth and feel for deep tissue recurrences. The scar is often thick and bulging at 6–12 weeks, so examine the patient a month or two later if growth is suspected.
  - On each visit examine all sun-exposed skin for new tumors.

Melanoma

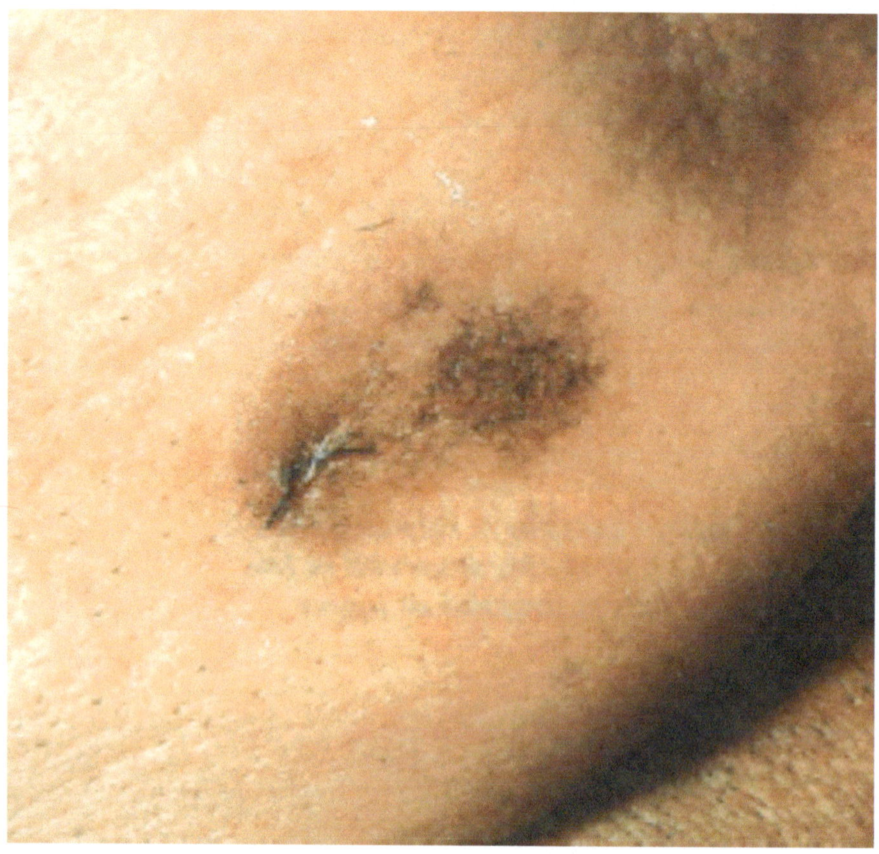

Typical lentigo maligna differs from a regular lentigo by having a feathered, poorly demarcated border and several shades of pigment.

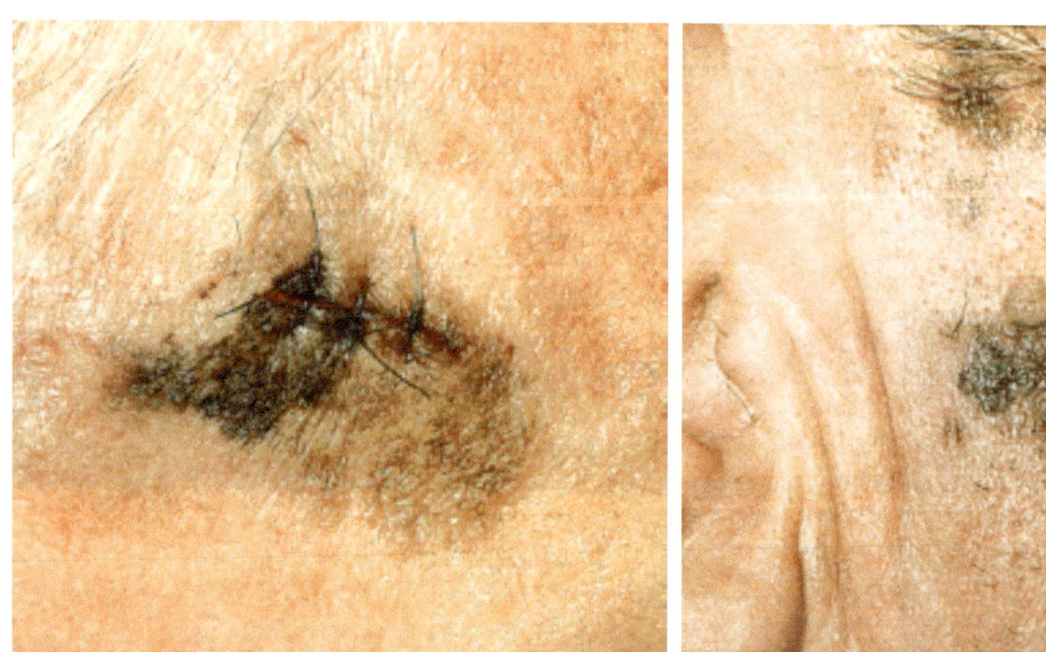

Dark lentigo maligna on cheek and in sideburn. Apparently clear area between the two sites was probably involved in the past but resolved. Seborrheic keratosis is present at upper edge of lower lesion.

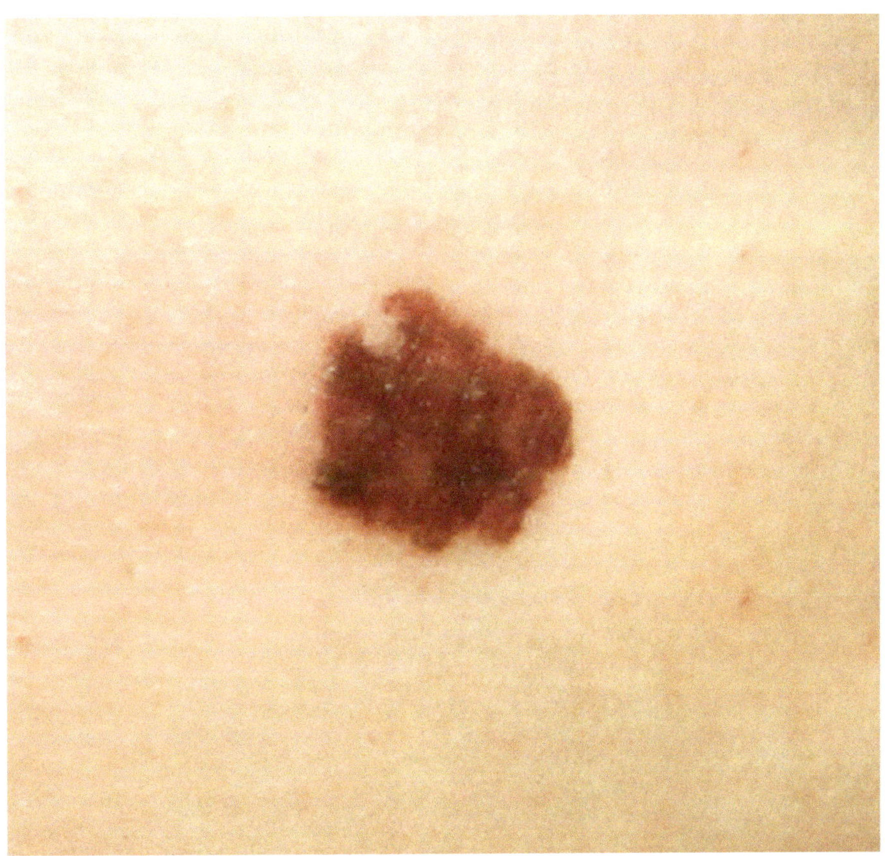

Superficial spreading melanoma: pseudopod-like irregular border and variegated pigment.

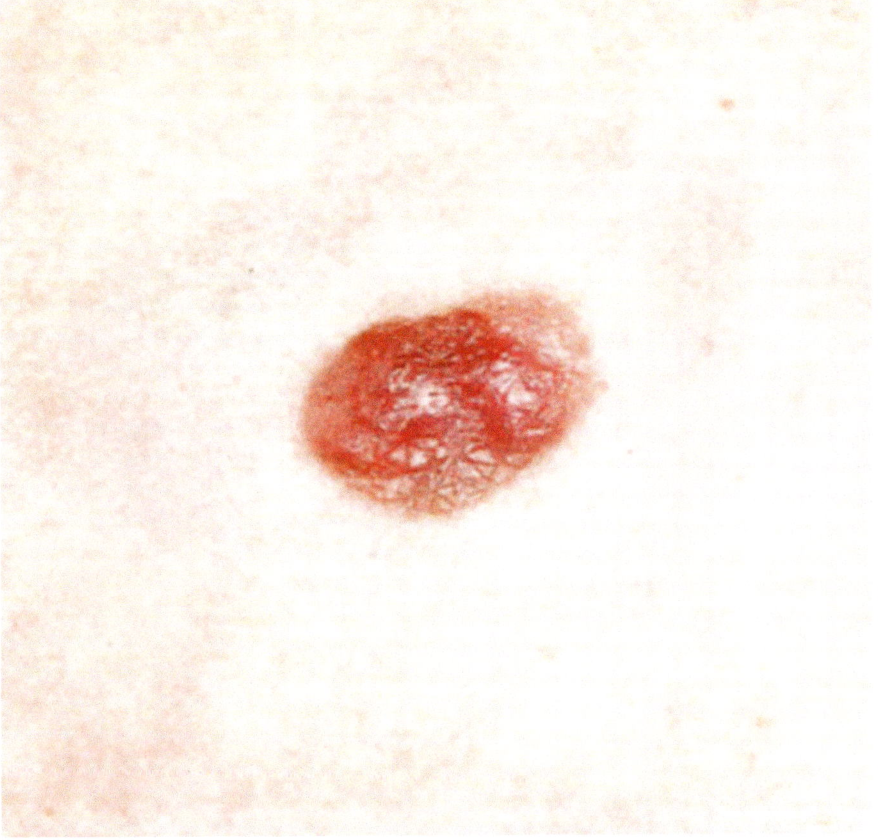

Nonpigmented superficial spreading melanoma, said to be present for 2 years.

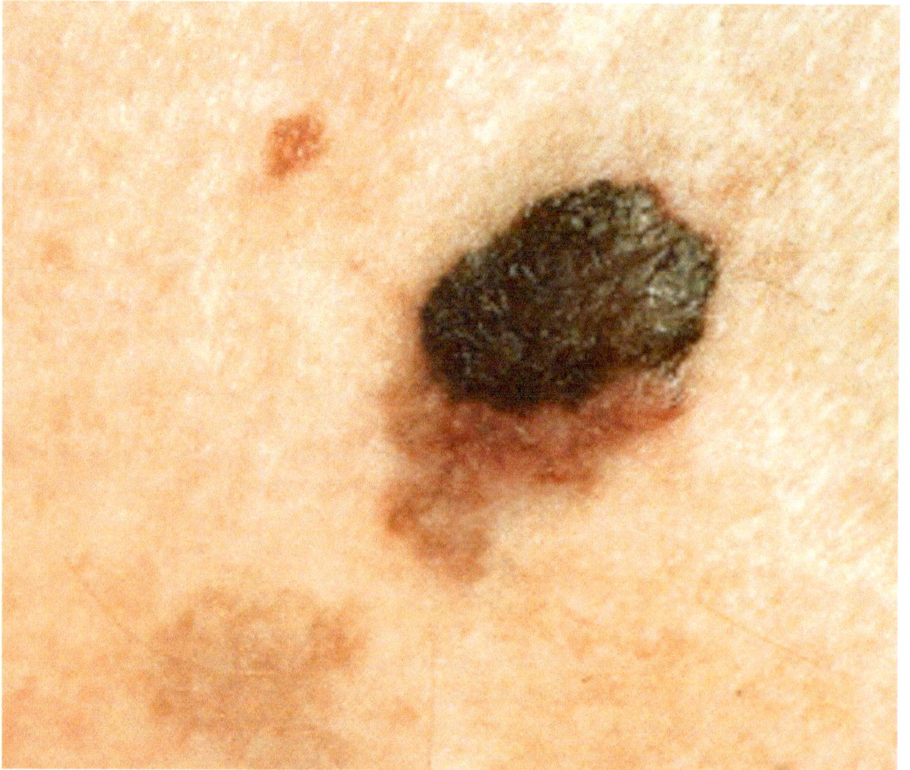

Superficial spreading melanoma still confined to upper dermis.

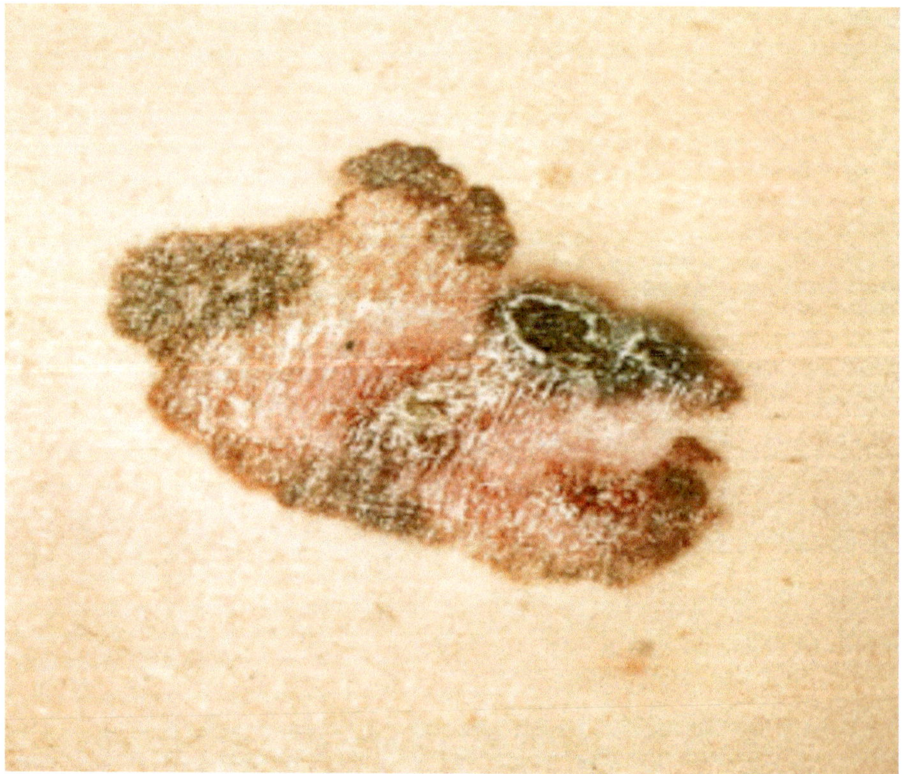

This superficial spreading melanoma measured 7 x 9 cm and had been present for several years. Healed areas in center were devoid of malignant cells.

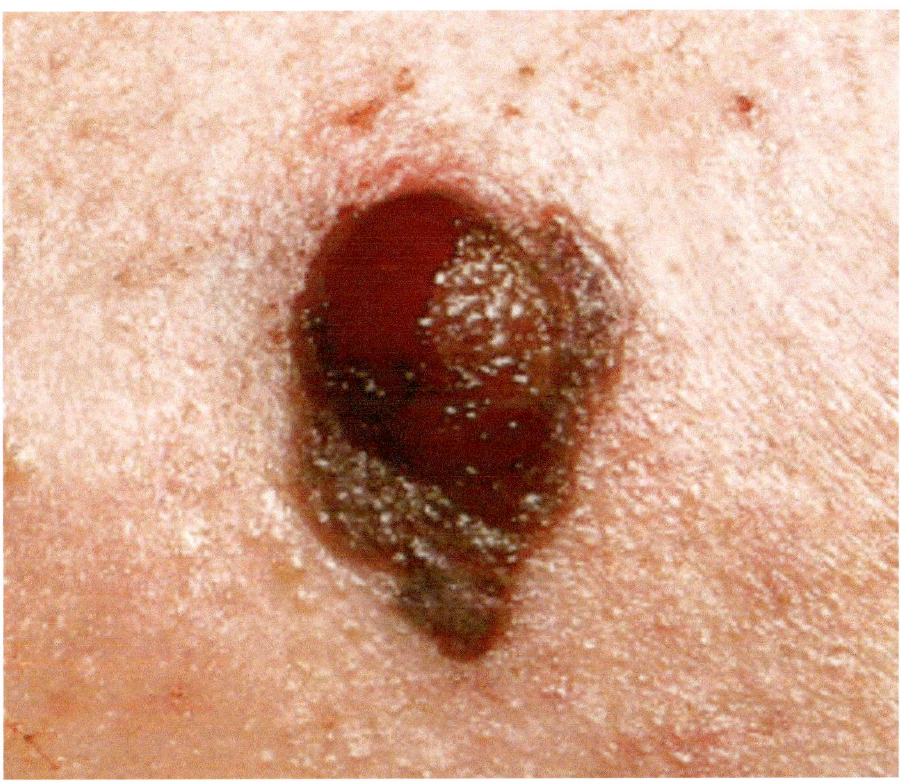

Nodular melanoma apparently arising from superficial spreading type. Fragility and bleeding are common.

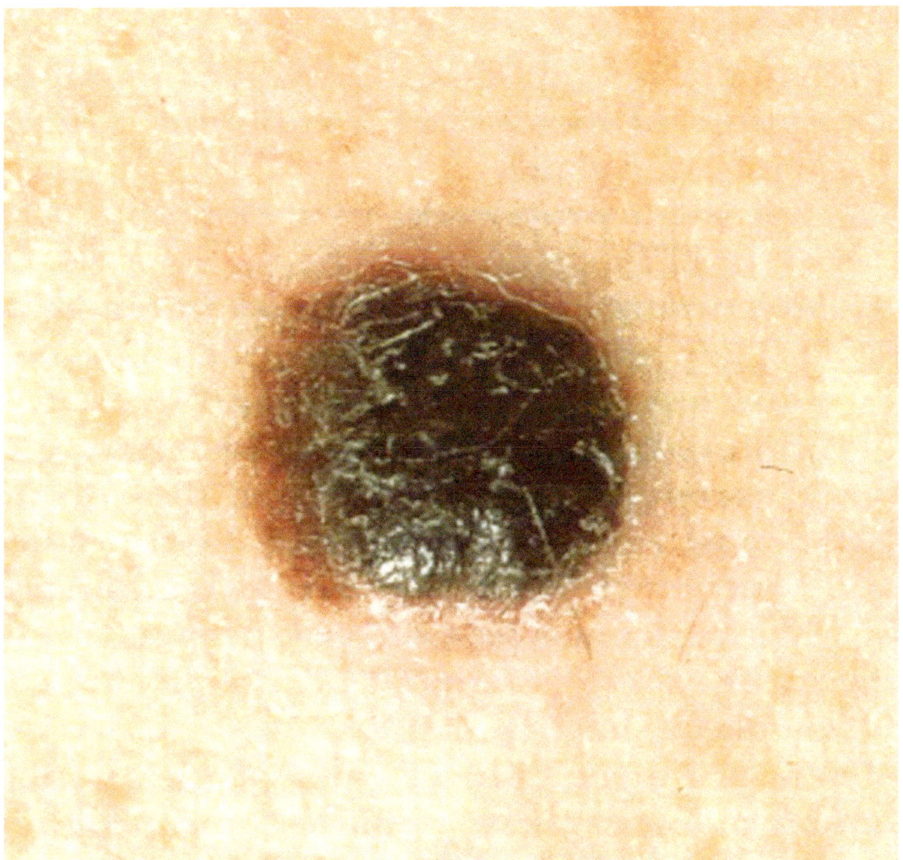

Nodular melanoma. Microscopic examination revealed that it arose in a mole.

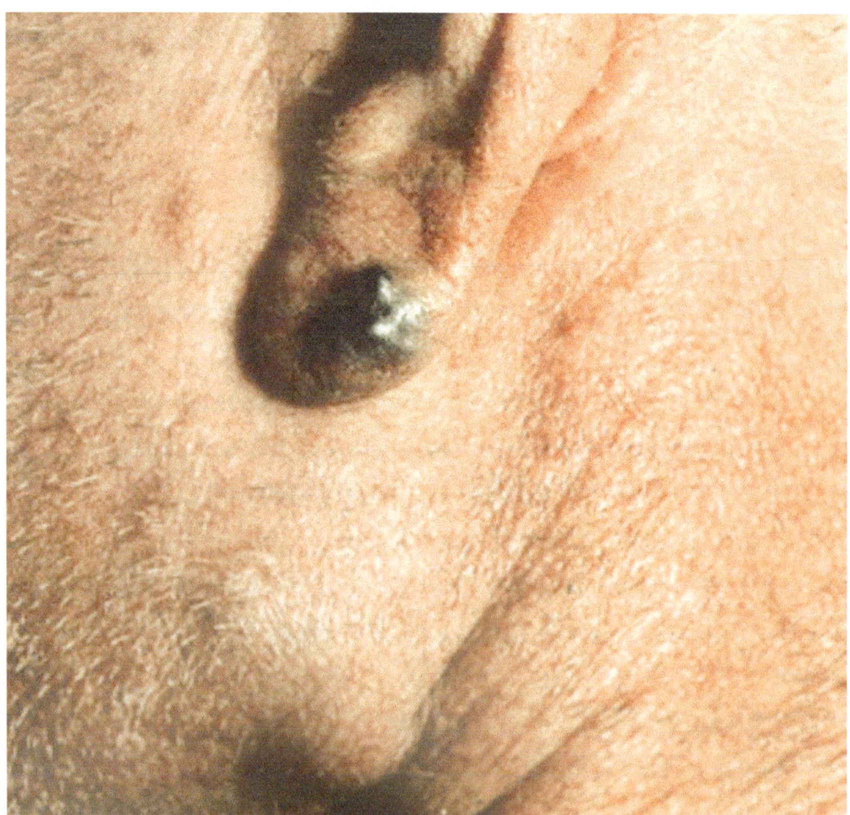

Nodular melanoma and involved cervical lymph node.

CLINICAL

- Melanoma is a malignant growth of pigment cells.
    - A large proportion of melanomas (70%) arise from normally pigmented skin.
        - A small proportion of melanomas (30%) arise from moles (*See* page 178).
    - Melanomas are most common in fair-skinned people.
        - They are rare in dark-skinned people, in whom they occur on less-pigmented palms and soles.
        - More frequent in geographic areas of high sun intensity but, except for lentigo maligna, they do not occur on skin sites most exposed to the sun. Some data suggest an increased incidence on areas burned by the sun in childhood and in adolescence (upper back in men and lower leg in women).
    - Rarely, there is familial occurrence, except in cases of familial dysplastic nevi (*See* page 181).
- There are three clinical types of melanoma, which differ considerably in appearance, behavior, and prognosis.
    - Lentigo maligna (about 10% of melanomas)
        - A slow-growing dark macule on the face of an elderly white person
        - Has an irregular border; indistinct edges; various shades of brown, tan, and black hyperpigmentation
        - May be present for many years as a macule (malignant cells confined to the epidermis) but may eventually develop an invasive nodule (lentigo maligna melanoma); may metastasize in the nodular stage but is less aggressive than the following types
        - Management by a specialist is recommended
    - Superficial spreading melanoma (about 70% of melanomas)
        - This grows as a slightly elevated plaque anywhere on the body.
        - It has an irregular border with areas of blurring of pigment into surrounding skin in various shades of black, brown, and white. It may have a rim of pink inflammation. The surface is slightly fragile and may bleed or ooze.
        - It grows as a small plaque (cells in epidermis and upper dermis) for 6–24 months and then develops a nodule, which is highly invasive.
        - There is a >90% cure rate with complete excision in the plaque stage, but prognosis is poor after the nodule develops.

- Nodular melanoma (about 20% of melanomas)
  - This arises suddenly as a papule or nodule on the skin or in a mole.
  - It is a blue-black or brown nodule that bleeds easily, often with a rim of inflammation. It is occasionally flesh-colored.
  - It takes only weeks or months for metastasis to occur (cells spread rapidly into dermis and blood vessels). Occasionally, nodular melanoma will involute after metastasis (10% of patients with metastatic melanoma have no remaining primary lesion).
  - Prognosis is poor without early and complete excision.

TREATMENT

- General
  - Learn to recognize benign lesions that can look like a melanoma.
    - Solar lentigines (*See* page 206)
    - Moles (*See* page 178)
    - Seborrheic keratoses (*See* page 185)
    - Dermatofibromas (*See* page 188)
    - Pyogenic granulomas (*See* page 192)
    - Pigmented basal cell epitheliomas (*See* page 213)
  - Perform biopsy on (*See* page 231) or excise "suspicious lesions."
    - Suspicious lesions have the characteristics described earlier, have appeared suddenly, or look peculiar to the patient or physician. A readiness to perform biopsy relieves the concern of patient and physician. Performing partial biopsy of a melanoma and re-excising the remainder later does not increase the incidence of metastasis.
  - The prognosis and treatment depend on the results of pathologic examination. In general, thin lesions (<0.75 mm) have a good prognosis when excised with a small margin. Thick lesions (>1.25 mm) have a worse prognosis. They are excised with a larger margin and may require lymph node dissection.
  - Except for thin lesions, check for metastasis.
  - Refer the patient to a center experienced in melanoma treatment.
- Surgical excision is recommended for all melanomas.
  - Lentigo maligna is excised with a narrow margin. If a nodule is present, a 1-cm margin is advised.
    - Large lesions in elderly patients may preclude surgery. Examine the patient every 6 months and perform biopsy if a papule develops.
  - Superficial spreading melanoma is excised with a 1-cm margin. If a nodule is present, a larger excision may be necessary, as well as regional node dissection.
  - Chemotherapy, now FDA-approved, is usually supervised by specialists.
  - Nodular melanoma is excised with at least a 2-cm margin. Regional node dissection is usually advised if the area drains to one group.
- Metastatic melanomas are usually poorly responsive to radiation therapy and chemotherapy. Prognosis is poor. Refer patients to an oncology center.
- Follow-up examinations after excision.
  - Sites of lentigo maligna or very thin superficial spreading melanoma should be checked at 6 and 12 months after excision and then yearly.
  - Thicker nodular lesions are followed up at 6-month intervals with physical examination for metastases.
- *See* Patient Guides on Moles and Melanoma, page 255.

7 CHAPTER Diagnostic Procedures

The Potassium Hydroxide (KOH) Examination and Culture for Fungi

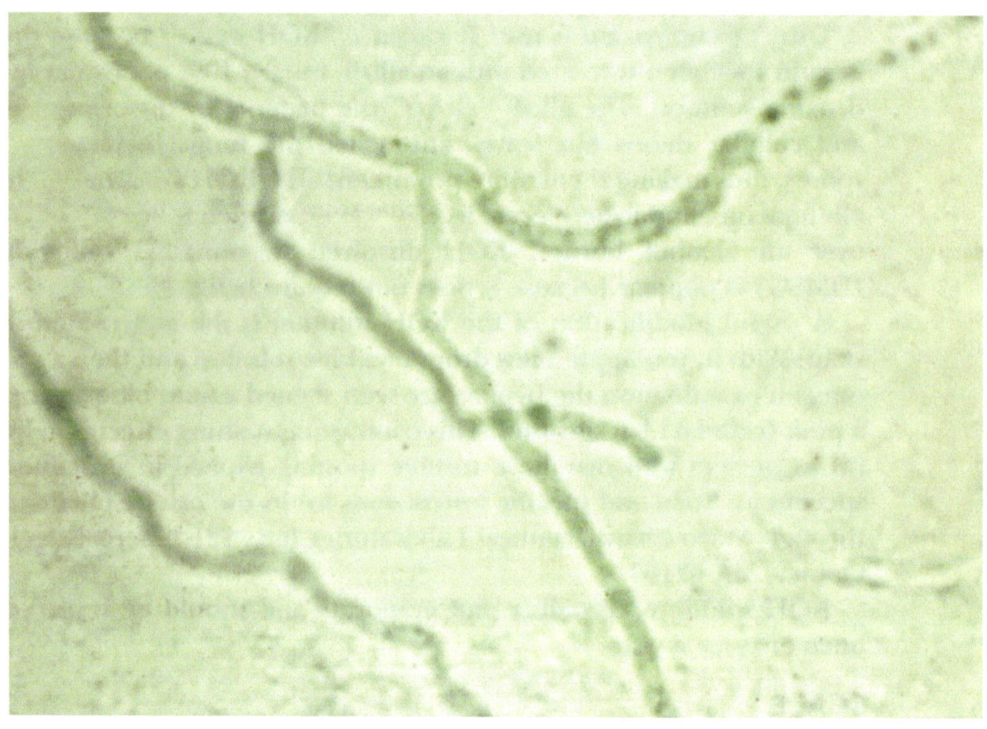

Branching hyphae of dermatophyte on skin scraping.

Fungi live on or in the keratin of the skin, hair, and nails. On the skin and nails they exist mainly as hyphae, but on hair they produce hyphae and spores. Direct examination of scale, nail, or hair may reveal the presence of fungi, thus immediately confirming a clinical diagnosis. Culture of the material may also confirm their presence, but cultures take 2–4 weeks to grow and require training and expertise to interpret.

The *absence* of fungi on examination and culture does *not* rule out the diagnosis of a tinea infection. Even in experienced hands, results of direct examination and cultures may often be negative in a single assessment of nail infections (*See* page 86) and some cases of vesicular tinea pedis (*See* page 82). Tinea cruris (*See* page 68) and tinea corporis (*See* page 156), however, usually yield positive results. The correct method of performing each examination so that it is most likely to produce positive results is discussed here.

Direct examination is usually called a "KOH exam" because the keratin specimen is treated with an alkali, usually 10% potassium hydroxide solution. The alkali "clears" the material by dissolving oils and cellular debris but leaves untouched the fungal hyphae and spores, thus making them more prominent. The KOH solution is usually aqueous, and to accelerate its effect the specimen is heated gently over an alcohol burner. KOH dissolved in dimethyl sulfoxide (DMSO) is popular because it does not require heating.

Potassium hydroxide solutions crystallize and evaporate and should be replaced once or twice a year.

SCALE

- Arrange patient so that the lesion skin is vertical.
- Place a microscope slide against the skin below the lesion.
    - Gently scrape (do not cut) scale from flaky areas of the lesion. In an annular or arcuate lesion, the advancing edge is most likely to yield a positive specimen. Try to obtain several large flakes.
- Add KOH. This can be done in two ways:
    1. Put 1–2 drops of solution on specimen; then add coverslip.
    2. Place coverslip on dry specimen and then carefully add solution at edge, allowing capillary attraction to spread the fluid. This method ensures that no excess solution will mar the microscope stage.
- Heat slide gently over alcohol burner for 10–15 seconds (except DMSO). Do not boil solution.
- Place slide on microscope stage. **Close condenser diaphragm and rack condenser way down:** This is essential to heighten detail of the specimen. If the condenser lens is up under the stage, fungal hyphae blend into the cellular background.
- Scan under × 10 magnification objective and locate a piece of scale.

  Examine it with × 10 magnification for hyphae. Look for a narrow, straight, sometimes branching walled structure that crosses epidermal cell walls (epidermal cell walls are in a honeycomb pattern and are not straight). Focus up and down to examine all levels of the specimen. If necessary, examine with × 43 magnification to confirm parallel hyphal wall structure (like a garden hose sliced end-to-end).
- Avoiding pitfalls and novice mistakes:
    - Get adequate scale.
    - Warm KOH and allow time for clarification.
    - Close condenser diaphragm and rack condenser down.
    - **Examine scale.** Most novices hunt futilely for hyphae floating free in solution between scales. The hyphae are embedded in the scale.
    - Focus up and down in all fields.
    - Learn to recognize oil droplets, dirt, and epidermal cell walls.
- Culture (*See* page 228 for interpretation)
    - Slice number 15 blade into agar. This makes blade sticky.
    - Loosen scale from lesion, carry on blade to agar, and slice it into the agar.
    - Plant several scales.

HAIR

- Fungal infections of hair are at scalp level and slightly into the follicle. The scalp, usually flaky, should be examined as described earlier. Hairs often break off a few millimeters above scalp level. Examine those broken stubs.
- With forceps, **gently** pluck stubble or intact hair. Try to remove hair with the bulb at its end; if it breaks, you might leave the fungus-bearing portion behind.
- Place the stubble or snipped-off proximal 1–2 cm of hair (the distal portion is negative and clutters the slide) onto the slide. Add KOH and coverslip, or infiltrate KOH under dry coverslip (*See* earlier). Warm the slide and let sit a few minutes.
- Place under microscope stage, **rack down condenser**, and examine under × 10 magnification objective.
- Hyphae are rarely seen. Look for clusters of small walled spores coating the hair shaft (ectothrix) or packed in the hair shaft (endothrix).
- Avoiding pitfalls:
    - Obtain a deep, proximal portion of hair.
    - Learn to distinguish between spores and epithelial cells clinging to bulb of hair.
    - Learn to distinguish hyphae from edges of cuticle plates on surface of hair (not long, straight, and branching).
    - Examine several hairs.
    - Results of examination of **kerion** are usually negative (inflammation kills fungi).

- Culture
  - With tweezers, obtain specimen as described earlier and embed on agar surface.
  - Plant several hairs. Be sure **proximal** end is embedded.
  - *Alternative method:* Scrub suspected scalp area with a sterilized toothbrush and then tap bristle tips into agar surface.

NAILS

- The rate of obtaining positive KOH or culture results on a single specimen is low. Also, saprophytic fungi often colonize infected nails and confuse the evaluation. Much skill is needed to obtain and interpret results. Repeat the examinations three times before considering the results negative.
- Wipe distal nail and toe surface with alcohol to remove dirt and oil. Allow the surfaces to dry.
- With number 15 blade or the edge of a pointed forceps, scrape crumbly debris from under the distal nail edge. If the nail is long, clip a generous portion off, scrape debris from the undersurface of the fragment and of the remaining nail.
- Place debris or nail clipping on the slide and add KOH; add the coverslip. The thick nature of the specimen holds the coverslip off the slide. Gently heat. Add more KOH, if necessary. Let specimen soften 5 minutes or longer. As it softens, gently compress coverslip onto specimen, flattening it as much as possible.
- Place the slide on the microscope stage. **Rack condenser down**. Examine as described earlier for scale. The thickness of the specimen makes examination of the center difficult, but the edges are thinner and may show hyphae. Focus up and down to examine all levels of the specimen.
  - If results are negative, re-examine in 30 minutes (may need to add more KOH), after further softening of specimen.
- Pitfalls are numerous. The debris is "messy" with dirt, keratin, and fibers. Hyphae are sparse.
- Culture:
  - Obtain debris by the method already outlined, and plant it on agar.
  - Interpretation is difficult because saprophytic overgrowth is common (*See* farther on).
- Additionally, histology with a PAS stain will be definitive.

CULTURE

- Dermatophytes will grow out on Sabouraud's agar generally as dry, folded white colonies in 2–4 weeks.
- The organism of tinea versicolor (*See* page 154) can be identified on KOH examination but will grow only on special media.
- *Candida* (yeast) will grow out on Sabouraud's agar in 2–6 days as a creamy and smooth colony.
- Saprophytic fungi (contaminants) grow out as dry, folded colonies, often in 1 week. They are often black or brown.
- Distinguishing true dermatophytes from contaminants require training and experience. One fairly reliable shortcut is dermatophyte testing medium (DTM). Specimens are placed on this yellow agar as described in the preceding sections. If a colony grows, the entire agar may turn red. This appearance almost always indicates a dermatophyte colony. If the agar stays yellow, the colony is most likely a contaminant (the test is based on the pH of the organisms).
- Avoiding pitfalls
  - Keep the media fresh; do not allow them to dry out.
  - Interpreting result is often difficult.
  - **Do not tightly cap culture after implantation**. Dermatophytes are aerobic and will not grow in sealed bottles. Novices often forget this and tighten caps too snugly. Leave the cap loose enough to rattle.
  - Do not declare a specimen result negative until after 4 weeks of incubation at room temperature. However, with DTM, late color conversion may yield a false-positive result.

Scabies Preparation

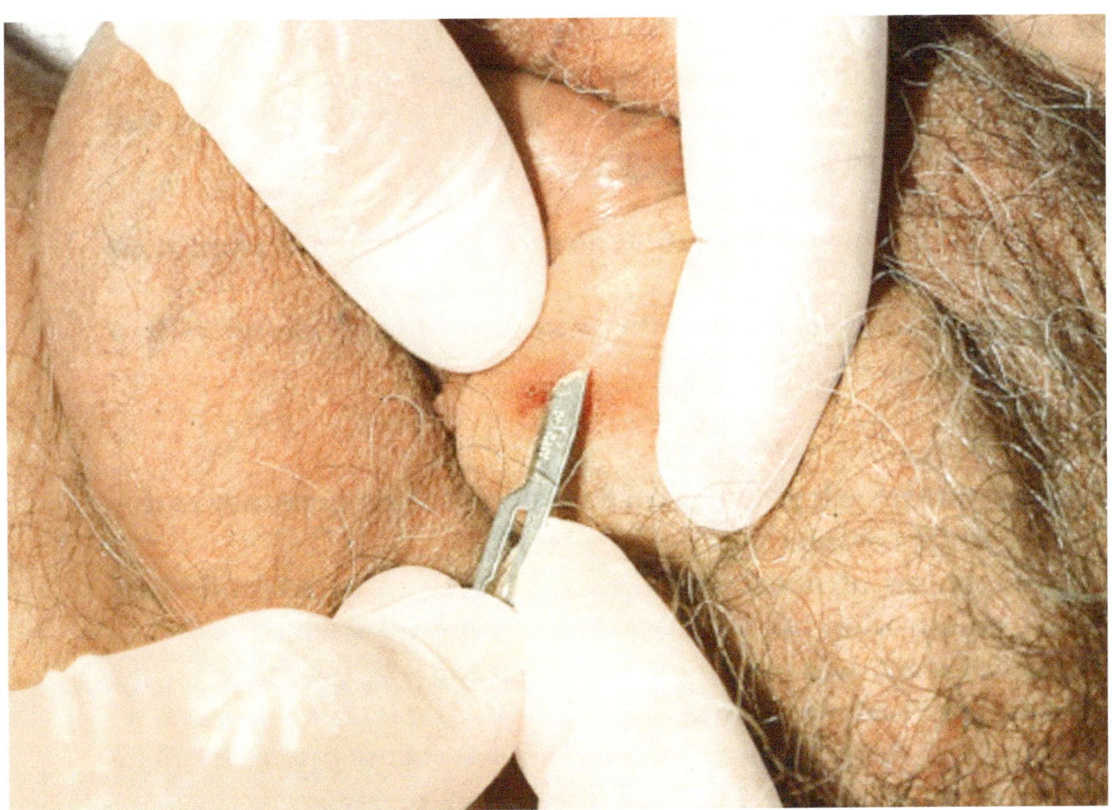

Specimens for scabies examination are obtained by superficial shave, not scrape.

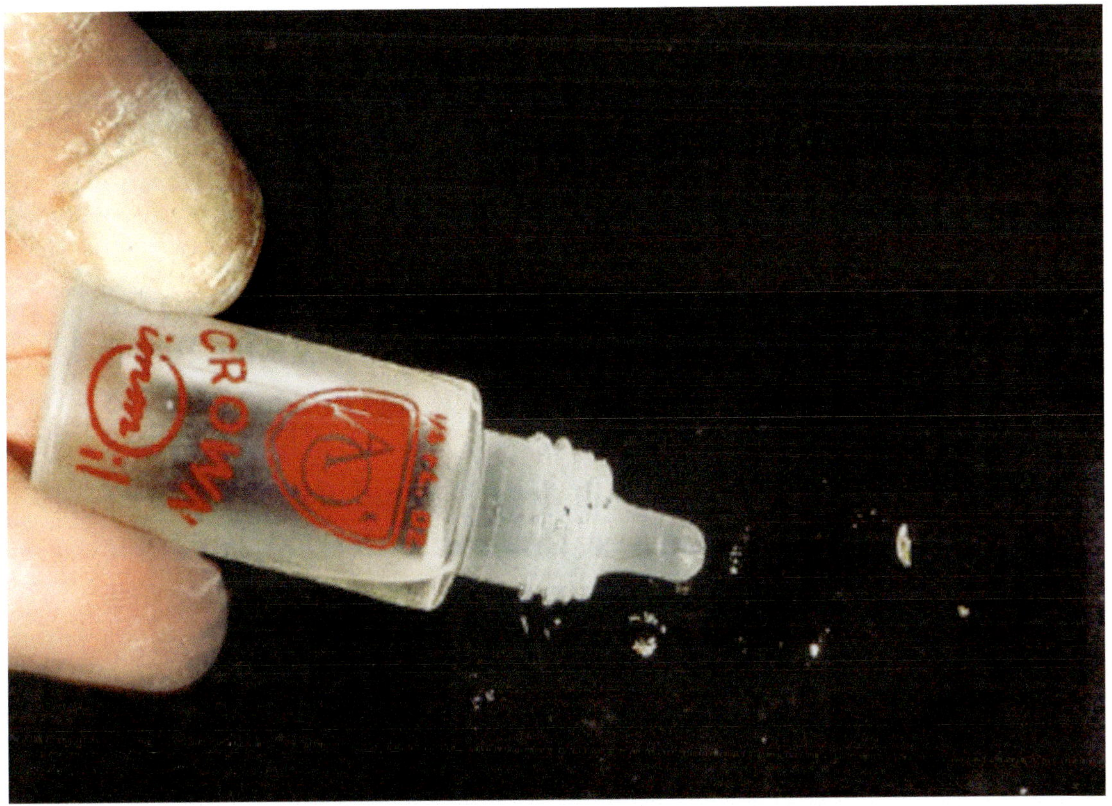

Several specimens are placed on a slide; oil is added, then a coverslip.

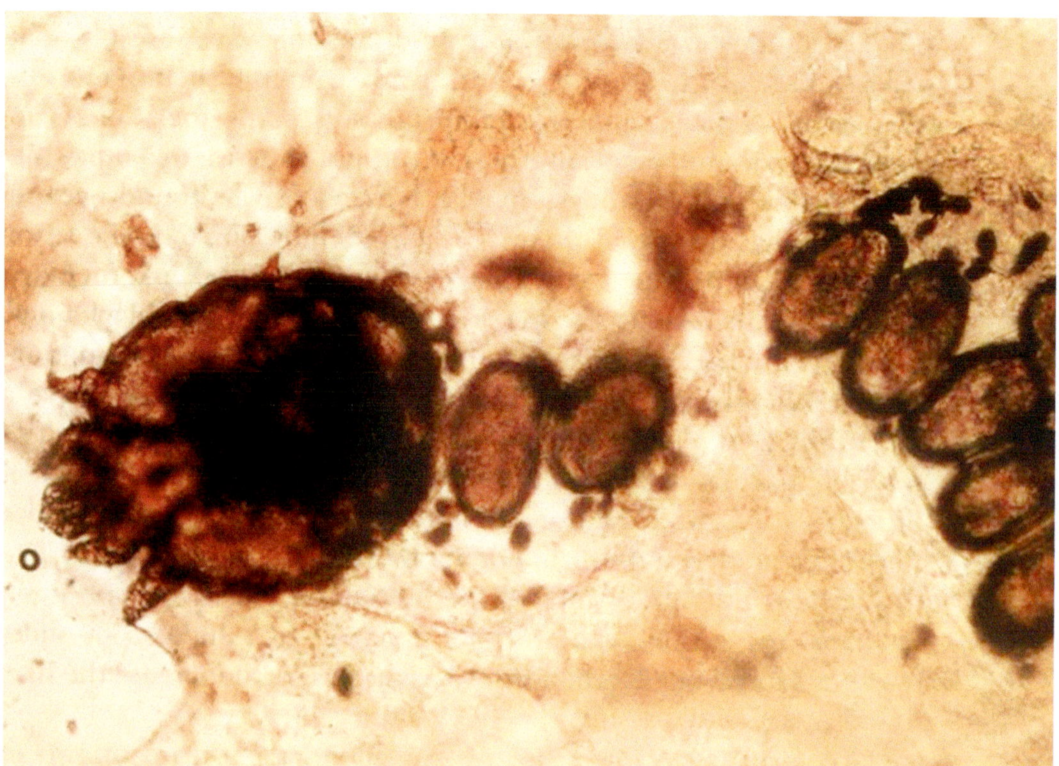

Adult mite, eggs, and feces in a burrow in a skin-shave specimen.

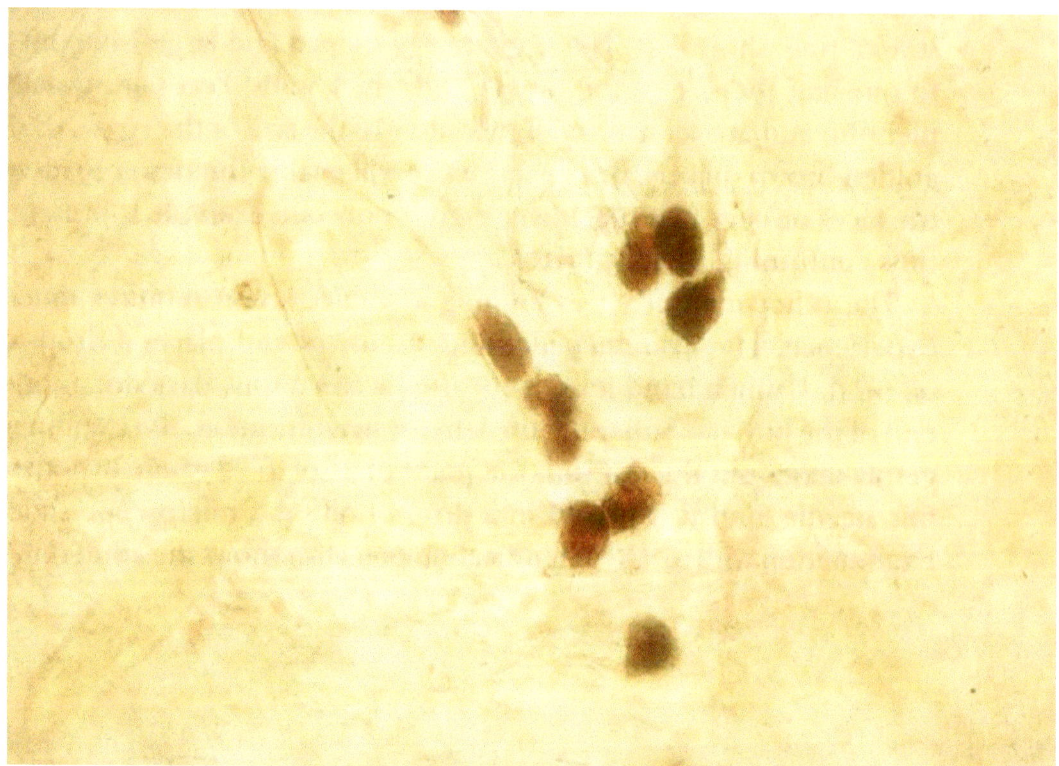

The diagnosis can be confirmed by finding the small, oval, honey-brown feces alone.

Most of the lesions in scabies are allergic in nature and do not contain organisms. In a full-blown rash, perhaps only 10 living mites are present, although dozens of lesions may contain eggs or feces. Identifying mites, eggs, or feces in a skin specimen confirms the diagnosis.

Selection of an appropriate lesion for examination is all-important. Infected lesions are likely to be in fold areas and are rare on open surfaces such as the arms, legs, and trunk. Examine the finger webs, wrist folds, axillae, nipples, umbilicus, and penis for intact (un-scratched) papules, especially those surmounted by a 1- to 5-mm white line (burrow). Often no lesions with burrows can be found because scratching has destroyed them. To help identify burrows, the suspicious areas can be wiped with a gauze soaked with black ink, then dry-wiped. Burrows take up the ink and stand out as distinct black lines.

Two techniques can be used to obtain a specimen for examination. Most commonly, a number 15 scalpel is used to carefully **shave** a paper-thin 3- to 5-mm wafer off the top of the papule. Scraping (instead of shaving) results in a rolled, crumpled specimen, which is difficult to interpret. Many practitioners prepare the lesion before shaving by placing a drop of mineral oil or immersion oil on it. The oil sharpens the appearance of the lesion and makes the specimen adhere to the scalpel blade for safe transport to a microscope slide. Shavings should be obtained from several lesions to increase the likelihood of a positive result.

Place the shaving on a microscope slide, add a drop or two of mineral or immersion oil, and then cover with a coverslip. Oil-mounting the specimen in this manner sharpens the microscopic image and does not kill mites (as KOH would), thus allowing their movement to be observed. Examine each shaving under × 10 magnification objective. Mites are easily recognized as oval, slightly spiny organisms with several fine, and short legs. The eggs are egg-shaped and large (one-third to one-half the size of the mites), with thick walls. Feces are usually plentiful and are seen as small (about 1/10 the size of the eggs), oval, and golden-brown objects. Brief experience will enable the viewer to identify feces or eggs in a specimen, even if only one example is present, thus confirming the diagnosis.

Anesthesia

When injection of local anesthesia is required in dermatology, almost always the agent used is lidocaine (Xylocaine) 1%, with epinephrine 1:100,000 or 1:200,000. This gives rapid anesthesia that lasts for 1.5–2 hours; the epinephrine significantly decreases bleeding. The presence of epinephrine requires an acidic pH for stability, so the patient feels considerable burning during injection. Many dermatologists buffer the local anesthetic with sodium bicarbonate 8.4%, mixed 1:10 with the anesthetic to decrease this burning. The shelf life of this mixture is only a few days, so often the mixing is done in the syringe as each product is drawn up.

Lidocaine without epinephrine is used on digits, where theoretically the presence of epinephrine may cause vasospasm for long enough to lead to anoxia and tissue damage. In practice this is very rare, but epinephrine is not advised and hemostasis can easily be achieved with a thick rubber band tourniquet during the procedure. Some physicians prefer to forgo epinephrine even on the nose and earlobes, fearing anoxia, but such events are extraordinarily rare (not to say unheard of) and surgery on those sites without epinephrine is quite bloody.

Superficial anesthesia can be achieved by the topical application of EMLA (eutectic mixture of local anesthetics) cream. This contains lidocaine 2.5% and prilocaine 2.5% in a vehicle that allows some penetration through the usually impermeable keratin layer. The cream is applied at home by the patient in a thick layer, occluded with plastic wrap for 2 hours, and removed just before the procedure. The resultant anesthesia is not deep enough for deep skin surgery but allows painless injection of local anesthesia for those procedures and allows for superficial procedures such as light curettage, cryotherapy, debridements, and pulsed dye laser therapy. In practice, injection of local anesthesia is well tolerated by most adults, and the somewhat complex preprocedure purchase and use of EMLA is mostly reserved for children.

Skin Biopsy

Histopathologic examination of some skin eruptions is helpful in confirming a diagnosis, but the main utility is in classifying growths, granulomas, and infiltrates. A small biopsy is simple, quick, and usually leaves little scarring. There are three techniques for doing small skin biopsies:

1. **Shave biopsy** is applicable only to elevated lesions. A papule or a portion of a plaque is anesthetized with an injection of local anesthetic. The papule or a portion of the edge of the plaque is shaved off with a number 15 scalpel or snipped off with small, curved scissors. It may be possible to control bleeding with pressure or a styptic (aluminum chloride, *See* page 244), but light electrocautery or electrodesiccation may be required. The resulting scab may be covered or left open, and it will come off in 1–3 weeks. The patient needs only to keep the area clean with routine bathing.

Shave biopsy should **not** be performed on a suspected melanoma (*See* page 220). Shave biopsy yields a partial specimen, which is not adequate for determining prognosis and method of treatment.

2. **Punch biopsy** is an easy way to obtain a full-thickness specimen. Biopsy punches are available in sizes from 2 to 10 mm, but 3- or 4-mm punches usually yield an adequate specimen with minimal scarring. The anesthetized lesion is cut with forceful, repeated turning of the circular biopsy punch. It is easy to feel when the soft subcutaneous fat layer is reached. The specimen is gently elevated with a fine forcep, and fine, curved scissors are used to snip the restraining subcutaneous fat. For best cosmetic results, close the defect with one or two sutures. In many cases, however, hemostasis with styptic or electrocautery and healing by secondary intention yield an acceptable appearance and save the patient a return visit for suture removal.

The round defect left by a punch biopsy may heal with an unsightly, depressed scar. To encourage healing as a linear scar along fold lines, forcefully stretch the skin at right angles to the intended scar line when making the biopsy. When the skin is released, the round hole assumes an oval shape oriented in the intended direction.

3. **Incisional scalpel biopsy** requires more time and skill than does a punch biopsy, and it almost always requires suture closure. However, incisional biopsies can be carefully aligned for good cosmetic closure, and they close with no dog-ear or depression (as punch ovals often do). They also allow angling of the incision edge outward to obtain a generous biopsy of deep dermal and subcutaneous tissue, which is important in certain conditions, such as erythema nodosum.

BIOPSY TISSUE PROCESSING

The biopsy specimen should be placed in 10% buffered neutral formalin solution, in a volume 10–20 times greater than the specimen. Small specimens are often difficult for the pathologist to orient for cutting. This should be discussed with your pathologist so that an identification system can be agreed on. A common one is to press the deep part of the specimen onto a small piece of filter paper or paper towel before placing them (stuck together) into the formalin. Dyes can also be painted onto certain surfaces.

8 CHAPTER Formulary

Principles of Topical Therapy

- Topical therapy is usually used to combat
  - Inflammation
    - Acute: Redness, edema, vesiculation, oozing, and crusting
    - Chronic: Lichenification (epidermal thickening and scaling) infection by bacteria, yeasts, fungi, and viruses
- Agents used for this purpose are:
  - Solutions
  - Lotions
  - Gels
  - Creams
  - Ointments
  - Aerosol sprays
  - Pastes
  - Occluding tapes or glazes (benzoin or collodion)
- The proper prescribing methods are detailed on the indicated pages; other agents (bleaches, soaps, shampoos, and so on) are covered in this chapter.

THE DERMATOLOGIC PRESCRIPTION

A typical prescription for a topical agent is as follows:

Hydrocortisone cream 1%
Dispense: 60 g
Signature: Apply thinly to itchy rash on face bid

Writing such a prescription requires knowledge of several components, described in the following paragraphs:

The **first line** describes the agent, the vehicle, and the concentration. The choice of the agent is discussed throughout this book. Vehicles determine the ease of application and delivery of the active agent; they are discussed in the clinical sections. The concentration of the active agent in the topical preparation is usually fixed or standard but is sometimes variable, in which case the concentration must be carefully stated for the pharmacist.

The **second line** directs the volume to be dispensed, expressed (depending on the country) in ounces, grams, milliliters, cubic centimeters, pints, and so on. One ounce = 28.5 g (approximately 30 g) = approximately 30 mL. Deciding on a volume to dispense requires experience and knowledge of the surface area and length of time to be treated, but it also depends greatly on how the medication is applied by the patient, which must be directed by the physician.

For almost all topical medications, **the thinnest possible application provides the maximum therapeutic effect.** Applying two or three times more material does *not* increase the therapeutic effect. If the medication is a cream or ointment, applying more of it may be more lubricating, but a less expensive way to achieve the same lubrication is by applying a thin layer of the medicated cream and then later applying a bland lubricant as necessary.

The patient should be taught how to apply a medication. Typically, the uninstructed patient applies a large bolus from a tube or jar and then tries to rub it in. This results in a layer of medication that is too thick at the center and too thin at the edges. While they are in the office, patients should be shown the correct way to apply a topical medication. Tiny amounts are dabbed on over the area to be treated and then rubbed in as a thin layer. The resulting treatment film is usually not unpleasantly sticky, even if an ointment is used; this allows the medication to be used most efficiently. When a cream or ointment is applied in this manner, 20–25 g can cover the entire body.

Estimates of coverage for specific sites can be made by using the rule of nines, in which the approximate surface area of the body is divided into 11 equal parts, each constituting 9% of the total body surface area. The areas are head, each arm, anterior chest, posterior chest, abdomen, lumbar/buttocks, and half of each leg. Each area can be covered with about 2 g of cream or ointment. Lotions and solutions go further per ounce than do ointments, creams, pastes, or gels.

The **third line**, the signature, determines the labeling instructions. Directing the patient to apply thinly reinforces the foregoing instructions. Most medications need to be applied only twice daily for maximum benefit; exceptions are discussed in the clinical sections.

The instructions should state what skin condition the medication is for, in terms the patient understands. The direction of "apply twice daily" or "apply as needed" may not be adequate for the forgetful patient. More importantly, as various creams and lotions accumulate in the patient's medicine cabinet, mention of the disease being treated by each cream or lotion becomes necessary. If, for example, a face rash returns, the patient may find a collection of tubes in the medicine cabinet, some perhaps for acne or athlete's foot, but all labeled only "apply twice daily." This possible confusion may be avoided by labeling creams and lotions according to the disease to which they apply. Also, use terms that are easily understood by the patient; do not use labels such as "tinea pedis" or "pityriasis rosea."

PRICING OF MEDICATIONS

It is difficult to estimate prices of medications because of widely varying markup policies among pharmacies and frequent updating of wholesale prices. We have estimated recent prices for certain medications or classes of medications.

Generic medications are often much less expensive than tradename medications, and they are usually just as effective. Equivalency is less certain, however, with topical than with oral medications because of the profound impact the medication's vehicle has on its stability, penetration, and efficacy. This is particularly true of corticosteroids; studies have shown some generic preparations to be markedly less potent than their brand-name equivalents.

Acne Medications

BENZOYL PEROXIDE

- Available in various concentrations and by prescription or over the counter (OTC)
- In general:
  - Gels, besides being more stable and more pleasant to use than solutions, are far more popular.
  - Water-based gels are less drying and less likely to be irritating than are alcohol-and acetone-based gels.
  - Because concentrations of 2.5–5% are adequate to sterilize follicles, a 10% concentration is probably unnecessary and is often irritating.
- Preparations available: Most are available in 45-, 60-, and 90-g sizes.
  - Alcohol-based
  - Water-based

TOPICAL ANTIBIOTICS

The liquid and gel preparations are usually available in 2-oz sizes, but some are available in 1-oz sizes.

COMBINATION OF ERYTHROMYCIN AND BENZOYL PEROXIDE

Various combinations are available.

RETINOIDS (VITAMIN A ACIDS)

- Tretinoin is available in solution (most irritating), gel, or cream (least irritating). The manufacturer states that all concentrations of the product are equally effective after 3 months of application, but this has not been confirmed independently. The solution and gel may penetrate better than the cream, so they are thought to be more potent even though they are in lower concentrations.

- Other available retinoids are adapalene (0.1% OTC and 0.3% on prescription), tazarotene (0.05% and 0.1% gel or cream, and 0.1% foam), and trifarotene 0.005% cream.
- *See* acne, page 27.

ADAPALENE

This is available as 0.1% gel OTC and 0.3% gel on prescription.

AZELAIC ACID

This is available as 10% OTC and 15% or 20% on prescription. It is available as a cream or foam.

Some Topical Antibacterials

- Gentamicin cream
- Mupirocin ointment

Combinations of antibacterial agents are available, but their use may lead to allergic contact dermatitis.

Treatment of Fungal Infections

See clinical sections for specific recommendations.

- Tinea capitis, *See* page 5
- Tinea faciei, *See* page 23
- Tinea corporis, *See* page 156
- Tinea cruris, *See* page 68
- Tinea pedis, *See* page 82
- Onychomycosis, *See* page 86
- Tinea versicolor, *See* page 154

TOPICAL ANTIFUNGAL AGENTS

- Small, uncomplicated fungal infections respond to topical antifungal agents listed in **Table 1**. General guidelines for use are as follows:
  - Apply thinly twice daily. *See* farther on for exceptions.
  - The usual duration of therapy is 1–2 weeks. Treat until the lesions flatten and stop scaling, then treat a few days longer.
  - Creams are best for dry areas.
  - Solutions, lotions, and aerosols are best for moist areas (groin or toe web) or hairy areas because they leave little residue and are drying.
  - Powders are poor vehicles for antifungal agents. As already mentioned, it is better to use solutions in moist areas; a bland powder should then be used if necessary to reduce chafing. Antifungal powders are effective for prophylaxis of interdigital tinea.

SYSTEMIC ANTIFUNGAL AGENTS

Systemic antifungal agents **(Table 1)** are indicated if the infection is:

- On the scalp or in a very hairy area
- Widespread
- Resistant to topical therapy
- In the nails (finger or toe)

Griseofulvin

Griseofulvin is a standard oral antifungal agent. The original preparation was of large particle size; doses required were 1–2 g daily. It has been superseded by materials of small particle size, which are absorbed better and are taken in smaller doses.

Table 1: Antifungal agents.

Agent	*Dermatophytes*	*Yeast*	*Tinea versicolor*
		Topical agents	
Ciclopirox	+	+	+
Clotrimazole	+	+	–
Econazole	+	+	+
Ketoconazole	+	+	+
Miconazole	+	+	+
Naftifine	+		
Oxiconazole	+	Uncertain	
Sulconazole	+	Uncertain	+
Terbinafine	+	Uncertain	
Tolnaftate	+		+
Undecylenic acid	+		
Amphotericin B		+	
Nystatin		+	
Iodoquinol	+	+	
Sodium thiosulfate			+
		Systemic agents	
Griseofulvin	+		
Itraconazole	+	+	+
Fluconazole	+	+	+

- Micronized, microsize, or ultra-fine form is taken in a dose of 500–1,000 mg daily (usually divided in a twice-daily dose).
- Ultramicronized form is taken in a dose of 250–750 mg daily in divided doses.

Response to griseofulvin is slow; clinical improvement is not seen for 1–2 weeks. Most infections require treatment for 4–6 weeks, or 1–2 weeks after apparent clearing. Topical corticosteroids may be given to relieve itching. It was originally thought that griseofulvin should be taken with fatty foods to enhance absorption, but absorption occurs just as completely, though somewhat more slowly, on an empty stomach. The slower absorption is not important to therapy. Fungal resistance to this product does exist. Griseofulvin is available in a generic form, and costs for generic forms are often lower than those for trade types.

Side effects of griseofulvin are common and numerous. They include the following:

- Gastrointestinal upset (common), which can be severe
- Headache, usually unresponsive to aspirin
- Mood changes, anorexia, insomnia, and nightmares
- Peripheral paresthesias
- Allergic rashes

Bone marrow suppression and photosensitivity were originally reported but have been inadequately documented. Griseofulvin induces liver microsomes and increases the metabolism of coumarin, phenobarbital, oral contraceptives, and other drugs. Chronic administration in rats has produced hepatoma.

Other Systemic Antifungals

Itraconazole is approved in the United States for deep fungal infections in the immunocompromised host and for onychomycosis, but it is also effective against dermatophyte (ringworm) infections and yeasts. For dermatophyte infections, a dosage of 200 mg daily for 1–2 weeks is common. For nail infections, a popular regimen is 200 mg twice daily for a week, once a month for 3 months. For scalp (hair) infections in children, some studies recommend 100 mg daily for 4–6 weeks. None of these treatments for dermatophytes has been approved in the United States.

Fluconazole is approved in the United States for systemic candidiasis, but it is also effective against dermatophytes. A brief dose is deposited into the keratin of the skin and nails, so benefit may increase after treatment is stopped. It does not appear to have the hepatic side effects occasionally seen with ketoconazole, and other types of side effects are few. Skin fungal infections are treated with 150 mg once weekly for 2–4 weeks. A common course for onychomycosis is 150 mg once weekly for 6–12 months or until the nails are clear. Approval for treatment of dermatophytes has not been obtained in the United States.

Topical Corticosteroid/Antifungal Combinations

These agents are useful when there is a dermatophyte or *Candida* infection with significant inflammation. The infected site is often flexural and thin-skinned (groin, axillae, and submammary), however, and potent corticosteroids may cause atrophy, making some of these combinations inappropriate.

- Hydrocortisone (1% or 1.9%) and iodoquinol (1%). These are available in 2-g and 30-g sizes (cream).
  - Mild corticosteroid that suppresses yeasts, bacteria, and dermatophytes. Good for "jock itch," intertrigo, and diaper dermatitis. Iodoquinol is occasionally irritating and occasionally sensitizing in the 3% concentrations.
- Betamethasone dipropionate 0.05% and clotrimazole 1% cream.
  - A strong corticoid makes this inappropriate for dermatophyte or *Candida* infections in fold areas or on the face, but it may be useful on thick-skinned areas such as the trunk and feet.

Pediculocides and Scabicides

- Permethrin: 1% cream rinse (available OTC), 5% cream prescription only
- Crotamiton: 30 g and 100 g
- Pyrethrin: Solution or gel
- *See* discussions of head lice (page 8), pubic lice (page 63), and scabies (page 149) for selection and administration of these agents.

Antiviral Agents

From a practical standpoint, these are agents for herpes simplex, varicella, and zoster. All of the agents useful in outpatient medicine are related to acyclovir but have some different pharmacologic qualities. These qualities may or may not make them more effective in comparable doses.

Available topically are acyclovir cream or ointment and penciclovir cream. Topical acyclovir is indicated only for primary herpetic lesions, but oral agents work much better, so it cannot be recommended. Penciclovir cream, if applied every 2 hours for 4 days to recurrent herpes lesions, reduces duration of outbreaks by only 1/2 day.

Acyclovir is poorly absorbed orally, so it has to be taken in large doses with frequency to be effective. Famciclovir is somewhat better absorbed orally and has a longer intercellular half-life than the other antiviral agents. Valacyclovir is absorbed very well orally and is metabolized to its active form, acyclovir. Blood levels from oral administration are comparable to those of intravenous administration of acyclovir.

Corticosteroids

Choosing a topical corticosteroid is confusing because of the vast selection of brands, concentrations, sizes, and vehicles. The process is actually fairly simple if one adopts a method of classification used in this book. However, when you choose a preparation for a particular patient you should consider:

- Size—*See* page 234 for the rule of nines
- Directions—*See* page 233 for the dermatologic prescription

Emphasize a thin application. This gives maximal therapeutic effect, least residual stickiness, and minimal cost. Twice-daily applications are usually adequate, especially just after bathing (to lubricate and achieve maximal penetration).

Table 2 lists the principal topical corticosteroids, ranked for relative potency from the strongest (group 1) to the mildest (group 7). Preparations within groups are comparable in therapeutic effect but may vary considerably in cosmetic qualities. Creams may vary immensely in thickness, for example, and may contain various amounts of propylene glycol, alcohol, or other additives that may be irritants in some people. Try to accumulate samples of these products and set aside a time to apply each of them to your skin to compare their properties.

A glance at the potency list may be daunting at first, but then it will be instructive. Potency is related to intrinsic qualities of the active molecule, but it may also be strongly affected by properties of the vehicle. Betamethasone dipropionate is the most striking example. In an optimized vehicle it is in the ultrapotent group 1. In more conventional vehicles, its potency ranges from group 2 to group 3 (cream) and even group 5 (lotion). In contrast, fluocinonide is in group 2 for all four of its vehicles. Topical corticosteroids prepared extemporaneously by a pharmacist or by a generic manufacturer are very unpredictable in potency, often being significantly weaker than their trade-name counterparts.

Selection of a potency is determined by the severity of the rash and its location. Rashes in a moist fold or on thin-skin areas (axillae, groin, or eyelid) usually require only mild or moderately potent corticosteroids because absorption there is good. Rashes on dry, thick skin (back or extremities) or rashes that are scaly or lichenified usually require potent corticosteroids. Although corticosteroids may behave more potently on the skin of children, especially infants, experimental proof of this is lacking.

Mild rashes on moist or thin-skinned areas may be treated initially with a mild corticosteroid (group 7, hydrocortisone 1%). More severe rashes, or rashes on other sites, may require a potent corticosteroid for initial therapy, but then a milder preparation may be used for maintenance. Prescriptions for both strengths can be given during the initial visit.

Most corticosteroid creams and ointments are available in sizes of 15, 30, and 60 g, but some (especially the generic and milder preparations) are available in 120 and 240 g. Triamcinolone is also available in 454 g.

For maximum efficiency of corticosteroid use, do not forget that **occlusion** greatly enhances potency, thus saving money. It is difficult and messy, but it can be simplified: Instead of adapting sheet plastic wrap for all uses, try disposable plastic gloves for hands, shower caps for the scalp, and plastic bags for other areas. The midportion of an extremity can be covered with a long, slender bag (such as used for bread) with the end cut off. Holding the plastic on with socks, T-shirts, or gauze wraps is often more comfortable than using tape. It is often most convenient to use occlusion only during sleep or for a few hours in the evening.

Occlusion, however, may cause adverse effects. Patients may experience heat rash and even overheating if large areas are covered. This increases cardiac demand and can be dangerous in elderly patients or in those with heart disease. Occlusion encourages or worsens bacterial infection in moist, oozing lesions. It is best used only on dry-eruptions. Also, occlusion of a corticosteroid increases the risk of systemic absorption or cutaneous atrophy.

SIDE EFFECTS

Side effects from topical corticosteroids are uncommon but can be avoided if the preparations are used correctly.

Systemic absorption is rarely a problem. Only small amounts of the applied material actually reach systemic circulation. Total body application of even group 4 corticosteroids (moderately potent) only occasionally results in lowered morning cortisol levels, and even then clinical changes are rare; the adrenals still respond to stress with endogenous cortisol production. A similar response can be seen with application of group 1 corticosteroids on 25–50% of the body. Actual cushingoid changes can result from prolonged application of group 1 materials to the entire body, from application of less potent corticosteroids with widespread occlusion (total body), or from group 1 materials with less-than-total-body occlusion. Children and infants are somewhat more sensitive to these effects, particularly those who are growth delayed. Systemic effects are rare and require prolonged and widespread application of strong corticosteroids. Skin conditions calling for such therapy are severe and are probably best managed by a dermatologist.

Cutaneous side effects from topical corticosteroids are somewhat more common but still unusual. They almost always result from incorrect use of corticosteroids, often from unauthorized refills or persons borrowing medications from friends. Basically they occur from the prolonged (>6 weeks and often >6 months) daily application of corticosteroids that are too potent for the area to which they are being applied, such as the face, eyelids, genitals, and flexors (in the groin particularly). **These side effects are related to the potency of the corticosteroid and not to whether or not the steroid molecule is fluorinated.** Fluorine or chlorine atoms are present in many potent corticosteroids, but some are not halogenated; fluorination should not be used to imply potency.

Group 1 corticosteroids are superpotent; their use should be restricted to 2 weeks, followed by a 1- to 2-week rest period to avoid skin atrophy. Group 2 corticosteroids can be used safely on thick-skinned areas (palms and back) without concern, but on thinner-skinned areas (antecubital and genital) they should be used for only a few weeks, at most, to avoid atrophy.

Table 2: Topical corticosteroids grouped by relative potency.

Agent/Concentration	*Vehicles*
Group 1	
Betamethasone dipropionate 0.05% (optimized vehicle)	o
Clobetasol propionate	c, l, o, g
Diflorasone diacetate 0.05%	c, o
Halobetasol propionate 0.05%	c, o
Group 2	
Betamethasone dipropionate 0.05%	c
Desoximetasone 0.25%	c, g, o
Diflorasone diacetate 0.05%	o
Fluocinonide 0.05%	c, g, l, o
Halcinonide 0.1%	c, o
Mometasone furoate 0.1%	o
Group 3	
Betamethasone valerate 0.1%	o
Betamethasone dipropionate 0.05%	l
Diflorasone diacetate 0.05%	c
Fluticasone propionate 0.005%	o
Triamcinolone acetonide 0.5%	c, o
Triamcinolone acetonide 0.1%	o
Group 4	
Desoximetasone 0.05%	c
Fluocinolone acetonide 0.2%	c
Fluocinolone acetonide 0.025%	o
Flurandrenolide 0.05%	o
Hydrocortisone valerate 0.2%	o
Mometasone furoate 0.1%	c
Triamcinolone acetonide 0.1%	c
Group 5	
Betamethasone valerate 0.025%	l
Betamethasone valerate 0.1%	c
Fluocinolone acetonide 0.025%	c
Flurandrenolide 0.05%	c
Fluticasone propionate 0.05%	c
Hydrocortisone butyrate 0.1%	c, o
Hydrocortisone valerate 0.2%	c
Mometasone furoate 0.1%	c, l, o
Prednicarbate 0.1%	c
Triamcinolone acetonide 0.1%	l
Group 6	
Alclometasone 0.05%	c, 0
Desonide 0.05%	c, 0
Flumethasone pivalate 0.03%	c
Betamethasone valerate 0.1%	l
Fluocinolone acetonide 0.01%	l
Group 7	
Topicals with hydrocortisone, dexamethasone, prednisolone, and methylprednisolone	

(c: cream; g: gel; l: lotion; o: ointment)

Source: Modified from Stoughton RB, Cornell RC. Review of superpotent topical steroids. Semin Dermatol. 1987;6:72-6.

Atrophic skin appears thin, shiny, and pink, with visible blood vessels. Even marked atrophy usually resolves in a few weeks or months after stopping corticoid therapy. Chronic potent corticosteroid applications on stretch areas, such as the upper thighs, axillae, and antecubital fossae, may eventually cause permanent striae.

Chronic potent corticosteroid application to the face can provoke a steroid rosacea (*See* rosacea, page 33) in which atrophy, telangiectasia, and acne-like papules and pustules are present. Another manifestation is perioral dermatitis (*See* page 37), consisting of many tiny acne-like papules around the mouth and on the chin. Inexplicably, young white women are most susceptible to these conditions. Steroid rosacea and perioral dermatitis clear when application of potent topical corticosteroids is discontinued, but days or weeks of rebound flare may occur before the eruption fades. Application of potent topical corticosteroids will suppress the flare, an effect that may induce the patient into starting their application again. However, cool soaks, lubricants, and mild topical corticosteroids (hydrocortisone 1%) may relieve the symptoms until they fade.

One last complication of topical corticosteroids is the possible development of glaucoma or cataracts if the material is applied on the eyelids. A few cases have been reported; most involved the use of potent corticosteroids, but in one case hydrocortisone was used. Experience with ocular corticosteroid drops suggests that this rare side effect tends to occur in persons predisposed to cataract or glaucoma development. If chronic corticosteroid application to the eyelids seems necessary, it is probably wise to obtain an ophthalmologic examination first, with slit-lamp examination and pressure determinations to identify susceptible individuals.

Use of potent corticosteroids is appropriate even on the face, genitals, and flexural areas if the clinical situation calls for it and if its use is monitored. Severe rashes require potent therapy, but usually patients can switch to a less-potent preparation in a few days. The patient should be cautioned against prolonged therapy (>3 weeks), and the possible consequences of this therapy should be explained. Fortunately, almost outrageous abuse of the medications is needed to produce adverse reactions.

TECHNIQUE FOR GIVING INTRALESIONAL CORTICOSTEROIDS

Materials

For most lesions triamcinolone acetonide 10 mg/mL from a 5-mL multidose vial is used. Many physicians dilute this with sterile saline to 2.5–5.0 mg/mL. When injecting this agent into keloids or hypertrophic scars, the more concentrated 40-mg/mL form may be used. All of the foregoing are suspensions, which must be shaken before use.

A small syringe allows accurate dosing and provides for injection into firm lesions with ease. The best may be a 1-mL insulin syringe with a swaged-on or integrated needle. A 1-mL tuberculin syringe is similar, but the needle is attached only with a compression fitting, which may pop apart if the injection is given under more pressure.

Although the suspension can be injected through a 30-gauge needle, which is most comfortable for the patient, it is almost impossible to draw the material into a needle of this small size. The suspension can be drawn through a larger needle, and then the needle can be changed. If an insulin syringe is used, then the attached 27-gauge needle must be used for both functions.

Technique

Intralesional corticosteroid injection is an invaluable treatment for many conditions. Correct technique is learned by doing. It is strongly advised that you initially perform the procedure with an experienced physician present to get a feel for the subtleties of volume and depth of dosing.

Conditions in which intralesional steroids are frequently used include acne, alopecia areata, psoriasis, lichen simplex chronicus, scars, and keloids. In all conditions, the suspension is injected directly into the lesion. In acne, injections go right into nodules and into the bases of cysts or pustules (injecting into the pus-filled cavity would yield no benefit). Psoriasis and dermatitis are treated by injection into the dermis of the lesions. In alopecia areata, the injections go into the junction of the dermis and subcutaneum. To minimize the number of injections required in large lesions, the needle is angled sharply beneath the lesion and a trail of triamcinolone is injected as the needle is withdrawn.

If a 10-mg/mL concentration is used, then tiny doses will suffice and pain is minimal. A volume of 0.05 mL would be typical for an acne nodule, for example, or 0.1–0.2 mL for a 1-cm patch of alopecia areata. The more dilute preparations would require commensurately larger volumes and would be somewhat more painful.

Injection of excessive material may result in atrophy or depression of the skin, but this complication resolves in a few months. In general, it is better to undertreat than to overtreat and to give a repeat injection if necessary. For acne and inflammatory conditions, benefit starts in 1–3 days and lasts at least 3 weeks. In alopecia areata, injections are given monthly; regrowth is usually not seen until 6–8 weeks, and the shots are continued for several more months.

Agents that Affect Pigmentation

For a discussion of the use of these materials, *See* the section on vitiligo (page 168).

Some cosmetic preparations are purported to produce a "tan" by application or ingestion. These preparations, which are either topical dyes or oral carotene derivatives, usually impart an unnatural orange hue to the skin.

Psoralens (which require prescription) are available as methoxsalen 1% lotion, 10-mg tablets, and trioxsalen 5-mg tablets.

HYPOPIGMENTING AGENTS

See the discussion of melasma (page 49). The only agent that effectively produces temporary pigment reduction is hydroquinone.

Monobenzone (Benoquin) produces **permanent** destruction of melanocytes and permanent depigmentation. Its uses are very limited and it should be administered only by a physician experienced in its use.

Hydroquinones are available in a range of strengths (4–10%) and vehicles (lotions, creams, and pastes) some containing para-aminobenzoic acid (PABA) and/or benzophenone.

Azelaic acid, described earlier, is available as 20% cream and 15% foam or gel (or 10% cream OTC). It should be applied twice daily if used alone or once daily when a topical retinoid is also used once a day at another time (applying them together may destabilize the tretinoin).

Cosmetic formulations of Kojic acid and tranexamic acid may be used.

Soaks, Baths, Dressings, Astringents, and Oils

Wet dressings and soaks are usually used in acute oozing or infected dermatoses, erosions, or ulcers. They soften and remove serum, debris, and bacteria and are soothing. For this debriding, flushing action to occur, the solutions should be washed over the lesions or the wet dressing changed frequently, rather than just leaving dressings on for long periods of time (which macerates surrounding tissue).

SOAKS AND BATHS

Soaks and baths can be performed in a washbowl, pan, bucket, or bathtub. The affected part, such as the foot, is placed in the partially filled container for 5–15 minutes. The solution is gently agitated over the lesion or repeatedly splashed up onto it, and debridement is gently encouraged with the fingers, cloth, or a gauze pad.

WET DRESSINGS

Wet dressings are used when it is difficult to get the patient to a tub or to immerse the affected area or when facilities are not available for soaks. Soft cotton cloth or gauze is used to apply the solution. The material is dipped in the solution and gently wrung so that it is still nearly dripping wet. The sopping dressing is applied to the lesion for a few minutes to soften the debris, perhaps rubbed gently across the lesion, and then removed, rinsed out in solution, gently wrung, and reapplied. By repeating this cycle several times in 15–30 minutes, serum and debris are loosened and carried away from the lesion. Merely applying and removing a wet dressing once is usually inadequate for debridement.

ASTRINGENT OR ANTISEPTIC SOLUTIONS

If the goal of a soak or dressing is to dry oozing tissue and prevent infection, then one may use an astringent or antiseptic solution. However, nearly equal results can be achieved with plain tap water, which many dermatologists routinely recommend. Prescribing astringents or antiseptics involves some risks. Astringents and antiseptics normally are dispensed as tablets, powders, or liquid concentrates, which the patient adds at home to a large volume of water. Unfortunate accidents have occurred in which the tablets were ingested, the liquid concentrate was used directly, or the tablets burned the skin in the bath before they dissolved completely. It is perhaps better to recommend saline solution or Epsom salt, both of which are relatively safe even if accidentally ingested.

- Saline solution is made by dissolving 1 tsp of salt in 500 mL of water.
- Epsom salt (magnesium sulfate) is added to water in a proportion of 60 g per 500 mL.

- Acetic acid, approximately 1%, can be made by diluting vinegar half and half with water.
- Aluminum acetate (Burow's solution), a widely available astringent and antiseptic, is usually diluted to a 1:20 or a 1:40 solution. It is commercially available in the form of tablets or as a powder in individual foil envelopes. Adding one tablet or one envelope of powder to 500 mL of water yields a 1:40 solution.
- Potassium permanganate 1:5,000 to 1:25,000 is sometimes used as a soak or bath but stains the skin purple. Find out from your local pharmacist how he or she dispenses it (it is available in generic tablets, crystals, or liquid concentrate of various strengths).
- Silver nitrate 0.25% solution is a strong astringent made by adding 1 tsp of 50% aqueous solution to 1 L of water. It stains skin, clothing, and (especially) metal utensils black.

OILS AND STARCHES

When soothing and cooling baths or soaks are desired, but the skin is dry and astringency would be irritating, then oil, protein, and carbohydrate substances are used. **Be aware that all oil-containing products make the tub so slippery that it becomes dangerous for even young, agile patients.** Oils in baths leave little residue on the skin. If lubrication of the skin is required, bathing in plain water is strongly recommended; apply the bath oil to the skin after bathing.

- Cold milk (not skim or low-fat) may be used as a soothing, non-drying soak for irritated areas such as first-degree burns or herpes simplex.
- Starch colloids apparently have a soothing effect of unknown mechanism. Starch baths are made by adding 2 cups of starch to a tub of water. Sometimes 2 cups of baking soda (sodium bicarbonate) are added as well. Oatmeal bath colloid is commercially available in powder form, plain or with oil added.

DRY SKIN PREPARATIONS

A lengthy discussion of these products appears on pages 110 to 125. Alpha hydroxy acid products are being widely used, with more appearing on the market all the time. Among these are:

- 12% ammonium lactate lotion
- 8% lactic acid in enhanced vehicle (over the counter)
- Urea

Soaps and Shampoos

Soaps help to remove oil and dirt from the skin. Antibacterial or deodorant soaps reduce the bacterial population of the skin. Soaps that are low in detergent properties or that have oil added may be less drying to the skin and may be used by people who tend to have dry skin (*See* page 109).

Contributing more to skin dryness than soap are the frequency and duration of bathing, water temperature, and failure to lubricate after bathing.

Shampoos remove oil, dirt, and scale from the scalp. Dandruff shampoos are perhaps keratolytic (soften scale) and possibly suppress inflammation and epidermal turnover (scale formation). More important than the specific shampoo chosen are the frequency and duration of use (*See* page 2 for treatment of seborrheic dermatitis).

Ingredients known to help control seborrheic dermatitis are chloroxine, selenium sulfide, sulfur/salicylic acid, zinc pyrithione, tar, and ketoconazole. Some of these shampoos are listed in **Table 3**. Chloroxine, ketoconazole, and selenium sulfide 2.5% require prescriptions. There is no evidence that they are superior to the OTC preparations, although the 2.5% selenium sulfide is probably more effective than the 1% form, which is available OTC.

Tar shampoos are particularly popular for psoriasis of the scalp, but thorough rinsing (which is recommended) removes all or most tar residue. Tar shampoos can stain white and light blond hair slightly yellow.

Some dandruff shampoos contain none of the aforementioned ingredients, and their effectiveness is questionable.

Table 3: Some commercially available dandruff shampoos.

Types of shampoo
Selenium sulfide (1–2.5%)
Sulfur and/or salicylic acid
Zinc pyrithione
Tar
Ketoconazole

Antihistamines

Antihistamines are often prescribed to counteract **itching**, but they are effective in that role only in histamine-mediated conditions such as hives (urticaria) and some drug reactions. For nonhistamine-mediated itching (dermatitis, dry skin, and jaundice), they are no better than a placebo. However, the placebo effect in itching exists in >40% of patients.

In **sedative** doses, antihistamines diminish the perception of itching, as would any central nervous system depressant. They are particularly useful to take at bedtime to encourage sleep in an itchy individual. Significant scratching occurs during sleep, and antihistamines in sedative doses reduce that scratching.

Individuals vary considerably in their responses to specific antihistamines, so various ones should be tried to find one that is effective but has minimal side effects. Listed in **Table 4** are the antihistamine families from which specific agents should be chosen. Dermatologists usually believe (with some experimental evidence) that hydroxyzine is the most effective single agent against hives (*See* page 134). Sometimes a combination of two antihistamines from different families will succeed.

Antihistamines often cause drowsiness, incoordination, gastrointestinal upset, dry mouth, or blurred vision. These side effects may vary considerably in prominence at different times when the same agent is taken. Patients may gradually become tolerant of the benefits and side effects of an antihistamine when taken regularly. Patients must be warned about the common occurrence of drowsiness and diminished coordination and must be advised not to drive or to operate dangerous machinery when taking antihistamines, especially at the onset of therapy, when the response is unpredictable.

Cetirizine, a metabolic product of hydroxyzine, is much less sedating than hydroxyzine but is somewhat more sedating than other nonsedating antihistamines.

Table 4: Some important antihistamines by chemical class.

Chemical class
Ethylenediamines
Hydroxyzine hydrochloride
Ethanolamines
Diphenhydramine hydrochloride
Carbinoxamine maleate
Doxylamine succinate*
Clemastine fumarate*
Alkylamines
Chlorpheniramine maleate*
Brompheniramine maleate*
Dexchlorpheniramine maleate
Triprolidine hydrochloride*
Phenothiazines
Promethazine hydrochloride
Methdilazine hydrochloride*
Propylamines
Cyproheptadine hydrochloride*
Azatadine maleate
Nonsedating antihistamines
Fexofenadine hydrochloride*
Loratadine*
Desloratadine
Cetirizine*
Levocetirizine*

*Available over-the-counter in the United States.

Keratolytics, Tars, and Destructive Agents

KERATOLYTICS

Keratolytic agents soften and/or remove keratin and scale. They are used to treat scaling disorders (e.g., psoriasis, *See* pages 3 and 117), warts, calluses, and so on.

- Salicylic acid is used alone or in combination with other medications for the treatment of psoriasis, seborrheic dermatitis, tineas, warts, and acne. Most preparations are sold OTC.
  - Salicylic acid 2–6% cream, ointment, or solution.
  - Propylene glycol is a keratolytic that, used as a vehicle, enhances the effect of salicylic acid. Tars and other compounds are also sometimes added. Salicylic acid 2–6% in propylene glycol or one of the proprietary equivalents may be prescribed.
  - Salicylic acid 5–20% in flexible collodion, often with equal parts of lactic acid, is used to treat warts and calluses. It may be prescribed as such or as a branded equivalent.
  - Salicylic acid plasters (40% on adhesive moleskin) are used for warts and calluses.
- **Urea compounds** are purported to be softening to keratin and are hydroscopic (draw water from the atmosphere), so they are used for dry skin (*See* page 109). Urea is sometimes combined with corticosteroids to enhance penetration. Urea creams can be compounded by a pharmacist but are relatively unstable, so commercial preparations are usually dispensed.
- **Lactic acid** is a potent keratolytic in an ointment base of 5–20% concentration made by a pharmacist. It is combined with salicylic acid in flexible collodion for the treatment of warts and calluses (*See* previously). In a 5% lotion form, it is used for dry skin. *See* also ammonium lactate, page 242.

TARS

Tar preparations are possibly keratolytic, antimitotic (slowing epidermal cell division of psoriasis), anti-inflammatory, and phototherapeutic. Tars are derived from petroleum, coal, shale, and wood. The most commonly used ones are coal tars.

- Crude coal tar can be compounded in ointment (1–5%), cream, oil, gel, or shampoo.
- Tar emulsions or bath oils are added to the bath or applied directly to the skin.
- Liquor carbonis detergens (LCD) is an extract of tar that is not as dark and, probably, is less potent. It is used in 5–10% concentrations in creams, oils, and shampoos, often in combination with corticosteroids, sulfur, or salicylic acid.

DESTRUCTIVE AGENTS

These are either caustics (which chemically **burn tissue)** or styptics (chemicals that stop bleeding). Mild caustics are often used as styptics.

- Monochloroacetic, dichloroacetic, or trichloroacetic acid can be compounded for use in the office. They are in 20–80% solutions, with 30–50% being the most common.
- Silver nitrate solution below 1% is used as a compress, but above 5% it is used as a cauterant. Silver nitrate sticks have a wad of nearly 100% silver nitrate at the end and are used as cauterants and styptics after moistening the wad.
- Ferric chloride solution 3–5% or ferric subsulfate 40% (Monsel's solution) is used as a styptic.
- Aluminum chloride in 1–3% concentrations is the active ingredient in antiperspirants and, in a 20% solution, is a potent antiperspirant and drying paint (*See* page 235). In a 30–80% alcoholic solution, it is a styptic and does not stain as the iron salts might.
- Negatol is a styptic that coagulates blood by enzymatic action.

Podophyllotoxin is purified extract of podophyllin, which can be applied to genital warts by the patient. It is less likely to irritate the skin than podophyllin. *See* the discussion of genital warts (page 57) for directions.

An anticancer drug, **5-fluorouracil (5-FU),** interferes with DNA synthesis. It is used topically as a cream or solution to treat actinic keratoses (*See* page 207).

- Imiquimod cream acts as a toll-like receptor 7 agonist and is available as a cream in various strengths.
- Tirbanibulin ointment is a microtubule inhibitor for the treatment of actinic keratoses.

9 CHAPTER Patient Guides

Seborrheic Dermatitis

It is normal to shed a few flakes of **dander** from the scalp every day, and regular shampooing will keep dander from building up in your hair. **Seborrheic dermatitis** is a severe scaling, usually with itching and inflammation. It occurs on the scalp and is also frequently seen in and behind the ears, on the face, in the brows, and even in the eyelashes. It often worsens with illness or emotional tension.

ANTI-DANDRUFF SHAMPOOS

Many anti-dandruff shampoos are available on the market, all of which are effective. The following points must be kept in mind about the use of anti-dandruff shampoos:

- The benefit of one shampooing lasts only 2–3 days, so washing must be at least that frequent.
- A severe case of dandruff may not respond to repeated shampooing for a week or more, so do not give up after one treatment. Maximum benefit takes 6 weeks of use.
- The medications in the shampoo must be in contact with the scalp long enough to work. Lathering and rinsing within a few seconds is not enough. The shampoo should be left on for several minutes. The longer it is left on, the more effective it will be.
- A severe flare-up of dandruff can occur despite shampoo use. Shampoos are just not strong enough to suppress all natural fluctuations of the disease.

To get the most benefit from an anti-dandruff shampoo, you should wash several times a week and leave the shampoo on for several minutes during each wash. If this schedule does not remove all the dandruff, then you may lather the shampoo, rinse it off, lather again, and cover your wet scalp with a plastic shower cap. Leave this in place for 30 minutes to 2 hours while you perform other activities; then rinse out thoroughly. This may be slightly irritating to the scalp but will usually remove all the scale.

Try many different brands of shampoo to find the one that is cosmetically acceptable to you. Some lather more than others, are more drying, or have different odors or textures. If you do not like the way the anti-dandruff shampoo makes your hair feel or smell, then you may perform a final wash with a regular-scented cosmetic shampoo, or you may use a conditioner or rinse. This will not reduce the potency of the anti-dandruff shampoo.

OTHER MEDICATIONS

Your doctor may prescribe an oil or gel to apply to the scalp to help remove excessive scaling. This should be rubbed into the scalp sparingly at bedtime, covered with a shower cap, and left on overnight. You should then shampoo in the morning, or sooner, if this treatment causes burning of the scalp. These treatments usually need to be performed once a week and sometimes even less often.

Your doctor may prescribe a cortisone solution to help reduce inflammation of the scalp. The easiest way to apply any liquid to the scalp is the following: Part your hair along the length of your scalp and apply a drop of medication about every 2 cm (a little less than an inch) along the part and rub it in; repart the hair about 2 cm parallel to the first part and again apply medication every 2 cm; keep reparting the hair and applying small amounts of the medication until the entire inflamed area is treated. This technique provides maximum medication to the scalp and minimum residue on the hair.

Acne

CAUSES

Most people have a few pimples during their teenage years; some people, however, have severe or long-lasting disease. Certain individuals will have acne regardless of their physical, social, or cultural upbringing. The sensitivity of the oil glands to becoming plugged (forming blackheads and whiteheads) and their tendency to rupture (form pimples) are inherited.

What We Know about Acne

Oil glands are inactive in childhood and develop at puberty. This explains why the face then becomes oily, pores become visible (pore size is related to oil gland size), and acne may develop. Pore size is unchangeable and is not affected by astringents, massage, saunas, facial packs, or cosmetics.

Blackheads, or pore plugs, the basic culprit in acne, are composed of dead skin produced by the cells lining the pore. The plug is not made of dirt or hardened oil. It is too deep to be scrubbed out. Its formation cannot be prevented by washing or using astringents.

A **pimple** is an inflamed area of tissue reacting to the rupture of an oil gland, a hair root, or both. The hair root ruptures at least partially because it is plugged. A pimple may contain some bacteria, but it is not a true infection and is not the result of touching the face with dirty fingers.

The occurrence of acne in some people may be influenced by:

- Stress, illness, or exhaustion
- Sunlight. Sun exposure sometimes improves acne but may worsen it in some individuals (especially those who sunburn easily).
- Hormonal changes. There are often slight flares of acne related to the menstrual cycle. Pregnancy usually improves acne. Birth control pills may or may not improve acne, depending on the estrogen content.
- Cosmetics. Certain ingredients in some cosmetics irritate the pore walls and worsen acne. It is advisable to choose noncomedogenic products.

The occurrence of acne is likely *not* influenced by:

- Diet. Chocolate, "junk food," and greasy food likely do not affect acne.
- Cleanliness
- Sexual activity

Scarring is the natural result of significant skin inflammation. It is usually not caused by picking. However, picking may worsen the inflammation of a pimple so that it is more likely to scar. The type of pimple especially sensitive to picking is the deep red bump without a pus head on top. This type has nowhere to drain and is fragile, so handling it is likely to cause more rupture and inflammation in the tissues.

TREATMENT

There is no "cure" for acne, but modern treatments help to keep acne under control until it clears with time. Your doctor will select the treatments that work best and have the fewest side effects, and he or she will follow your progress and change treatments if your response to treatment changes. General rules about acne treatments follow; your doctor will tell you specifically how to use various medications.

Except for cortisone treatments given by doctors, all treatments for acne work primarily by preventing new pimples from forming; they do little to speed the healing of existing pimples. As a result, at least 2–4 weeks of constant treatment are necessary before improvement begins. Things will continue to improve even more for up to 12 weeks before leveling off. Also, treatment must be given constantly to all acne-prone areas, not just to individual existing pimples.

Washing excessively with regular soap, special acne soaps, or abrasives has little impact on acne. More often they dry out, chap, and irritate the skin. Then, when effective anti-acne creams or lotions are used, they are likely to burn and irritate more. Just washing once or twice a day with a mild soap is best. If parts of the face feel oily during the day, they can be wiped with a mild alcohol-and-water astringent.

Acne Treatment with Topical Antibiotics, Benzoyl Peroxide, and/or Topical Retinoids

These are external anti-acne medications. All are applied regularly to the areas likely to break out with acne. They work slowly to stop the appearance of new pimples. No benefit may be seen for a month or more, and the benefit may increase over 2–3 months. About two-thirds of patients get a good response from these medications.

Benzoyl peroxide and topical retinoids, especially, may be irritating. To minimize irritation they should be applied thinly, with care taken to avoid puddling in folds around the eyes, nose, and mouth. They are more irritating on moist skin, so they should not be applied within 15 minutes of washing. Washing should be infrequent (no more than twice a day) and with mild soap. Washing with strong acne soaps tends to increase irritation. Your doctor may prescribe a soothing medication if irritation cannot be avoided.

Benzoyl Peroxide

This product helps to reduce inflamed pimples and may also reduce blackheads. Benzoyl peroxide is available in various topical formulations and as a cleanser. It may be applied twice a day, to the point that the skin feels slightly dry and tight but not to the point of redness and irritation. Some people can use it only once a day. Find the schedule that suits your skin. Occasionally, an allergy to benzoyl peroxide develops, so if an itchy red rash occurs, stop treatment. Be careful to keep benzoyl peroxide away from dark clothing and towels because it has a mild bleaching action.

Topical Antibiotics

Like benzoyl peroxide, topical antibiotics (antibiotics that are applied to the skin) help to prevent new pimples. They have no effect on blackheads. Most are in alcohol solutions and may be slightly drying but usually do not irritate, as benzoyl peroxide might. They do not bleach clothing. They are applied twice daily to acne-prone areas.

Topical Retinoids

Topical retinoids, or vitamin A acids, work best against blackheads but also reduce pimples. They are ideally applied once a day in the evening but it is advisable to start two to three times weekly and gradually increase their use as tolerated. After a few weeks your skin may be able to tolerate them more often. Mild redness often occurs. It may make your skin more sensitive to the sun, so be cautious when getting your first sun exposure of the year. Sunscreens should be used.

Using Topical Retinoids with Benzoyl Peroxide or Topical Antibiotics

Using benzoyl peroxide or topical antibiotics and topical retinoids together is often more beneficial than using either alone. The retinoid is used at night, and the other medication is applied in the morning or afternoon. They must not be put on at the same time, as such mixing could neutralize the retinoid, unless a combined benzoyl peroxide-retinoid formulation is used.

Isotretinoin Therapy for Acne

Isotretinoin is a derivative of vitamin A that is taken by mouth for severe acne. It works by greatly reducing oil gland output and possibly by decreasing inflammation and pore plugging. It completely clears facial acne in the majority of patients and usually clears acne of the chest and back as well. Isotretinoin is unique among all acne medications in that its effect continues for weeks, months, or even years after its use is discontinued.

Isotretinoin is usually taken for 3–5 months. The dose (number of tablets per day) varies, depending on the patient's body weight and any side effects noted. If the first 3–5 months of treatment are not completely successful, then isotretinoin may be given again at a later time. Although side effects are numerous and common, none is permanent. Because oil gland output is reduced so much, skin dryness is a common problem. Up to 80% of people taking the drug may develop dry, chapped skin; itching; a dry nose, mouth, or both; or even nose bleeds. Most people (90%) develop dry, cracked lips, and 40% develop dry or irritated eyes. Fewer than 10% experience dry, lifeless hair and breaking or thinning of hair. Fewer than 5% experience peeling of the palms and soles. Other symptoms that may be caused by the drug include muscle or joint aches and pains (15%). Occasionally, patients taking this drug get headaches or become fatigued.

Isotretinoin is very damaging to unborn babies, so it should not be taken during pregnancy or while nursing. Women taking the drug must use reliable birth control methods. In the United States, isotretinoin prescribing is controlled by the Food and Drug Administration (FDA)—under iPLEDGE—see website for details.

Up to 25% of persons taking isotretinoin develop elevated blood fat levels, and 10% may have mild liver test changes or changes in blood cells. The practical significance of these findings is unknown, but blood tests should be taken before therapy and at least once during treatment.

Because these side effects are similar to those of vitamin A over-dose, vitamin supplements containing vitamin A should ***not*** be taken during isotretinoin therapy. Other medications may also exaggerate side effects, so be sure to clear those medications with your physician.

Isotretinoin is an effective, exciting drug for severe acne. Because of its side effects and expense, however, it should not be used casually, and close supervision by a dermatologist is necessary.

Herpes Simplex

Herpes simplex is a viral infection unique in its ability to reappear repeatedly. It can do so because viral particles lie dormant in the nuclei of nerve cells located near the spinal column, where the body's natural immune reaction cannot destroy them. The dormant virus may "awaken" spontaneously or be provoked by fever, illness, sun-burn, injury, or stress.

Herpes simplex occurs repeatedly at the same site in an individual, most often on the lips, genitals, and buttocks. The virus causing the lip eruption is usually a slightly different one than the one causing the genital rash, so it is rare, but possible, to have fever blisters in both places.

The frequency and duration of attacks are difficult to predict. Fewer than one in four persons has recurrent episodes. Attacks may occur as often as a dozen times yearly or as rarely as twice in a lifetime. The attacks are more frequent in young adulthood and diminish with age. Attacks often start with a tingling and burning sensation for a few hours before the skin breaks out. A red and swollen area appears, which usually becomes studded with tiny blisters after 1 or 2 days. After another few days, the blisters dry up to become scabs, which are shed in a few more days. There may be redness without blisters or tiny ulcers without blisters. The attack may last 2–3 days one time and 7–10 days the next, with varying amounts of discomfort.

Herpes simplex is passed by skin-to-skin contact and is contagious during the blistering phase until dry, hard scabs are present. During that time, skin contact should be avoided. A condom probably prevents spread of infection during intercourse. Herpes simplex present in the vagina during childbirth may be dangerous to the newborn infant, so the obstetrician should be informed if attacks occur there so that precautions can be taken at birth. Brimmed hats and sunscreen lotions for the lips may prevent sunburn-induced cold sores. You should avoid touching cold sores and then rubbing your eye, because occasionally the eye will become seriously infected.

With time, attacks of herpes simplex may diminish and die out on their own. Right now there is no medical cure for the condition. Various medications, vitamins, and vaccines have been tried but have proved ineffective in preventing recurrent attacks. Accelerating the drying and healing of a current attack is possible, and your doctor may recommend a lotion, cream, or compress for that purpose.

The drug acyclovir, which can suppress the multiplication of the herpes simplex virus, is available as tablets or ointment. Acyclovir ointment may be helpful during the first attack of your life, when the virus is multiplying on the skin, but is useless in later attacks, when the virus is multiplying in nerve cells. Taking acyclovir, famciclovir, or valacyclovir tablets every day, before attacks occur, prevents herpes outbreaks, but if you wait to begin taking them until a herpes attack begins, the benefit is much less. If you have six attacks or more per year in a predictable pattern, then it may be reasonable to consider taking antiviral tablets every day to prevent outbreaks.

Pubic Lice ("Crabs")

"Crabs" are tiny insects that live on humans, usually on body hair in the pubic area and occasionally on body hair on the trunk or in the armpit. Occasionally they even inhabit eyelash hair. These insects grasp the hair firmly with a pincer, periodically bite the skin for food, and attach eggs (nits) to the hairs. These insects are small (3 mm), gray, flat, and slow-moving. They are often mistaken for flakes of dry skin. They may cause intense itching or no itching at all.

"Crabs" are passed between humans who sleep together. Sometimes they fall off the person who had them and can survive in bedding or clothing for up to 4 days. Although it is possible for them to infest others from those sources, this rarely happens.

TREATMENT

To treat "crabs," use the shampoo or lotion prescribed by your doctor and follow his or her instructions: Some types of shampoo or lotion are left on for minutes; other types, for hours. Usually the area from the waist to the knees is treated to ensure coverage of all affected areas. One treatment kills the "crabs" and their nits, but itching from the bites may last for a few more days. The dead nits may remain tightly attached to the hairs after treatment, but this is usually of no concern.

After treatment, you should dress in clean clothes and put fresh sheets on the bed. The old bedding and clothes worn during the last day should be washed, cleaned, or hot-ironed. It is not necessary to clean your entire wardrobe or to clean the mattress and the bedroom. Persons sleeping together should be treated at the same time to prevent spread from one to the other.

Eyelash Infestation

If the eyelashes are infected, your doctor will prescribe an ointment that should be applied thinly with a cotton swab twice a clay. Your doctor may gently remove the organisms from the lashes with fine tweezers. Do not attempt to do this yourself, as absolute stillness, good light, and magnification are needed.

Head Lice

Head lice infestation occurs in epidemics among children and may be passed to adults in their families. The tiny insect bites the scalp and attaches its eggs (nits) to the hairs with a strong "glue." A person with head lice may have no itching at all or may have a lot of itching, especially toward the back of the scalp and the nape of the neck. He or she may be aware only of the tiny nits beading the hairs. The lice are passed from one person to another by close personal contact (children wrestling or sleeping together) or through infested hats, collars, pillows, upholstered furniture, or combs and brushes.

To kill the lice, use the shampoo or lotion that your doctor prescribes or recommends. The shampoo is generously lathered in, left on for 5 minutes, and then rinsed. The lotion is generously rubbed in and left on for 15 minutes, then washed out. Avoid contact with the eyes and make sure that children do not have the opportunity to drink the materials, as they are strong poisons. The bites may itch for several days after successful treatment, so do not treat again unnecessarily, and do not refill the prescription until you have consulted your doctor. Everyone in the family who may have lice should be treated at the same time.

The shampoos and lotions kill the nits but do not remove them from the hairs. If the dead nits do not comb out easily and are annoying, then:

- Soak the hair thoroughly with a solution made up of equal parts of water and white vinegar.
- Wrap the wet scalp in a towel or put on a shower cap for at least 15 minutes to soften the attachment of the nits to the hairs.
- Comb gently but thoroughly with a fine-toothed comb. Flea combs, available at pet stores, are well-suited to this task.
- Thoroughly rinse or shampoo the hair.
- Repeat periodically if necessary for stubborn nits.

Note: After adequate treatment, the lice and nits are dead and no longer contagious. Children may return to school even if nits are still present.

Doing certain things at home will prevent the lice from spreading to others in the family or reinfesting the same children. Wash combs and brushes in hot, soapy water. Hats, coat collars (especially fur), sheets, and pillowcases should be washed, dry-cleaned, or pressed with a hot iron. Vacuum or clean possibly infected pillows, mattresses, and upholstered furniture. The adult lice can live away from humans for only a few days, so cleaning of all articles of clothing and furniture is unnecessary.

Hand Dermatitis

The hands of some people are sensitive to normal daily activities and easily become dry, cracked, and scaly. Water, soap, detergents, and cleansers are the most common culprits in triggering this problem, so "dishpan hands" occur in healthcare workers, cooks, hairdressers, beauticians, bartenders, waiters, and others whose hands are repeatedly wetted. The rash caused by these exposures is a mild to severe irritation, not an allergy.

Blistering eczemas, psoriasis, and other rashes may occur on the hands. They may look like "dishpan hands" and are irritated and worsened by water and cleanser exposure. The treatment of these "hand eczemas" of whatever cause is the same.

TREATMENT

An important part of treating these problems is preventing further irritation. You should decrease your exposure to water and cleansers as much as possible. This might mean asking another household member to do some of these chores or being temporarily transferred to another sort of job at work. How often your hands are wet and dry is more important than the duration of wetting, so washing one large load of dishes a day would be better than doing several small ones during the day. If you can use tongs and long-handled brushes when practical, this decreases water exposure. Unfortunately, rubber or plastic household gloves are not of great benefit in protecting you from common household exposures, because it is the wetting that is most damaging, and gloves trap sweat and make the hand completely wet after a few minutes. Gloves flocked with cotton take only a few more minutes to do this. A truly protective system is to use a thin cotton glove under a loose vinyl one and to change to a fresh, dry cotton glove whenever the current one becomes moist, but this is so complicated and bulky as to be impractical for many activities. Avoiding wetting is much more effective than trying to protect against wetting.

Moisturizing the skin is important, to replace natural skin oils removed by wetting. You should stop using all commercial hand lotions and moisturizing creams and use only the products your doctor recommends, because many of the commercial products contain fragrances and other chemicals that are irritants. Plain greases, such as mineral oil or petroleum jelly, are the safest. These should be rubbed in thinly after every water exposure and whenever the skin feels dry. This may require applications as often as 10 times a day, especially at the beginning, but overmoisturization is impossible and undermoisturization is harmful.

Treatment of the inflamed skin itself is by cortisone creams or ointments. Strong ones are usually necessary because penetration through the thick skin of the palm is poor. The cortisone cream or ointment is applied thinly one to two times a day, especially after water exposure. If the topical cortisone alone does not stop redness and itching, then a much greater effect can be obtained by covering it with a disposable plastic glove. This greatly increases penetration of the medication and softens and humidifies dry skin. After wearing the gloves overnight, for a few hours, or as long as possible, the hands should be rinsed and a topical cortisone or lubricant applied to prevent drying. If only the palm of the hand has a rash, then the fingers of the gloves can be cut off to make wearing the glove more comfortable. After the rash has improved or is under control, a mild cortisone cream or ointment is used instead of a strong one. Prolonged use of strong topical cortisones, especially under plastic gloves, may cause temporary thinning of the skin. If the rash has healed, just a lubricant should be enough. A cortisone cream can be used again if the rash returns.

If the hand inflammation does not respond to external therapy, then your doctor may recommend cortisone pills or shots. These usually improve the rash but may have internal side effects, and the rash may reappear when they are stopped, so they are used with caution for only short periods.

Atopic Dermatitis ("Eczema")

Atopic dermatitis (also called *atopic eczema*) is an inherited condition. It often occurs in individuals who have allergic hay fever or asthma or in whose families those conditions occur, although atopic dermatitis itself is not an allergy. Atopic dermatitis is a condition of sensitive skin that is easily provoked to itch, and, when the skin is rubbed or scratched, an itchy rash quickly appears. Dry weather, soaps, bathing, sweating, rough clothing, and common industrial agents (automotive greases, ceramic clays, and so on) may provoke severe itching in an atopic person, whereas these factors usually have less effect on other people. Another example is that, although most people can scratch an insect bite for a few days with no lasting consequences, an atopic person may scratch for only a day or two and develop a stubborn, itchy rash.

Atopic dermatitis usually starts in childhood and flares and subsides repeatedly for several years before resolving. The trend is for the rash to improve before adolescence, but it may flare in adulthood, especially on the hands if they are frequently exposed to water, detergents, and chemicals. Occasionally, atopic dermatitis appears only briefly in a lifetime, but for a few people it lasts continuously into adulthood.

TREATMENT

Until it improves spontaneously, atopic dermatitis can be controlled by medication. Treatment has two goals: (1) prevention of itching and (2) treatment of the rash itself.

Prevention of itching is important. Try to determine what conditions in your life stimulate itching. In temperate climates, dryness of the skin is a major provoking cause. Dryness is often worst in the winter when central heating causes low humidity in buildings. Bathing, even with mild soap, removes natural moisturizing oils from the skin and makes it drier. It is nearly impossible to make interior winter air humid in large homes (large central humidifiers are necessary; pans of water have no effect). Therefore, the only practical way to minimize skin dryness is to bathe relatively infrequently (every other day) with a mild soap and then to moisturize the skin immediately with an oil or cream. Lotions are pleasant to use but contain too little oil to be effective and are occasionally even more drying. Applications of moisturizers once or twice a day on particularly dry skin (usually the arms and legs) may be necessary.

Heat and humidity make some atopic persons itch. If that is true of you, wear lightweight, loose clothing and **avoid** thick greases and oils, as they may plug your sweat pores. In general, most atopic people itch when they wear heavy, unlined wool or polyester clothing. They are not allergic to wool, but the rough fibers of those materials lightly scrape and irritate the skin, causing itching. Wear cotton and cotton-blend clothing as much as possible to minimize such irritation.

Atopic persons are not allergic to soap but they are often irritated by exposure to soaps, detergents, cleansers, and chemicals. Wearing plastic gloves is recommended when using strong cleansers, but they provoke sweating, which itself may be irritating. Minimize exposure to water, detergents, and cleansers as much as possible and apply your medication immediately after each exposure.

Your doctor will probably give you a cortisone-type cream or ointment to treat and prevent your eczema. Rub it in thinly to all susceptible areas about twice daily. Your doctor will tell you if certain creams are too strong to use on thin-skinned areas, such as the face and groin. Do not apply these creams to the eyelids without specific recommendation from your doctor.

People inaccurately say that atopic dermatitis is caused by nervousness, and much guilt can result from such statements. Eczema is inherited, not "caused" by anything. However, tension can provoke itching, just as dryness and detergents can. Atopic eczema is not the only disease provoked by tension; almost all diseases can be. In eczema, however, the consequences are apparent. Itching and scratching can occur subconsciously and during sleep. Your doctor may prescribe an "itch pill," usually an antihistamine, to reduce the urgency of itching. These pills often cause drowsiness, so they are best taken at bedtime. If you take them during the day, do not drive or operate dangerous equipment until you know how your body reacts to them.

Dry Skin

Dry skin afflicts many people. It can be annoying because of its rough, scaly appearance, and it can cause severe itching. In dark-skinned individuals, "chapping" can cause vague areas of decreased pigment (light color). This is particularly common on the face in children. After puberty, heavy oil production on the face usually corrects that dryness. Adults usually find that their legs and arms are the driest areas; the tendency to skin dryness increases in the elderly.

Warm, humid weather will usually completely control dry skin. Hot and dry weather is moderately drying to the skin, but the most drying occurs in cold climates. When cold air is heated in buildings, its humidity drops drastically, drawing water from the skin, lips, and nasal membranes, as well as from plants and wood (which is why doors often become loose in their frames during periods of low humidity). It is difficult to make such indoor air humid again; gallons of water must be added (by a central humidifier on the furnace) to each room each day. Putting open pans of water on the radiator is useless unless used in a very small room.

The only ways to treat dry skin are to avoid removing normal skin oils and to add oil (moisturization) to the skin. **Putting water on the skin is actually drying** because water leaches out the natural skin oils that keep the skin soft and smooth. Soaps and detergents leach oil out even more. Bathing, therefore, can result in "dishpan body," with dry, rough skin. In dry weather, bathe only once a day or less often, and avoid long, hot baths or showers with lots of soap. Oilated or superfatted soaps are probably less drying than regular and deodorant bath soaps.

After bathing, and at other times if necessary, apply a lubricant to dry skin areas. Lotions are pleasant to use but contain a lot of water and little oil, so usually they are not adequate for moisturization.

Creams and ointments are good moisturizers. Creams containing urea are sometimes used as moisturizers, but they may cause a temporary burning sensation on dry, cracked skin. All moisturizers are best applied immediately after bathing.

Moisturizers containing alpha hydroxy acids (glycolic acid and lactic acid) may soften dry skin that does not respond to conventional moisturizers. They do not moisten the skin but rather change the way the dead skin layer is being formed, so that slowly a softer, more pliable dead skin layer is produced. They are applied once or twice a day for up to about a month to achieve maximum benefit and then applied perhaps one to three times a week to maintain the benefit. They may sting during the first few days of application. Some individuals with very sensitive skin may have so much burning from alpha hydroxy acid creams that they may not be able to use them at all.

Certain myths about dry skin should be laid to rest. Dryness of the skin does not lead to permanent wrinkling, and moisturizers will not prevent wrinkling. Dryness occurs only on the top, dead skin layer and is seen as fine lines. The dead skin layer is constantly shed and renewed, so no surface dryness lines are permanent. Wrinkles are due mostly to sun exposure (which damages deeper skin layers) and aging. Another myth is that diet affects dry skin; it does not. Unless the patient is literally starving, his or her skin's oil glands produce the same quantity and type of oil regardless of diet, and consuming less or more oil has no impact on them.

Pityriasis Rosea

Pityriasis rosea is a mysterious condition that erupts on the skin, lasts a short time, and disappears. It is unsightly and may itch, but it does no harm. Its characteristics are:

- It occurs mostly in young adults but may appear in children or older adults.
- It often starts with one large patch, which is followed in a few days by increasing numbers of smaller spots.
- It usually lasts about 6 weeks and then clears. Occasionally, it lasts 8 to 10 weeks. Many spots occur during the first few weeks; few spots appear during the last 2 to 3 weeks.
- The spots are usually concentrated on the trunk and the upper portions of the arms and legs. The rash rarely occurs on the face, wrists, and hands.

The cause of pityriasis rosea is unknown, but a virus is considered the most likely culprit. The condition occurs in a certain age group, erupts suddenly, lasts a certain length of time, clears completely, and rarely occurs again in the same individual. There is also a slight "epidemic" quality to the occurrence of pityriasis rosea; it occurs more frequently in the spring and autumn. However, arguing against a viral cause of this disease is the fact that it is not contagious (it is rarely seen in family or school groups), and no viruses have been found.

There is no treatment that shortens the duration of pityriasis rosea. Ultraviolet light temporarily suppresses or heals some of the rash, but treating this condition effectively with ultraviolet light is impractical. Itching is usually sporadic and mild. When itching becomes bothersome, it can be soothed by baths, lotions, or creams, which your doctor will recommend. Antihistamine pills may relieve itching but often cause drowsiness, so they are best used at bedtime. If you have severe itching, your doctor may prescribe cortisone pills for a week or two.

All in all, the appearance of pityriasis rosea is at first alarming, but you can take comfort in the knowledge that it will not last long, it will not harm internal organs or leave scars, it is not contagious, and it is unlikely to recur.

Tinea Versicolor

This is a harmless, noncontagious, mild yeast infection of the skin. The yeast that causes this condition normally lives on everybody's skin in small numbers, but in young adults it occasionally grows profusely and causes a discolored rash. We do not know why this sudden growth and rash occurs, but it does not indicate that the person has low resistance or internal disease.

The name *tinea versicolor* means "fungus that changes color." The rash may last for years, worsening and improving over the months. It often becomes more noticeable during the summer with sun exposure and tanning. Washing with regular soap will abolish the scaling of the rash for a few hours, but the rash itself cannot be washed away that easily. However, the yeast is on the surface of the skin, not in it, so treatment with medication that causes mild peeling of the top, dead skin layer will remove it.

The most commonly used medication is a dandruff shampoo (sometimes available only by prescription), which softens and removes the "dandruff" or top, dead layer of skin found on everyone. Apply the shampoo as a lotion thinly over the entire trunk from neck to waist and down the arm to the elbow. Put it on a generous margin of normal skin around the rash, just to be sure you get all the yeast. Leave it on a few hours or overnight, if you can, but remove it sooner if your skin begins to burn or itch. Then wash in a bath or shower, using more of the shampoo as a soap, and rub the area briskly with a facecloth to help to remove the loosened dead skin. If you tend to have dry skin, apply a moisturizing oil or lotion after bathing.

This treatment should be repeated once a week for 6 weeks. The ashy scale of the rash will disappear after a few treatments, but it may take months for your skin color to return to normal. This slow return of color is a normal healing process and does not mean that treatment has failed. The rash may return in months, and a repeat treatment may then be necessary. If the rash does not seem to respond well to this treatment or if it returns immediately after each treatment, return to your doctor for another type of medication.

You will outgrow this condition eventually, but usually it is easy to cure or keep under control. Your skin is not harmed or scarred by this infection, and you cannot give it to other people, so do not let tinea versicolor blemish your peace of mind.

Scabies

Scabies is caused by the human itch mite, which is too tiny to see with the naked eye. When a mite gets onto human skin, it burrows into the top layer of dead skin and lays eggs. The eggs hatch in 5 days; those mites then burrow in and produce more eggs. During this initial phase of reproduction, while a few hundred mites are produced, the human host experiences no itching or rash but can spread the mites to others. Finally, after 2 or 3 weeks, the person becomes allergic to the mites and an itchy rash develops. Curiously, only a dozen or so mites are now present, as the allergic response kills many of them.

The rash is usually extremely itchy, especially at night. Dozens to hundreds of tiny bumps are present all over the body, with greater concentrations in the fold areas, such as finger webs, wristfolds, armpits, belly button, under the breasts, and between the buttocks. There is often a rash on the nipples and genitals. Older children and adults rarely have a rash above the neck or on the palms and soles, but infants frequently have rash in those areas. Some people have only a mild allergic reaction and develop only a few faint bumps with only mild itching.

Scabies is passed by skin-to-skin contact, usually among people sleeping together and to children who are hugged and carried by adults. Casual contact such as shaking hands or contact in a crowd does not pass the organism. Mites live in the skin and do not come off easily, but occasionally a mite is shed into clothing or bedding, where another human may come in contact with it. Mites are rarely passed in this way, however, partially because they can survive away from a human host for only 12–24 hours (usually less).

Treatment of scabies is simple and effective. Children and adults apply a cream or lotion (prescribed by the doctor) to their entire skin surface below the neck. Do not apply just to the rash or itchy areas, and do not skip the buttock folds, genitals, toe webs, or other difficult treatment areas. The medication is applied at bedtime and washed off in the morning. One or two treatments are adequate, depending on the medication prescribed. Bed partners should be treated at the same time. Infants may be given a different treatment medication than that used by adults, and they should be treated on the face and scalp as well as elsewhere.

Itching usually persists for 2–3 weeks or longer after treatment, because it takes time for the allergic reaction to subside. Your doctor may prescribe creams or pills to relieve the itching. Do not increase your frequency of bathing or use the antiscabies cream over and over, because that further irritates the skin and can increase itching. If you think you still have scabies or have acquired it again, you should return to the doctor for examination.

Simple precautions should be taken to prevent the spread of scabies in the home. All occupants who are in intimate contact with each other should be treated at the same time (whether or not they are itchy). The morning after treatment, the bedding, nightclothes, and clothes worn the previous day should be washed. No other clothes or furnishings need to be cleaned. If some clothing is difficult to clean, just set it aside for a day or two. Because scabies mites are rarely shed into the environment and can survive <24 hours without human contact, clothes treated in this way will then be safe to use again.

Sun Protection

The considerable energy in the sun's rays can significantly penetrate and damage skin. The effect can occur immediately after exposure, as a sunburn, but the most common and serious damage accumulates over years of repeated exposure. Many changes occur as a result of exposure years before, even if the skin has been protected more recently. These late effects of sun exposure include wrinkles, freckles, light spots, coarsened surface texture, dilated capillaries, scaly growths, and tumors. Most affected are light-skinned individuals, somewhat affected are darker persons who tan easily, and least affected are the very dark skinned. Some skin changes just mentioned can be treated, but the results are never as satisfactory as avoiding their development. Simple precautions greatly reduce sun damage without really interfering with work or recreational activities. A few facts about sun intensity form a basis for these precautions:

- Almost two-thirds of the sun's energy strikes the earth between 10 AM and 3 PM. At other times the rays come to the earth at such a sharp angle that the atmosphere filters out much of their energy.
- Less energy is filtered out by the thin air at high altitudes. About 5% more energy is present for each 300-meter (1,000-feet) increase in altitude. For this reason, even short sun exposures at high altitudes can be damaging.
- Much energy is reflected by water, sand, and snow. So even being in the shade at pools, at beaches, and in the snow can result in significant exposure if the reflection goes under a sunshade.
- Sun penetrates water and wet (especially white) clothing, so being in the water or wearing a T-shirt while swimming is not completely protective.

Knowledge of these facts about the sun can help to minimize sun damage. If convenient, plan outdoor activities before 10 AM and after 3 PM, and take extra precautions between those hours or at high altitudes and around water, sand, and snow.

The best precaution against sun damage is complete shading from the sun by clothing and hats. The frequent wearing of a widebrimmed hat is a simple way to greatly reduce sun damage to the face, ears, and back of the neck, the areas most commonly affected by the sun. Even a very lightweight long-sleeved shirt or blouse will protect the arms and trunk.

When fixed shade and clothing are impractical, sunscreens should be worn. These materials filter out 70–95% of the damaging energy of the sun. Do not confuse a sunscreen with a sunbathing oil or cream. The latter are merely moisturizers to minimize drying and, if anything, actually **increase** sun penetration into the skin.

Sunscreens are ranked by a sun protective factor (SPF) from 5 to 50 (or above). An SPF 15 sunscreen blocks 93% of the burning rays of the sun, and an SPF 30 blocks 98%, so using a sunscreen above SPF 15 is only moderately more protective. Some new sunscreens block a wider range of ultraviolet light wavelengths and may be more protective against the "aging" changes caused by the sun. Most sunscreen products are clear, easy to apply, and effective. Because they are available in creams, gels, lotions, and alcohol solutions, anyone should be able to find one that is acceptable and convenient. These products are safe to use but some chemical sunscreens may occasionally cause an allergic rash.

All in all, you can enjoy the sun but, by taking a few simple precautions, you can greatly minimize its consequences. Learn to do this now and teach your children so that they can wear still-young skin for the rest of their lives.

SUNTANNING PARLORS

The form of ultraviolet light used in suntanning parlors tends to promote tanning without burning, except with extremely prolonged exposures. This would seem to be an ideal way to obtain a tan, but it is these ultraviolet rays that are responsible for wrinkling and "aging" changes of the skin, and people who have used suntanning parlors for many years have definite damage to their skin and an increased risk of skin cancer. Their use can cause significant skin damage and eye damage without adequate eye protection.

EYE PROTECTION

Ultraviolet light is a major cause of cataracts and it may even damage the retina of the eye. It is recommended that sunglasses capable of screening out ultraviolet light be worn as much as possible when outdoors or where there is great reflection of sun into shaded areas. Older plastic sunglasses often did not filter ultraviolet light at all, even though they may have been very dark in color. Most newer sunglasses filter out ultraviolet light quite successfully, but when purchasing a pair, you should look specifically for a tag attached to the glasses stating that they provide "complete" or "maximal" protection. When having prescription sunglasses made, ultraviolet filters can easily be added for only a small additional cost. Suntanning booths have such a high intensity of ultraviolet light that parlors should provide goggles that filter out all ultraviolet light rays and should insist that they should be worn at all times.

Psoriasis

Psoriasis is a red, scaly rash that often occurs on the scalp, over joints (elbows, knees, and knuckles), and on the lower back. It usually appears first in teenagers and young adults, and in common mild cases it waxes and wanes with a few patches here and there over many years.

Psoriasis is not an infection or allergy; it is familial. One-third of people with the condition know that it runs in their families. In another third, examination of relatives reveals mild cases. In the remaining third, inheritance cannot be proved and it is possible that these people represent new genetic cases. Nonetheless, psoriasis is inborn and is not "caught" or caused by certain foods or emotional behavior. However, its development or severity may be influenced by several things. A profuse eruption, for example, may occur a week or two after a streptococcal throat infection. Fortunately, this type often heals by itself in a few months. Patches of psoriasis may occur at sites of skin injury, such as scrapes or bruises. Sunlight tends to improve the rash; illness or emotional upset may worsen it.

Occasionally, psoriasis is severe. The scalp may become inflamed and caked with thick scale. The palms and soles may erupt with scales and cracks or even blisters. The nails may become pitted, thickened, and crumbly. A rash may occur on the genitals. So much rash may develop on the body that flakes are shed profusely, and the person may feel chilled from loss of body heat. Arthritis sometimes develops, especially in the fingers and back.

Several effective treatments exist to control psoriasis. Prolonged cures are not expected, but the condition tends to wax and wane, so there are often periods when no treatment is needed. Most treatments require a doctor's supervision. Cortisone, tar, and vitamin D-related creams are easy to use at home. Ultraviolet light treatments are an excellent treatment option. They are usually administered in a hospital or clinic, but sunlight can be used, or an ultraviolet "light box" can be used at home under the doctor's supervision. PUVA is a treatment involving a drug taken by mouth (psoralen) and a special-wavelength ultraviolet light. It is available only in clinics and doctors' offices.

For more severe cases, various systemic medications are available, which are either taken by mouth or injected into the skin or veins. These require supervision by a dermatologist.

In summary, psoriasis is an inborn condition that can manifest itself in different ways and in varying severity. It can be controlled fairly well with treatment, but a doctor's supervision is necessary for many cases. Much research is being conducted, and new treatments can be expected.

All about Warts

Warts are benign growths of the skin caused by a virus. The virus gets into the skin from the outside through cuts, scratches, or cracks and does not go into the bloodstream. The time between the penetration of the virus and the appearance of the wart (the incubation period) is a few months.

As with most viral infections, warts occur more commonly in children, and they go away when immunity develops. In young children warts may last just a few months, in older children they may last a few years, and in adults they may last for many years. Some people never develop complete immunity to warts and may have them intermittently for most of their lifetime. However, most warts do go away and heal without scars.

Warts may behave differently in different locations. Warts around the fingernails and on the palms and soles are particularly long-lived and stubborn. Warts in hair-bearing areas are particularly troublesome because shaving often spreads them around. In the same way, picking or chewing of warts on the hands may spread them, especially under the fingernails. Warts may grow profusely on the genitals of adults and be passed back and forth between sexual partners.

Treatment of warts is not always satisfactory. Genital warts often respond to an antiviral liquid (podophyllotoxin), but repeated treatments are often necessary. The callus like dead skin on warts elsewhere can be reduced with repeated application of wart softeners or corn plasters. They reduce the bulk of the wart and may speed healing.

Warts can be cured by destroying them by freezing, burning, or surgical removal, but all of these treatments may leave scars. Freezing is the preferred method, as a rule, because it tends to be the least scarring, but it can sometimes cause dyspigmentation.

These treatments also are painful and may fail. Regrowth of warts occurs probably 30% of the time on the hands and up to 70–90% for warts around the nails and on the soles. Repeated treatments usually clear the wart, but often the wart disappears on its own. Because the incubation period of warts is several months, often a "cure" becomes a relapse as time goes on, requiring more treatments. What treatment, if any, is selected for warts depends on the age and needs of the patient and on the location of the wart.

Note: Warts on the soles of the feet are called "plantar warts" because they occur on the plantar surface of the foot (similar to the palmar surface of the hand).

Moles and Melanoma

Babies are usually born without moles. They start appearing in early childhood and develop rapidly in adolescence, but new ones continue to appear into the 20s and 30s. By adulthood the average light-skinned patient has about 40 of them while dark-skinned patients tend to have fewer. Later in life many of them become more elevated and prominent. We do not know what causes moles, but the number of them in an individual is generally hereditary and may vary from few to dozens.

Moles are collections of pigment cells, or melanocytes, in the skin. They appear first as small, flat dots that may grow larger in diameter and either in childhood or in adult life may grow to elevated bumps, although they may also remain flat throughout life. The surface of moles may vary from smooth to pebbly or even raspberry-like. They may contain heavy, dark hairs or no increased hairiness at all. The color may vary from flesh-colored to darker shades but, in general, light-skinned people have light-colored moles and darker-skinned people have very dark moles. Asians generally have fewer moles than do light-skinned people, and dark-skinned have fewer still. Moles do not signify any internal diseases. They can be removed by a variety of surgical techniques if the individual desires.

Melanoma is a cancer of pigment cells. Perhaps 30% of melanomas arise in moles, and the other 70% arise in previously normal skin without a preceding mole. Melanoma is most common in light-skinned individuals, particularly those who are redheaded and freckled. It is fairly uncommon in darker-skinned persons and Asians and occurs in dark-skinned people more on the palms and soles (which are the lightest skin on the body) or in the mouth. Occasionally, melanomas arise in the eye or nervous system, where pigment cells also occur normally.

Hundred years ago melanomas occurred in about 1 out of 1,000 light-skinned Americans. This rate has now increased to about 1 out of 40, a change thought to be due to increased sun exposure, although some melanomas occur on parts of the body that are never exposed to the sun and affect people living in areas of the world that receive very little sunlight. Possibly sunburns suffered in childhood or adolescence are more responsible for the later development of melanoma than is the total accumulated amount of sun received on any given area of the skin.

There is a slight family tendency for melanoma, but that may reflect an inherited light skin color. However, there are some families whose members grow many large and bizarre moles called "dysplastic moles," and those individuals have perhaps a 50% lifetime chance of developing melanoma. Interestingly, the melanomas grow more often from normal skin between these unusual moles than in the moles themselves.

The finding of a few small dysplastic moles on an individual with no other family members involved perhaps increases that person's risk of melanoma slightly. It has been noted that persons with an unusually large number of regular moles also have an increased risk of melanoma. The exact number is debatable, but probably a person with >75 regular moles should be watched closely for the possible development of melanoma.

Melanomas usually appear as very dark, flat growths that may become elevated bumps. They often are black, blue-black, or brownblack, which makes them considerably darker than the tan or medium-brown moles of the average light-skinned person. However, melanomas are sometimes also skin-colored to red. Moles usually have a round or oval shape, but melanomas may have an irregular shape with a jagged border. Colors within the melanoma may be uniform or may be speckled or varied in some manner, and redness or swelling may be present in the area. In addition, melanomas may be fragile and bleed spontaneously or with minor irritation. Any of these signs in a growth on the skin calls for an immediate examination by a physician trained to recognize skin cancers.

Surgical removal of the melanoma and about 0.5 inch of the surrounding normal skin cures 85% of melanomas. Unfortunately, melanomas that have been present longer or that have grown deeper may already have spread into nearby lymph nodes or throughout the body, which may result in death. For that reason it is extremely important to have unusual growths examined and treated early. It is wise to examine his or her skin at least every 6 months and to have a companion examine hard-to-see places on the body so that suspicious-looking areas can be detected early and treated while they are still completely curable.

Index

C

D

I

J

K

L

R

S